Clinical Pharmacokinetics:

Concepts and Applications

Clinical

Pharmacokinetics:

Concepts and Applications

Malcolm Rowland, Ph.D.
Department of Pharmacy
University of Manchester
Manchester, England

Thomas N. Tozer, Ph.D.
School of Pharmacy
University of California
San Francisco, California

LEA & FEBIGER PHILADELPHIA

Library of Congress Cataloging in Publication Data

Rowland, Malcolm.
  Clinical pharmacokinetics.

  Bibliography: p.
  Includes index.
  1. Pharmacokinetics. 2. Chemotherapy.
I. Tozer, Thomas N., joint author. II. Title.
[DNLM: 1. Drug therapy. 2. Kinetics.
3. Pharmacology. QV38.3 R883c]
RM301.5.R68 1980   615'.7   79-10735
ISBN 0-8121-0681-4

Printed in the United States of America
Print Number   3

To Margaret and Dawn

preface

FOR EIGHT years we jointly shared responsibility for teaching basic courses in pharmacokinetics at the University of California. The students were from a variety of persuasions, including professional students in pharmacy, clinical pharmacology fellows, and graduate academic students. Their feedback on the courses resulted in our making a dramatic shift in the way we presented the material. Over the years the emphasis shifted from kinetics and modeling to providing a conceptual base for applying pharmacokinetics to rational drug therapy. We firmly believe that the reoriented content of these courses goes much further in relating to the needs of students and of practitioners of pharmacotherapeutics. One of the major difficulties in teaching the subject has been the lack of a book that teaches the application of pharmacokinetics in drug therapy. This deficiency prompted the writing of this book.

The title of the book was chosen because it emphasizes the bedside application of pharmacokinetics. The book, in fact, is a primer on pharmacokinetics with clinical applications. It should be useful to any student, practitioner, or researcher who is interested or engaged in the development, evaluation, or use of drugs in man. It is an introductory text and therefore presumes that the reader has had little or no experience or knowledge in the area. Previous exposure to certain aspects of physiology and pharmacology would be helpful, but is not essential. Some knowledge of calculus is also desirable.

In our experience, the average student has felt very uncomfortable with kinetic principles and mathematics. Indeed, in many cases there is a strong mental block. Our desire is to teach the application of pharmacokinetics in therapeutics. We believe we are achieving this goal by applying the essential concepts through problem solving with only the essence of required mathematics. This approach is a theme throughout the book. In this respect this book is a programmed learning text. Every attempt is made at the beginning of each chapter to present objectives that identify the more important points to be learned. To further aid in the learning process, examples are worked out in detail in the text. At the end of many chapters there are two kinds of problems. The first is study problems, which allow the reader to test his grasp of the material in the chapter. The second kind is unifying problems, which build upon the material of previous chapters. For the interested reader there is a list of suggested further reading located at the back of the book.

An attempt has been made to establish uniformity for symbols and units throughout the book; definitions of symbols begin on p. 280. The liter is used as the standard measure of volume and hour as the standard unit of time. A special comment should be made on the choice of mg/liter for the

viii   PREFACE

units of drug concentration. Although molarity has considerable utility and has been strongly advocated for common use, the dosage of drugs is most often expressed in milligrams. Until doses are given in molar units, we feel that mg/liter is the more convenient unit for concentration.

The book is divided into four sections: Concepts, Disposition and Absorption Kinetics, Therapeutic Regimens, and Individualization. Section I contains the fundamental concepts in drug absorption, distribution and elimination. Section II covers the kinetics of drug and metabolites following drug administration and integrates kinetics with the fundamental concepts. Section III deals with the basic elements of the design and evaluation of therapeutic regimens, while Section IV examines the causes of variability in human drug response, the adjustment of dosage based on age, weight, and renal function, explores the kinetic consequences of drug interactions, and presents principles for the monitoring of drug therapy using plasma concentrations. The sequence is intended to give the reader the basic underlying concepts, the quantitative tools, and the essence of the kinetic basis for variability in human drug response.

The content of the book, by design, has been limited. There are many important areas of pharmacokinetics either touched on only lightly or not covered at all. Most of these areas are more specialized, dealing with such topics as distribution dynamics, including multicompartment systems, dose and time dependencies, turnover concepts, dialysis, and kinetic considerations in the treatment of drug overdose. These and other specialized topics and a more detailed examination of the clinical pharmacokinetics of selected drugs, including digoxin, theophylline, and phenytoin, form the basis of a sequel to this book entitled Clinical Pharmacokinetics: Specialized Topics and Selected Drugs.

We wish to express our gratitude to Jere E. Goyan, Dean, and Sidney Riegelman, Associate Dean for Research Services, School of Pharmacy, University of California, for their encouragement. We also wish to acknowledge Paul Bailey of Manchester, England, for his preparation of the illustrations. We particularly wish to thank our past students whose comments have been so useful in formulating our ideas.

To the reader of the book we hope that we have succeeded in helping you develop kinetic reasoning that will be of personal value in your practice. In general perspective, we hope we have made some contribution to the development of a more rational management of drug therapy.

Manchester, England

San Francisco, California

MALCOLM ROWLAND

THOMAS N. TOZER

contents

1
why clinical pharmacokinetics?

THOSE patients who suffer from chronic ailments such as diabetes and epilepsy may have to take drugs every day for the rest of their lives. At the other extreme are those who take a single dose to relieve an occasional headache. The duration of drug therapy is usually between these extremes. The manner in which a drug is taken is called a *dosage regimen.* Both the duration of drug therapy and the dosage regimen depend on the therapeutic objectives, which may be either the cure, the mitigation, or the prevention of the disease. Because all drugs exhibit undesirable effects such as drowsiness, dryness of the mouth, gastrointestinal irritation, nausea, and hypotension, successful drug therapy is achieved by optimally balancing the desirable and the undesirable effects. To achieve optimal therapy, the appropriate "drug of choice" must be selected. This decision implies an accurate diagnosis of the disease, a knowledge of the clinical state of the patient, and a sound understanding of the pharmacotherapeutic management of the disease. Then the questions how much, how often, and how long, must be answered. The question "how much" recognizes that the magnitude of the response (therapeutic or toxic) is a function of the dose given. The question "how often" recognizes the importance of time, in that the magnitude of the effect eventually declines with time following a single dose of drug. The question

"how long" recognizes that there is a cost (in terms of side effects, toxicity, economics) incurred with continued drug administration. In practice, these questions cannot be divorced from one another. For example, the convenience of giving a larger dose less frequently may be more than offset by an increased incidence of toxicity.

In the past, the answers to many important therapeutic questions were obtained by trial and error. The clinical investigator selected the dose, the interval between doses, and the route of administration and followed the patient's progress. The desired effect and any signs of toxicity were carefully noted, and if necessary the dosage regimen was adjusted empirically until a maximal desired effect with minimal toxicity was achieved. Eventually, after considerable experimentation on a large number of patients, reasonable dosage regimens were established (Table 1-1), but not without some regimens producing excessive toxicity or proving ineffective. Moreover, the above empirical approach left many questions unanswered. Why, for example, does theophylline have to be given every 6 to 8 hours to be effective, while digoxin can be given daily? Why must oxytocin be infused intravenously? Why is morphine more effective given intramuscularly than when given orally? Furthermore, this empirical approach contributes little, if anything, toward establishing a safe, effective

Table 1-1. Empirically Derived Usual Adult Dosage Regimens of Some Representative Drugs[a]

Drug	Indicated Use	Route	Dosage Regimen
Theophylline	Relief of asthma	Oral	160 mg every 6 hours
Digoxin	Amelioration of congestive heart failure	Oral	1.5–2 mg initially over 24 hours, thereafter 0.25–0.5 mg once a day
Oxytocin	Induction and maintenance of labor	Intravenous	0.2–4 milliunits/min infusion
Morphine sulfate	Relief of severe pain	Intramuscular Oral	10 mg when needed Not used because of reduced effectiveness
Phenobarbital	Prevention of epileptic seizures	Oral	120–200 mg daily

[a]Taken from American Medical Association: Drug Evaluations. 2nd Edition. Publishers Science Group, Inc., Acton, Mass. 1973.

dosage regimen of another drug. That is, our basic understanding of drugs has not been increased.

To overcome some of the limitations of the empirical approach and to answer some of the questions raised, it is necessary to delve further into the events that follow drug administration. *In vitro* and *in vivo* studies show that the magnitude of the response is a function of the concentration of drug in the fluids bathing the site(s) of action. From these observations the suggestion might be made that the therapeutic objective can be achieved by maintaining an adequate concentration of drug at the site(s) of action for the duration of therapy. However, rarely is a drug placed at its site of action. Indeed, most drugs are given orally, and yet they act in the brain, on the heart, at the neuromuscular junction, or elsewhere. A drug must therefore move from the site of administration to the site of action. Simultaneously, however, the drug distributes to all other tissues including those organs, notably the liver and the kidney, that eliminate it from the body. After a dose is administered, the rate at which a drug initially enters the body exceeds its rate of elimination; the concentrations of drug in blood and in tissue rise, often sufficiently high to elicit the desired therapeutic effects and sometimes even to produce toxicity. Eventually, the rate of drug elimination exceeds the rate of its absorption, and thereafter, the concentration of drug in tissues declines and the effect(s) subsides. To administer drugs optimally, therefore, knowledge is needed not only of the mechanisms of drug absorption, distribution, and elimination but also of the kinetics of these processes, that is, *pharmacokinetics*. The application of pharmacokinetic principles to the therapeutic management of patients is *clinical pharmacokinetics*.

The problem of drug administration can now be divided into two phases, a *pharmacokinetic phase* that relates dose, frequency, and route of administration to drug level–time relationships in the body, and a *pharmacodynamic phase* that relates the concentration of drug at the site(s) of action to the magnitude of the effect(s) produced (Fig. 1-1). Once both of these phases have been defined, a dosage regimen can be de-

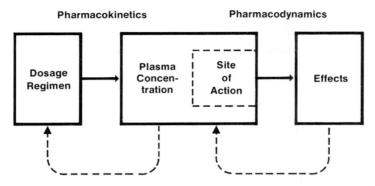

Figure 1-1. *An alternative approach to the design of a dosage regimen. The pharmacokinetics and the pharmacodynamics of the drug are first defined. Then either the plasma drug concentration-time data or the effects produced, via pharmacokinetics, are used as a feedback to modify the dosage regimen to achieve optimal therapy.*

signed to achieve the therapeutic objective. Despite the greater amount of information required with this approach, it has several advantages. First, and most obvious, distinctions can be made between pharmacokinetic and pharmacodynamic causes of an unusual drug response. Second, the basic concepts of pharmacokinetics are common to all drugs; information gained about the pharmacokinetics of one drug can help in anticipating the pharmacokinetics of another. Third, understanding the pharmacokinetics of a drug often explains the manner of its use; occasionally such an understanding has saved a drug that otherwise may have been discarded or has suggested a more appropriate dosage regimen. Lastly, knowing the pharmacokinetics of a drug often aids in anticipating the outcome of a therapeutic maneuver.

Before examples are given of the application of clinical pharmacokinetics, the situation depicted in Figure 1-2 should be considered. Assuming the hypothesis that both the magnitude of the desired response and the degree of toxicity are a function of the drug concentration at the site(s) of action, two reasons for therapeutic failure are evident. Either therapy is ineffective because the concentration is too low or there is an unacceptable degree of toxicity because the concentration is too high. Between these limits of concentration lies a

region associated with therapeutic success; this region may be regarded as the "therapeutic window." Rarely can the concentration of the drug at the site of action be measured directly; instead the concentration is measured at an alternative site, *the plasma.* Besides being a more convenient and accessible site of measurement, the concentration of a drug in plasma also probably reflects the drug concentration at the site of action.

Based on the foregoing considerations, an optimal dosage regimen might be defined as one that maintains the plasma concentration of a drug within its therapeutic window. For many drugs, this therapeutic objective is met by giving an initial dose to

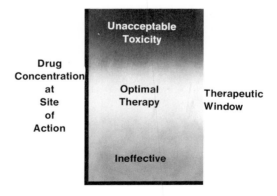

Figure 1-2. *Between certain limits of concentration lies a region associated with therapeutic success, the therapeutic window.*

achieve a plasma concentration within the therapeutic window and then maintaining this concentration by replacing the amount of drug lost with time. One popular and convenient means of maintenance is to give a dose at discrete time intervals. Figure 1-3 illustrates the basic features associated with this approach by depicting the events that follow the administration of two regimens, A and B; the dosing interval is the same but the dose given in regimen B is twice that given in regimen A. Because some drug always remains in the body from the preceding dose, accumulation occurs until, within a dosing interval, the amount lost equals the dose given; a characteristic saw-toothed plateau is then achieved. With regimen A, several doses had to be given before drug accumulation was sufficient to produce a therapeutic concentration. Had therapy been stopped before then, the drug might have been thought ineffective and perhaps abandoned prematurely. Alternatively, larger doses might have been tried, e.g., regimen B, in which case, although a therapeutic response would have been achieved fairly promptly, toxicity would have ensued on continued administration. Once again, the drug might have been abandoned. This almost happened with the synthetic antimalarial agent, quinacrine. Developed during World War II to substitute for the relatively scarce quinine, quinacrine was either ineffective against acute attacks of malaria, or, if a sufficiently high

dose regimen to be effective acutely was given, eventually produced unacceptable toxicity. Only after its pharmacokinetics was defined was this drug used successfully. Quinacrine distributes extensively into various tissues and is eliminated slowly; hence it accumulates extensively on prolonged administration. As now expected, the answer was to give a large initial dose, which immediately achieves therapeutic success, followed by smaller doses that maintain the concentration within the therapeutic window.

An examination of the plateau situation in Figure 1-3 also shows that the size of the maintenance dose and the frequency of administration are governed by two factors: the width of the therapeutic window and the speed of drug elimination. When the window is narrow and the drug is eliminated rapidly, small doses must be given often to achieve therapeutic success. Both theophylline and digoxin have a narrow therapeutic window, but because it is eliminated much more rapidly than digoxin, theophylline has to be given the more frequently. Oxytocin is an extreme example; it also has a narrow therapeutic window, and it is eliminated within minutes. The only means of adequately ensuring a therapeutic concentration is therefore to infuse oxytocin at a precise and constant rate directly into the blood. Control is too erratic with any other mode of administration. Besides, had it been given orally, oxytocin would have

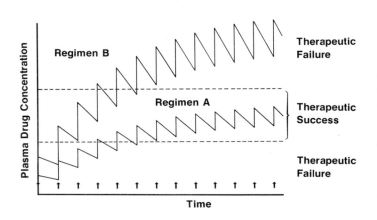

Figure 1-3. *When a drug is given at fixed time intervals (denoted by the arrows), it accumulates within the body until a plateau is reached. With regimen A, therapeutic success is achieved although not initially. With regimen B, the therapeutic objective is more quickly achieved but the plasma drug concentration is ultimately too high.*

been destroyed by the proteolytic enzymes in the gastrointestinal fluids. Morphine, given orally, is also substantially destroyed before entering the general circulation, but for a different reason than oxytocin. Morphine is rapidly metabolized in the liver, an organ lying between the gastrointestinal tract and the general circulation.

Figure 1-4 illustrates an important problem in drug therapy, variability. There is a wide range of daily dose requirements of the oral anticoagulant, warfarin, needed to produce a similar prothrombin time (an index of blood coagulability). Sources of variability in drug response include the patient's age, weight, degree of obesity, type and degree of severity of the disease, and the patient's genetic make-up, other drugs concurrently administered, and environmental factors. The result is that a standard dosage regimen of a drug may prove therapeutic in some patients, ineffective in others, and toxic in still others. The need to adjust the dosage regimen of a drug for an individual patient is evident; this need is clearly greatest for drugs that have a narrow therapeutic window, that exhibit a steep concentration-response curve, and that are critical to drug therapy. Examples are digoxin, used to treat congestive heart failure; phenytoin, used to prevent epileptic convulsions; theophylline, used to diminish chronic airway resistance in asthmatics; and

lidocaine, used to suppress ventricular arrhythmias. With these drugs, and with many others, variability in pharmacokinetics is a major source of total variability in drug response. Accounting for the variability in pharmacokinetics more readily permits improved individual dosage adjustment.

Coadministration of several drugs to a patient, prevalent in clinical practice, is fraught with problems. Each agent may have been chosen rationally but when coadministered, the outcome can be unpredictable. Phenylbutazone, for example, devoid of anticoagulant activity, markedly potentiates the hypoprothrombinemic effect of the oral anticoagulant, warfarin. The possible causes of this change are many. Often, such drug interactions involve a change in the pharmacokinetics. Some drugs stimulate drug-metabolizing enzymes and hasten drug loss; others inhibit these enzymes and slow elimination. Many others displace a drug from plasma and tissue binding sites or interfere with its absorption. Such interactions are graded; the change in the pharmacokinetics of a drug varies continuously with the plasma concentration of the interacting drug and hence with time. Indeed, given in sufficiently high doses, any drug will probably interact with another drug. It is always a question of degree. Understanding the quantitative

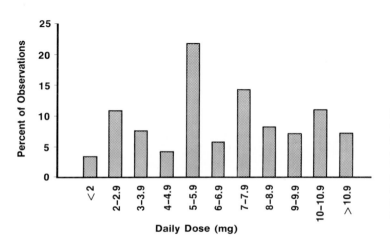

Figure 1-4. *The daily dose of warfarin, required to produce similar prothrombin times in 200 adult patients, varies widely. (Redrawn from Koch-Weser, J.: The serum level approach to individualization of drug dosage. Eur. J. Clin. Pharmacol., 9: 1–8, 1975.)*

elements of interactions ensures the more rational use of drugs that may have to be coadministered.

Figure 1-5 illustrates a situation in which monitoring of the drug concentration may be beneficial. Over the narrow range of the daily dose of the antiepileptic drug, phenytoin, the plateau plasma drug concentration varies markedly within the patient population. Yet the therapeutic window of phenytoin is very narrow, 7 to 20 mg/liter; beyond 20 mg/liter, the frequency and the degree of toxicity increase progressively with concentration. Here again, pharmacokinetics is the major source of variability. A pragmatic approach to this problem would be to adjust the dosage until the desired objective is achieved. Control on a dosage basis alone, however, has proved difficult. Control is achieved more readily and accurately given plasma drug concentration data and a knowledge of the pharmacokinetics of the drug.

Drug selection and therapy have traditionally been based solely upon observations of the effects produced. In this chapter, the application of pharmacokinetic principles to decision making in drug therapy has been illustrated. Both approaches are needed to achieve optimal drug therapy. This book emphasizes the pharmacokinetic approach. It begins with a consideration of the concepts basic to pharmacokinetics.

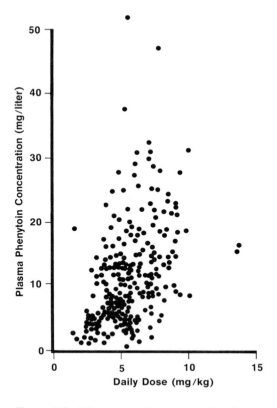

Figure 1-5. *Although on the average the plateau plasma drug concentration of phenytoin increases with the daily dose, there is considerable variation at any given daily dose. (Redrawn from Lund, L.: Effects of phenytoin in patients with epilepsy in relation to its concentration in plasma. In Biological Effects of Drugs in Relation to Their Plasma Concentration. Edited by D.S. Davies, and B.N.C. Prichard. Macmillan, London and Basingstoke, 1973, pp. 227–238.)*

SECTION ONE

concepts

2

basic considerations

Objectives

The reader will be able to define the following terms:

1. **Pharmacokinetics**

2. **Intravascular and extravascular administration**

3. **Absorption**

4. **Disposition**

5. **Distribution**

6. **Metabolism**

7. **Excretion**

8. **First-pass effect**

9. **Enterohepatic cycling**

Useful clinical applications of pharmacokinetics can be made from basic principles and concepts. In this and subsequent chapters, these concepts are developed. It should be noted, however, that the concepts are only valid to the extent that they can then explain observations or that they can serve as a basis for making predictions.

Anatomic and Physiologic Considerations

Measurement of a drug in the body is limited usually to the blood, or plasma, and to the urine. Nonetheless, the limited information obtained has proved very useful. Such usefulness can be explained by ana-tomic and physiologic considerations of the events that occur to a drug following its administration.

Blood or plasma, in addition to being a practical and convenient site of measurement, is the most logical one for determining drug in the body. Blood both receives a drug from the site of administration following its absorption and carries the drug to all the tissues including the sites of action and the organs that eliminate it from the body.

The fate of a drug as it moves from the site of administration to the site(s) of elimination is depicted schematically in Figure 2-1. This scheme includes the processes of absorption and disposition. Disposition may be further subdivided into distribution, elimination, and enterohepatic cycling.

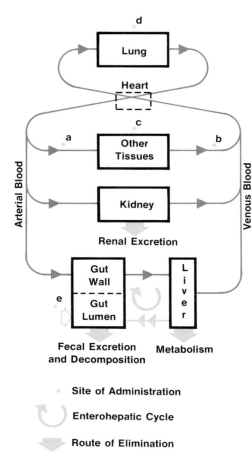

d

Lung

Heart

c

a   b

Other
Tissues

Arterial Blood

Venous Blood

Kidney

Renal Excretion

Gut
Wall   L
i
v
Gut   e
Lumen   r

e

Fecal Excretion   Metabolism
and Decomposition

＊   Site of Administration

Enterohepatic Cycle

Route of Elimination

Figure 2-1. *Once absorbed from any of the many sites of administration, a drug is distributed by blood to all sites within the body including the eliminating organs. Sites of administration are: a, artery; b, peripheral vein; c, muscle and subcutaneous tissue; d, lung; and e, gastrointestinal tract. The red and the blue lines with arrows refer to the mass movement of drug in blood and in bile, respectively. The absorption and disposition of virtually any drug can be followed from site of administration to site of elimination.*

Absorption

There are several sites at which drugs are commonly administered. These sites may be classified as either intravascular or extravascular. *Intravascular* administration refers to the placement of a drug directly into the blood, either intravenously or intra-arterially.

Extravascular modes of administration include the oral, sublingual, buccal, intramuscular, subcutaneous, pulmonary, and rectal routes. To enter the blood, drug administered extravascularly must be absorbed: No absorption step is required when a drug is administered intravascularly.

Distribution

Once absorbed, a drug is distributed to the various tissues of the body. The rate and the extent of distribution are determined by how well each tissue is perfused with blood, the binding of drug to plasma proteins and to tissue components, and the permeability of tissue membranes to the drug.

Elimination

The two principal organs of elimination, the liver and the kidney, are shown separately. The kidney is the primary site for excretion of the chemically unaltered, or unchanged, drug. The liver is the usual organ for drug metabolism; however, the kidney and other organs can also play an important metabolic role for certain drugs. The liver may also excrete unchanged drug into the bile. The lungs are, or may be, an important route for eliminating substances of high vapor pressure, for example the gaseous anesthetics. Another potential route of elimination is a mother's milk. Although not a significant route of elimination for the mother, the drug may be consumed in sufficient quantity to affect the suckling infant.

Enterohepatic Recycling

Once excreted into the bile, a drug may be reabsorbed from the gallbladder or from the intestinal tract. By doing so, the drug completes a cycle, the *enterohepatic cycle*. If all the drug is reabsorbed in this manner, biliary excretion is not a route of elimination; the cycling is then a component of distribution. The situation is analogous to one in which water is pumped from one reservoir into another, only to drain back into the original reservoir. Biliary excretion is truly a route of elimination only to the extent that the excreted drug fails to be reabsorbed. This failure may result from either decomposition in the intestinal lumen, poor absorption characteristics, or other complications. Unchanged drug that is neither reabsorbed nor decomposed is excreted in the feces.

Definitions

Although the processes of absorption and disposition are descriptive and their meaning is apparent at first glance, one must keep in mind that it is only within the context of experimental observation that they can be quantitated (Chaps. 7 to 10) or even given qualitative definition.

Absorption

To illustrate one complexity in defining absorption, consider the validity of the following statement: "The drug must have been completely absorbed; the metabolites in the urine account for the oral dose." The drug may have been absorbed, metabolized in the body, and the metabolites excreted in the urine. Alternatively, the drug may have been completely destroyed or metabolized before entering the body; the metabolites were then absorbed and excreted in the urine. Absorption of *drug* occurred in the former case, but not in the latter. Absorption might have been defined in terms of the amount or the moles administered. Then, absorption would have been considered complete in both cases. However, in the context of this book, absorption relates to an individual chemical species, generally the drug, and not to the amount administered. A basic lesson is learned here—distinguish carefully between drug and its metabolites. Although metabolites may also be of interest, especially if they are active or toxic, each chemical entity must be considered separately.

To illustrate another complexity in defining absorption, consider the events depicted in Figure 2-2, as a drug, given orally, moves from the site of administration to the general circulation. There are several possible sites of loss. One site is the gastrointestinal lumen where decomposition may occur. Suppose, however, that a drug survives destruction in the lumen only to be completely metabolized as it passes through the membranes of the gastrointestinal tract. One would ask, Is the drug absorbed? Even though the drug leaves the gastrointestinal tract, it would not be detected in the general circulation. Taking this one step further, Is the drug absorbed if all of the orally administered drug were to pass through the membranes of the gastrointestinal tract into the portal vein only to be metabolized completely on passing through the liver? In an experiment performed *in vitro* in which the passage of a drug across the intestinal membranes is studied separately, the answer would be positive. If, however, as is common, blood or plasma in an arm vein is the site of measurement, then, because no drug would be detected, the answer would be negative. Indeed, loss at any site prior to the site of measurement contributes to a decrease in the apparent absorption of the drug. The gastrointestinal tissues and the liver, in particular, are often sites of elimination. The requirement for an orally administered drug to pass through these tissues prior to reaching the site of measurement, makes absorption dependent on elimination. The loss of drug as it passes through the gastrointestinal membranes and the liver, for the first time, during the absorption process is known as the *first-pass effect*.

Absorption is not restricted to oral administration. It is equally applicable to events following the intramuscular or the subcutaneous administration of drugs. Monitoring the intact drug in blood or plasma offers a useful means of assessing the entry of drug into the body from any site of administration.

Some drugs are intended to act locally. A

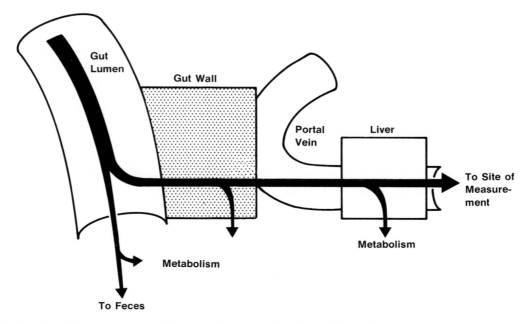

Figure 2-2. *A drug, given as a solid, encounters several barriers and sites of loss in its sequential movement during gastrointestinal absorption. Dissolution, a prerequisite to movement across the gut wall, is the first step. Incomplete dissolution or metabolism in the gut lumen or by enzymes in the gut wall is a cause of poor absorption. Removal of drug as it first passes through the liver further reduces absorption.*

mydriatic drug instilled into the eye to dilate the pupils and a drug injected subcutaneously to produce local anesthesia are examples. In such instances, monitoring the drug in the general circulation may be inappropriate; in fact, a more useful index of drug absorption would be monitoring changes in the pharmacologic response. Even if the mydriatic drug were given intravascularly instead of by local instillation, absorption would still be a prerequisite for action. The site of administration and the site of measurement are clearly not the same.

For the preceding reasons, *absorption* is defined here as the process by which a drug proceeds from the site of administration to the site of measurement within the body.

Disposition

As absorption and elimination of drugs are interrelated for physiologic and anatomic reasons, so too are distribution and elimination. Once absorbed, a drug is de-

livered simultaneously to all tissues, including organs of elimination. Distinction between elimination and distribution is often difficult. Disposition is the term used when distinction is not desired or is difficult to obtain. *Disposition* may be defined as all the processes that occur subsequent to the absorption of a drug. By definition, the components of disposition are distribution and elimination.

Distribution. Distribution is the process of reversible transfer of a drug to and from the site of measurement, usually the blood or plasma. Any drug that leaves the site of measurement and does not return has undergone elimination, not distribution.

Elimination. Elimination is the irreversible loss of drug from the site of measurement. Elimination occurs by two processes, metabolism and excretion. *Metabolism* is the conversion of one chemical species to another. *Excretion* is the irreversible loss of the chemically unchanged drug.

Basic Model for Drug Absorption and Disposition

The complexities of human physiology would appear to make it difficult, if not impossible, to model how the body handles a drug. Reasonably complex models to describe the pharmacokinetics of certain drugs have been developed. Perhaps surprisingly then, it is a simple pharmacokinetic model, depicted in Figure 2-3, that has proved most useful in application and that is emphasized throughout the book. The model could apply to any route of extravascular administration.

The boxes in the figure can be thought of as *compartments* that logically fall into two classes, transfer and chemical compartments. Drug at the site of administration, drug in the body, and that excreted are clearly in different places. Each place may be referred to as a location or transfer compartment. In contrast, metabolism involves a chemical conversion and the metabolite is therefore in a chemical compartment.

The model is based on amounts of drug. However, only the amount of drug in the urine can be measured directly. The amount of drug metabolized includes metabolites in the body as well as metabolites that have been eliminated. Drug in the body is usually determined from measurement of the blood or plasma concentration. Estimates of drug in the absorption compartment are also made indirectly from either blood or urine data. Drug at the absorption site includes drug that is never absorbed, for example, drug that is decomposed in the gastrointestinal tract or is lost in the feces.

The model is readily visualized from mass balance considerations. The dose is accounted for at any one time by the molar amount of substance in each of the compartments:

$$\text{Dose} = \begin{array}{l}\text{Amount at} \\ \text{absorption site}\end{array} + \begin{array}{l}\text{Amount in} \\ \text{body}\end{array} \\ + \begin{array}{l}\text{Amount} \\ \text{metabolized}\end{array} + \begin{array}{l}\text{Amount} \\ \text{excreted}\end{array} \qquad 1$$

The material balance accounting for a drug is shown in Figure 2-4. Since the sum of the molar amounts of drug in the transfer and the chemical compartments is equal to the dose, the sum of the rates of change of

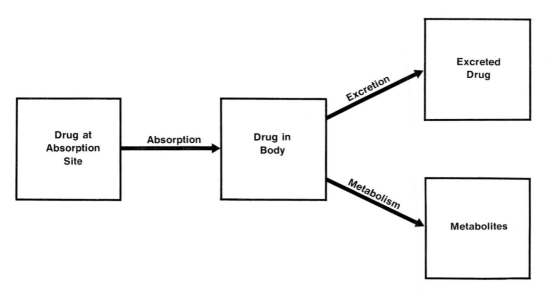

Figure 2-3. *A drug is simultaneously absorbed into and eliminated from the body. The processes of absorption, renal excretion, and hepatic metabolism are indicated with arrows and the compartments with boxes.*

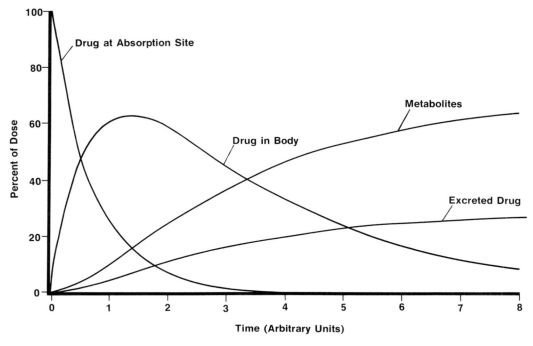

Figure 2-4. *Time course of drug in each of the compartments shown in Figure 2-3. The amount in each compartment is expressed as a fraction of the dose administered.*

the drug in these compartments must be equal to zero so that:

$$\text{Rate of change of drug in body} = \text{Rate of absorption} - \text{Rate of elimination} \qquad 2$$

These relationships, expressed in Equations 1 and 2, apply under all circumstances regardless of the nature of the absorption and the elimination processes. They are particularly useful in developing more complex models for quantitating drug absorption and disposition. Quantitation of the time course of a drug and its metabolites in the body and the development of appropriate models is *pharmacokinetics*.

To appreciate the model presented, consider the following questions:

Q. Does a 100 percent recovery of unchanged drug in the urine following oral administration indicate that the drug is completely absorbed and not metabolized?

A. It must, since the amount ultimately excreted equals the dose. An exception might be the renal excretion of an unstable metabolite which, during storage of the urine or under assay conditions, reverts back to the original drug. In this case, excretion of unchanged drug is not being measured; the observation is an artifact.

Q. When does the drug in the body reach a peak following an oral dose?

A. When the rate of absorption equals the rate of elimination. Prior to that time, absorption is the faster; subsequently, elimination is the faster.

Q. Can the amount of drug absorbed up to a given time be determined?

A. Yes, if the amount of drug in the body and the amount of drug eliminated are both known.

Q. When is the rate of change of drug in

the body equal to the rate of drug elimination?

A. When the rate of absorption is zero. This is the case following intravascular administration or following extravascular administration when absorption has stopped.

Q. When is the rate of change of drug in the body equal to the rate of absorption?

A. When the rate of elimination is virtually zero. This condition exists when there is no drug in the body. It occurs initially following extravascular administration and is essentially the case during most of the absorption phase if absorption is much faster than elimination.

Study Problem

(Answer to Study Problem is found in Appendix G.)

1. Define the terms listed in the objectives at the beginning of this chapter.

3

absorption

Objectives

The reader will be able to:

1. **Describe the steps involved in the absorption process.**

2. **Define passive and facilitated diffusion, active transport, permeability, dissolution, a rate-limiting step, and availability.**

3. **Distinguish between perfusion and diffusion rate-limited absorption from solution.**

4. **Distinguish between dissolution and transmembrane rate limitations in absorption.**

5. **Describe the role of pH in drug absorption from solution.**

6. **List the factors influencing the dissolution rate of a drug.**

7. **Anticipate the role of gastric emptying in the absorption of an orally administered drug.**

DRUGS are most frequently administered extravascularly. The majority are intended to act systemically, and for these, absorption is a prerequisite for activity. Delays or losses of drug during absorption may contribute to variability in drug response and, occasionally, may result in failure of drug therapy. It is primarily in this context, as a source of variability in systemic response, and as a means of controlling the concentration–time profile of drug in the body, that drug absorption is considered here and throughout most of the book. It should be kept in mind, however, that even for those drugs intended to act locally (e.g., mydriatics, local anesthetics, nasal decongestants, topical agents, aerosol bronchodilators), systemic absorption influences the time of onset, the intensity, and the duration of effect.

Figure 2-2 depicts the steps involved in the absorption of a drug given orally. Passage of drug across the membranes dividing the absorption site from the blood is a prerequisite for absorption. To do so, the drug must be in solution. Even then absorption is variable. Drugs pass through membranes with differing facilities. The physicochemical properties of the molecule and the nature of the membrane are controlling factors. Absorption is also influenced by such physiologic factors as the pH of the solution at the absorption site and local blood flow.

Some drugs pass readily through membranes but are still poorly absorbed, especially when given orally because they are unstable in gastrointestinal fluids, metabolized by intestinal microflora or by epithelial enzymes, or are extensively removed by the liver, an organ that lies between the gastrointestinal tract and the systemic circulation where the drug is measured.

Most drugs are taken orally in solid dosage preparations. Common examples are tablets and capsules. Because solid particles cannot pass through membranes, a drug has to dissolve to be absorbed. The rate and extent of dissolution depend in part upon the physicochemical properties of the drug and in part upon the manufacturing process. Besides the active ingredient, other substances are incorporated into the dosage form to improve drug stability, ease of manufacture, and patient acceptability. These "inert" ingredients may have a profound effect on the dissolution performance of the active ingredient and, occasionally, can make the difference between ineffective and effective therapy.

This chapter deals with the general principles governing the rate and extent of drug absorption. Emphasis is placed upon absorption following oral administration. This is not only because the oral mode of administration is the most prevalent for systemically acting drugs, but also because it illustrates essentially all the sources of variability encountered in drug absorption. Where important, distinctions are made between absorption from the gastrointestinal tract and absorption from other sites.

The term *availability* is used to express the completeness of absorption. Thus, availability is generally defined as the fraction or percent of the administered dose of drug that is ultimately absorbed intact. The influence of rate of absorption and availability on the kinetics of drug in the body and methods of assessing these parameters are discussed in Chapter 9. *Biopharmaceutics* is a comprehensive term denoting the study of the influence of pharmaceutical formulation variables on the performance of a drug *in vivo*.

Absorption from Solution

Several physiologic and physical factors control drug absorption from solution.

Movement Through Membranes

The movement of a drug across a membrane is known as *drug transport*. Membranes at absorption sites have properties in common with other membranes. They appear to be composed of an inner, predominantly lipoidal matrix covered on each surface by either a continuous layer or a latticework of protein. The hydrophobic portions of the lipid molecules are oriented toward the center of the membrane, while the outer hydrophilic regions face the surrounding aqueous environment. The hydrophobic inner region permits the passage of lipophilic drugs. Small water-soluble molecules, including urea and methanol, move through membranes faster than anticipated. This has led to the idea that membranes also contain small aqueous-filled pores, but these have never been observed. The following discussion is applicable to the movement of any drug through all membranes of the body.

Passive Diffusion. Most drugs pass through membranes by *diffusion*. Diffusion is the natural tendency for molecules to move from a region of high to one of low concentration. Movement results from the kinetic energy of the molecules, and since no work is required by the system, the process is known as *passive diffusion*.

One can imagine a simple system in which a membrane separates two well-stirred aqueous compartments. The driving force for drug transfer is the difference between the concentration of the diffusing species in the compartments on either side of the membrane:

$$\text{Rate of penetration} = \text{Permeability constant} \times \text{Surface area} \times \text{Concentration difference} \quad 1$$

The dependence of the rate of penetration on the surface area of the membrane is readily apparent. For example, doubling the surface area doubles the probability that a drug molecule will collide with the membrane and increases the absorption rate twofold. Some drugs readily pass through a membrane while others do not. This difference in ease of penetration is quantitatively expressed in terms of the *permeability constant*. This constant, a characteristic of both the molecule and the membrane, is defined by:

$$\text{Permeability constant} = \frac{\text{Diffusion coefficient} \times \text{Partition coefficient}}{\text{Membrane thickness}} \qquad 2$$

The major source of variation in the permeability constant is the partition coefficient of a drug between the lipid membrane and the aqueous environment. Lipid-soluble drugs have high permeability constants and penetrate membranes with ease. Polar neutral molecules (e.g., mannitol) and ionized compounds partition poorly into lipids. They are either unable to pass through membranes or do so with much greater difficulty than do lipophilic compounds. The molecular weights of most drugs lie within the narrow range of 100 to 350. Accordingly, being related to the square root of the molecular weight, the diffusion coefficient is only a minor source of variation in the permeability constant. The thickness of the membrane varies with the membrane and is the distance between the absorption surface and a blood capillary. This distance is generally only a few microns.

Diffusion continues until equilibrium is achieved, at which time the concentration of the diffusing species is the same in the aqueous phases on either side of the membrane. Movement of drug between regions still continues at equilibrium but the net flux is zero. The speed at which equilibrium is achieved depends upon the permeability constant and the surface area of the membrane. Equilibrium is achieved much more rapidly with highly permeable drugs and when there is a large surface area of contact with the membrane.

Initially, when all the drug is placed on one side of the membrane, the rate of drug transport is directly proportional to the concentration (Fig. 3-1). For example, the rate of transport is increased twofold when

the concentration of drug is doubled. Stated differently, each molecule diffuses independently of the other and the system cannot be saturated. Unless a drug alters the nature of the membrane, the last statement also applies when the other molecule is a different drug. Both the absence of competition between molecules and the lack of saturation are characteristics of a passive diffusion process.

Carrier-Mediated Transport. Membranes are not inert barriers; they have a specialized function. Membranes maintain the internal cellular environment, excluding toxic materials while sequestering or selectively retaining vital substances. Many of these compounds are polar, with low lipid solubility. Yet they penetrate membranes much faster than anticipated assuming only passive diffusion through an inert lipoidal barrier. Specialized carrier-mediated transport systems appear to be operative. The substrates are often endogenous compounds, or close analogs.

The concept of a carrier stems from the observation of a limited rate of transport at increased substrate concentrations (Fig. 3-1). Two types of specialized transport processes have been proposed, namely, passive facilitated diffusion and active transport.

Passive facilitated diffusion is exemplified by the movement of glucose into erythrocytes. It is a passive process; glucose moves down a concentration gradient without expenditure of energy and, at equilibrium, the concentrations in and surrounding the red blood cell are equal. At high plasma glucose concentrations, however, the rate of transport of glucose into the erythrocyte reaches a limiting value or *transport maximum*. Furthermore, in common with other carrier-mediated systems, glucose transport is reasonably specific and is inhibited by other substrates. Few drugs undergo passive facilitated diffusion. An example is vitamin B_{12}, which is transported across the gastrointestinal epithelium.

Examples of *active transport* are the renal

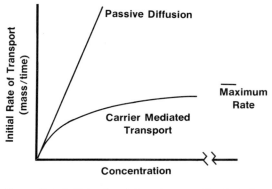

Figure 3-1. *Initial rate of drug transport is plotted against the concentration of drug placed on one side of a membrane. With passive diffusion, the rate of transport increased linearly with concentration. With carrier-mediated transport systems, the rate of transport reaches a maximum value at high concentrations.*

and biliary secretion of many acids and many bases, the secretion processes of certain acids out of the central nervous system, and the intestinal absorption of 5-fluorouracil. Characteristics in common with passive facilitated diffusion are saturability, specificity, and competitive inhibition. Active transport is distinguished from facilitated diffusion by the net movement of substance against a concentration gradient. The maintenance of this gradient requires metabolic energy. Active transport can therefore be affected by metabolic inhibitors.

Blood Flow—A Potential Rate-Limiting Step

Blood flow assures continuous absorption by removing drug that passes through membrane. The concentration gradient across the membrane is, thereby, continuously maintained. With highly lipid-soluble drugs, or those that pass freely through the aqueous-filled pores, penetration through a membrane may be so rapid that equilibrium is established between the drug in the blood and that at the absorption site by the time the blood leaves the membrane. Under these conditions the slowest or *rate-limiting step* controlling drug absorption is blood flow, not penetration through the mem-

brane. This is seen in Figure 3-2. Tritiated water moves freely through the aqueous pores, and its rate of absorption increases with blood flow. Absorption of ethanol and many lipophilic drugs is similarly perfusion rate-limited. In contrast, with ribitol and many other polar compounds, absorption is controlled or rate-limited by diffusion through the membrane. Here, absorption is insensitive to changes in perfusion; the problem now lies in penetrating the membrane, not in removing the drug from the other side of the membrane. Some compounds, like urea, have intermediate permeability characteristics. At low blood flow rates, the compound has sufficient time to diffuse across the membrane so absorption is perfusion rate-limited. At higher blood flow rates, however, membrane permeabil-

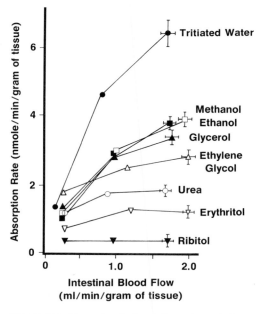

Figure 3-2. *The rate of absorption of a substance from the jejunum of the rat was determined by measuring its rate of appearance in the intestinal venous blood. Absorption is blood flow-limited when, like tritiated water, the molecule freely permeates the membrane. With poorly permeable substances, like the polar molecule ribitol, absorption is limited by transmembrane penetration, not by blood flow. (Redrawn from Winne, D., and Remischovsky, J: Intestinal blood flow and absorption of non-dissociable substances. J. Pharm. Pharmacol., 22: 640–641, 1970.)*

ity becomes the rate-limiting step, and absorption is insensitive to blood flow (Fig. 3-2).

Absorption of drugs in solution from muscle and subcutaneous tissue is normally perfusion rate-limited. Increases in blood flow increase absorption. Here the impedance to absorption is the capillary wall. At these sites, the capillary wall, a much more loosely knit structure than the epithelial lining of the gastrointestinal tract, permits the rapid passage of all molecules below a molecular weight of about 5000, whether ionized or un-ionized. This molecular weight range includes essentially all drugs. For example, whereas neomycin, a relatively water-soluble polar base, has difficulty penetrating the gastrointestinal mucosa, it is rapidly absorbed from the intramuscular site.

Ionization and Absorption—
A Hypothesis

Most drugs are weak acids or weak bases and exist in solution as an equilibrium between the un-ionized and the ionized forms. Increased accumulation of drug on the side of membrane whose pH favors a greater ionization of the drug has led to the *pH partition hypothesis*. According to this hypothesis, only un-ionized nonpolar drug penetrates the membrane, and at equilibrium the concentration of the un-ionized species is equal on both sides of the membrane. The majority of evidence supporting the pH partition hypothesis stems from studies of the gastrointestinal absorption, renal excretion, and gastric secretion of drugs. The pH of the gastric fluid varies between 1.5 and 7.0, while urinary pH fluctuates between 4.5 and 7.5. Elsewhere in the body, changes in pH tend to be much smaller. Because both ionized and un-ionized solutes readily pass across the capillary wall, the influence of pH on intramuscular and subcutaneous absorption of drugs is likely to be far less significant. The influence of pH on the renal excretion of drugs

is considered in Chapter 5. The following discussion examines the role of pH on gastrointestinal drug absorption. The un-ionized form is assumed to be sufficiently lipophilic to transverse the membrane. If it is not, theory predicts that there is no absorption, irrespective of pH.

The fraction un-ionized at the absorption site is controlled by both the pH and the pKa of the drug, according to the Henderson-Hasselbalch equation. Thus, for acids,

$$pH = pKa + \log\left(\frac{\text{Ionized concentration}}{\text{Un-ionized concentration}}\right) \quad 3a$$

and for bases

$$pH = pKa + \log\left(\frac{\text{Un-ionized concentration}}{\text{Ionized concentration}}\right) \quad 3b$$

Since $\log 1 = 0$, the *pKa* of a compound is the pH at which the un-ionized and ionized concentrations are equal. The *pKa* is a characteristic of a drug (Fig. 3-3). Consider, for example, the anticoagulant warfarin. Warfarin is an acid with *pKa* 4.8, that is, equimolar concentrations of un-ionized and ionized drug exist in solution at pH 4.8. Stated differently, 50 percent of the drug is un-ionized at this pH. At one pH unit higher, 5.8, by appropriate substitution into the Henderson-Hasselbalch equation, the ratio is 10 to 1 in favor of the ionized drug, i.e., 10 out of 11 total parts or 91 percent of the drug now exists in the ionized form and only 9 percent is un-ionized.

Figure 3-4 shows changes in the percent of un-ionized drug with pH for acids of different *pKa* values. The pH range 1.0 to 8.0 encompasses the changes in pH seen in the gastrointestinal tract and at other absorption sites. Several considerations are in order. First, very weak acids, such as phenytoin and many barbiturates, whose *pKa* values are greater than 7.5, are essentially un-ionized at all pH values. For these acids absorption should be independent of pH. Second, the fraction un-ionized only changes dramatically for acids with *pKa* values in the range 2.5 to 7.5, and for these compounds a change in the rate of absorp-

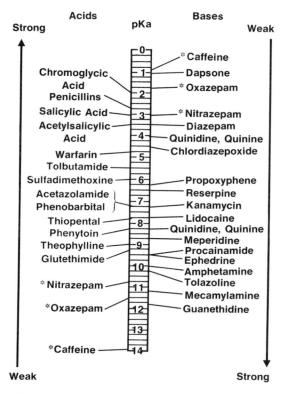

Figure 3-3. *The* pKa *values of acidic and basic drugs vary widely. Some drugs are amphoteric (*).*

alkaline environment. All evidence supports these expectations.

Despite its general appeal, the pH partition hypothesis fails to explain certain observations. A variety of quaternary ammonium compounds, which are always ionized, elicit systemic effects when given orally. Absorption occurs, although at a slow and erratic rate. Animal studies also indicate penetration of the ionized form of many acids and many bases through the intestinal epithelium, though more slowly than the un-ionized form. Whether these ionized species transverse the membrane through the aqueous pores, through channels between the cells, or by some carrier-mediated transport process is not fully understood. Whatever the mechanism, however, these observations suggest that quantitative predictions of the influence of pH on drug absorption, assuming the pH partition hypothesis, are unlikely to be accurate.

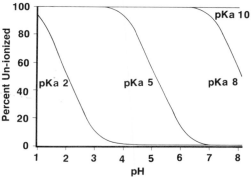

Figure 3-4. *Very weak acids, pKa values greater than 8, are predominantly un-ionized at all pH values between 1 and 8. Profound changes in the fraction un-ionized occur with pH for an acid whose pKa value lies within the range 2 to 8. Although the fraction un-ionized of even stronger acids increases with hydrogen ion concentration, the absolute value is low.*

tion with pH is expected and has been observed. Third, although the absorption of still stronger acids, those with *pKa* values less than 2.5, should theoretically also depend upon pH, in practice the fraction unionized is so low that absorption may be slow even under acidic conditions.

A similar analysis indicates that a base must be very weak, *pKa* less than 5, for absorption to be independent of pH. Caffeine (*pKa* 0.8), an example of a very weak base, is rapidly absorbed, and no pH-dependent absorption has been observed. Only with stronger bases, those with *pKa* values between 5 and 11, is pH-dependent absorption expected. At the low pH of the gastric fluid, these bases exist almost exclusively in the ionized form, and for these, gastric absorption should be slow. Absorption of these bases should be more rapid from an

Gastric Emptying—Another Rate-Limiting Step

In accordance with the prediction of the pH partition hypothesis, weak acids are absorbed more rapidly from the stomach when the pH of the contents is 1 than when the pH of the contents is closer to 8, and the converse holds for weak bases (Table 3-1). Absorption of acids, however, is always much faster from the more alkaline intestine (pH 5–7) than from the stomach (Fig. 3-5). How are these apparently conflicting observations reconciled? Surface area and, for perfusion rate-limited absorption, blood flow are important determinants of the rapidity of absorption. The intestine, especially the small intestine, is favored on both these accounts. The total absorptive area of the small intestine, composed largely of microvilli, has been calculated to be about 200 m^2, and an estimated 1 liter of blood passes through the intestinal capillaries each minute. The corresponding estimates for the stomach are only 1 m^2 and 150 ml/min. These increases in both surface area and blood flow more than compensate for the decreased fraction of un-ionized acid in the intestine. Indeed, the absorption of *all* compounds, be they acids, bases, or neutral compounds, is faster from the (small) intestine than from the stomach. The rate of gastric emptying, therefore, is a controlling step in the speed of drug absorption. Food, especially fat, slows stomach emptying, which explains why drugs are frequently recommended to be taken on an empty stomach when a rapid onset of action is desired.

Retention of drug in the stomach will increase the percentage of drug absorbed through the gastric mucosa but the majority of drug is still absorbed through the intestinal epithelium. In this regard, the stomach may simply be viewed as a repository organ from which pulses of drug are ejected onto the absorption sites in the small intestine.

Causes of Low Availability

As stated previously, an important parameter in drug therapy is availability, that is, the completeness of absorption. So far, the assumption has been made that, if a drug is given in solution and passes readily across membranes, absorption is complete. This assumption is reasonable for drugs placed at most sites of administration, but it is not always so for drugs placed into the gastrointestinal tract. The explanation lies in any one or combination of the following: insufficient time at the absorption site, the presence of a competing reaction, and the removal of drug by the liver. These events are depicted in Figure 2-2, but before examining each of them in detail the general situation is considered.

A drug must pass sequentially from the gastrointestinal lumen, through the gut wall, and through the liver, before entering the general circulation. This sequence is an anatomic requirement because blood perfusing virtually all the gastrointestinal tis-

Table 3-1. Influence of pH on the Gastric Absorption of Acids and Bases from Solution in the Rat

Drug	pKa	Percent Absorbed in 1 Hour	
		pH 1	pH 8
Acids			
Salicylic acid	3.0	61	13
Thiopental	7.6	46	34
Bases			
Quinine	8.4	0	18
Dextromethorphan	9.2	0	16

Abstracted from Schanker, L.S., Shore, P. A., Brodie, B.B., and Hogben, C. A. M.: Absorption of drugs from the stomach. I. The rat. J. Pharmacol. Exp. Ther., *120:* 528–539, 1957.

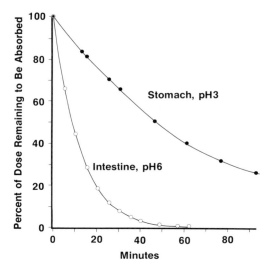

Figure 3-5. *Despite an environment favoring a greater percentage of un-ionized drug, absorption of salicylic acid (pKa 3) is slower from the rat stomach at pH 3 (●) than from the rat intestine at pH 6 (○). (Modified from Doluisio, J.T., Billups, N.F., Dittert, L.W., Sugita, E.G., and Swintosky, J.V.: Drug Absorption I. An in situ* rat gut technique yielding realistic absorption rates. J. Pharm. Sci., 58: 1196–1199, 1969. Adapted with permission of the copyright owner.)*

sues drains into the liver, via the hepatic portal vein. If the only cause of loss is incomplete time for absorption, then the availability would be the fraction of the administered dose, F_F, that passes through the gut wall and the liver to reach the systemic circulation. The remaining fraction, $1 - F_F$, a measure of luminal retention, would appear in the feces as unchanged drug. If drug is also lost by decomposition in the lumen or in the walls of the gastrointestinal tract, then the fraction of the dose reaching the liver is $F_F \cdot F_G$, where F_G is the fraction of the drug not lost in the feces that escapes destruction in the gastrointestinal tract. If drug is also eliminated in the liver, an additional fraction, F_H, of that reaching the liver escapes extraction there. The measured overall availability, F, clearly is then

$$F = F_F \cdot F_G \cdot F_H \qquad 4$$

For example, if 50 percent of the drug is lost at each step, then the availability of the drug, measured systemically, would be $0.5 \times 0.5 \times 0.5$ or 12.5 percent. Moreover, the availability of the drug is zero if at any stage the drug is rendered totally unavailable.

The lungs are excluded from the foregoing considerations of availability even though they may occasionally be an important site of elimination. As discussed in greater detail in Chapter 9, drug given intravenously is used as a standard to measure availability, and the calculation of availability is based, for example, upon the measurement of drug at a peripheral venous site distant from the site of the intravenous injection. Since to reach this site of measurement, both intravenously and orally administered drug must first pass through them, the effect of the lungs on the measurement of availability need not be considered.

Insufficient Time for Absorption. Ingested drug is exposed to the gastrointestinal mucosa for no more than 1 to 2 days, and for much less time at the main absorption site, the small intestine. If a drug is poorly permeable, for example, neomycin and quaternary ammonium compounds, there is insufficient time for complete absorption. There may be insufficient time for complete absorption of the vitamin, riboflavin, and of other substances absorbed by a carrier-mediated transport process. The site of the transport process is usually restricted to a select part of the gastrointestinal tract; the system for absorbing riboflavin is located in the upper part of the small intestine. At the doses taken, the concentration of riboflavin reaching the site of absorption saturates the transport process. The oral availability of riboflavin can be increased by taking the vitamin with small amounts of food. The resultant slowing of stomach emptying both extends the duration and diminishes the rate of delivery of riboflavin and hence its concentration at the absorption site; both factors favor more complete absorption.

The rectum has a small surface area and a drug given rectally is not always retained for a sufficient length of time to ensure complete absorption. No time limitation exists for a drug injected into muscle or subcutaneous tissue; complete absorption is anticipated unless destruction occurs at the site of administration.

Competing Reactions. Any reaction that competes with absorption may reduce the oral availability of a drug. Table 3-2 lists various reactions that can occur within the gastrointestinal tract. Reactions can be both enzymatic and nonenzymatic. Acid hydrolysis is a common nonenzymatic reaction. Enzymes in the intestinal epithelium and within the intestinal microflora metabolize

some drugs. The reaction products are often inactive or less potent than the parent molecule. Interactions with constituents of the gastrointestinal fluids also occur; The result may be poor drug availability. For example, one reason why tetracycline is incompletely absorbed when coadministered with milk and with certain antacids is that this antibiotic forms sparingly soluble and poorly permeable complexes with the polyvalent cations (e.g., Ca^{2+}, Mg^{2+}, Al^{3+}) contained in these preparations.

The degree of reduction in absorption due to a competing reaction is a function of the relative rates of the various processes involved. Unfortunately, the complexity of events that occur *in vivo* precludes accurate prediction of the contribution of the competing reaction to a decrease in drug availability. Sometimes the problem of incomplete absorption can be circumvented by

Table 3-2. Reactions Within the Gastrointestinal Tract that Compete for Drug Absorption from Solution

Reaction	Drug	Comment
Acid hydrolysis	Penicillin G	Loss of activity: product inactive
	Erythromycin	Loss of activity: product inactive
	Digoxin	Product probably inactive
Enzymatic hydrolysis	Aspirin	Salicylic acid formed, active anti-inflammatory compound
	Pivampicillin	Active ampicillin formed: pivampicillin (ester) is inactive
Complexation	Tetracycline	Unabsorbed insoluble complexes with polyvalent metal ions, e.g., Ca^{2+}, Al^{3+}
Conjugation		
Sulfate formation	Isoproterenol	Loss of activity; product inactive
Glucuronidation	Salicylamide	Loss of activity: product inactive
Oxidation	Chlorpromazine	Loss of activity: product inactive
Reduction (microflora)	Cyclamate	Cyclohexylamine formed, carcinogenic in animals
	Sulfasalazine	Intended for local (intestinal) anti-inflammatory action; parent drug inactive; product, 5-amino salicylic acid, active
Decarboxylation	Levadopa	Loss of activity: product active but not absorbed

physically protecting the drug from destruction in the stomach (see enteric coating, p. 30) or by synthesizing a more stable derivative, which is converted to the active molecule within the body. These derivatives are generally referred to as *prodrugs* if they are inactive.

Hepatic Extraction. Aspirin (acetylsalicylic acid) was one of the first prodrugs marketed. It was synthesized at the turn of the century to overcome the bitter taste and the gastrointestinal irritation associated with the parent drug, salicylic acid. Aspirin was originally thought to be inactive, being designed to be rapidly hydrolyzed within the body to salicylic acid. Only subsequently was aspirin shown to be also pharmacologically active. Yet the original design worked; upon ingestion, aspirin, a labile ester, is rapidly hydrolyzed, particularly by esterases in the liver. Indeed, hepatic hydrolysis is so rapid that a significant fraction of aspirin is converted to salicylic acid in a single passage through the liver, resulting in a substantial "first-pass effect."

Drugs that show a significant first-pass effect in man due to hepatic elimination are listed in Table 3-3. Apart from this feature, they have little in common. They are of diverse chemical structure, possess different pharmacologic activities, and are metabolized via a number of pathways. When the metabolite(s) formed during the first pass through the liver are less potent than the parent drug, the oral dose is larger than the intravenous or intramuscular dose required to achieve the same therapeutic effect. This occurs for many of the drugs listed in Table 3-3. In some instances, e.g., lidocaine, hepatic extraction is so high as to essentially preclude the oral route; no amount of pharmaceutical formulation helps. Either the drug must be given by a parenteral route, or it must be discarded in favor of another drug candidate. A method of estimating the maximum likely decrease in oral availability due to this first-pass effect is discussed in Chapter 6.

Table 3-3. Drugs Showing Low Oral Availability due to Extensive First-pass Hepatic Elimination

Aspirin	Morphine
Desipramine	Nitroglycerin
Hydralazine	Pentazocine
Isoproterenol	Propoxyphene
Lidocaine	Propranolol
Methylphenidate	Salicylamide

Avoiding the first pass through the liver probably explains the activity of nitroglycerin administered sublingually. Blood perfusing the buccal cavity bypasses the liver and enters directly into the superior vena cava. This anti-anginal drug is almost completely metabolized as it passes through the liver, and any drug swallowed is not systemically available. The metabolites seen in blood are only weakly active.

The rectal route has a definite advantage over the oral route for drugs that are destroyed by gastric acidity or by enzymes in the intestinal wall and microflora. Potentially, the rectal route may also partially reduce first-pass hepatic loss. Part of the rectal blood supply, particularly the inferior and middle hemorrhoidal veins, bypasses the hepatic portal circulation and dumps directly into the inferior vena cava. Achieving a reproducible availability, which is important in drug therapy, may be difficult, however, since availability is strongly dependent upon the site of absorption within the rectum.

Absorption and Dissolution from Solids

Formulation—An Added Variable

Solubility and stability limitations, taste, and convenience often argue against administration of solution; hence the use of solid medicaments. Tablets and capsules are the most common examples. Equality of drug content was once assumed to assure equality of efficacy. Evidence now exists that questions this assumption. Therapeutic failures have been reported when one manufacturer's brand of prednisone tablet was substituted by another's. Increased side effects associated with phenytoin have occurred upon switching formulations of this drug. In each case, the amount of drug in the dosage form was the same. The problem was due to differences in absorption of drug from the different formulations. The magnitude of the problem is poorly defined, but extends beyond these two drugs. Other drugs that have shown marked differences in absorption from various marketed products of the same dosage form include: digoxin, tolbutamide, tetracycline, oxytetracycline, phenylbutazone, chloramphenicol, and dicumarol.

Generally, when problems arise in drug therapy because of differences in absorption, availability is the major consideration. Occasionally variations in absorption rate may also be important. Much depends upon whether the drug is taken occasionally or continuously (Chap. 13). The major cause of differences in absorption of a drug from various formulations is dissolution. How such differences in dissolution arise

and why dissolution is such an important variable in absorption are now examined.

Marketed products must meet pharmacopeial standards. These standards, however, have been primarily for content and purity of the active ingredient(s). Few standards exist for the inert ingredients (excipients) used to stabilize the drug and to maintain the integrity of the dosage form upon handling and storage. Just how many excipients are used in a typical tablet is shown in Table 3-4. Intended, or otherwise, each ingredient can influence the rate of dissolution of the drug, as can the manufacturing process. The result is a large potential for variability in absorption of a drug between generic products. Sometimes, these differences in absorption can be correlated with differences in the dissolution rate of the drug measured in an *in vitro* apparatus. There are dissolution requirements for certain important drug products. However, on occasion, *in vitro* dissolution tests fail to distinguish between products showing inequivalent absorption profiles. At present, evaluation in humans appears to be the best way of discriminating between good and poor formulations. The cost, however, is high. Perhaps *in vitro* tests will eventually be developed to screen out poor formulations of most drugs.

Table 3-4. Composition of a "Typical" Tablet

Ingredient	Amount	Function
Drug, defined quality and particle size	60 mg	
Lactose	26 mg	Diluent—increases tablet to practical size
Starch	20 mg	(1) Binder—prevents tablet from crumbling (2) Disintegrant—facilitates breakup on contact with water
Talc Magnesium stearate	20 mg 0.3 mg	Lubricant—improves flow properties of granules prior to compression and reduces sticking of tablet to punches and dies of tablet machine
Coloring agent	1 mg	Esthetic and identification

Dissolution—A Rate-Limiting Step

The answer to why dissolution is so important may be gained by realizing that absorption following administration of a solid is a two-step process:

Solid $\xrightarrow{\text{Dissolution}}$ Drug in $\xrightarrow[\text{the body}]{\text{Entry into}}$ Absorbed
drug   solution   drug

Two situations are now considered. The first, depicted in Figure 3-6A, is one in which dissolution is much faster than the rate of entry of drug into the body. It should be noticed that most of the drug has dissolved before an appreciable amount has been absorbed. Here, there is clearly transmembrane rather than dissolution rate-limited absorption. An example is the gastrointestinal absorption of neomycin. This polar antibiotic dissolves rapidly but has difficulty penetrating the gastrointestinal epithelium; little is absorbed. Differences in rates of dissolution of neomycin from dif-

ferent tablets have little or no effect on the speed of absorption of this drug.

In the second, and much more common, situation shown in Figure 3-6B dissolution proceeds relatively slowly, and any absorbed drug readily traverses the gastrointestinal epithelium. Absorption cannot proceed any faster than the rate at which the drug dissolves. That is, absorption is dissolution rate-limited. In this case, changes in dissolution profoundly affect the rate, and sometimes the extent, of drug absorption. Evidence supporting dissolution rate-limited absorption comes from the slower absorption of most drugs from solid dosage forms than from a simple aqueous solution.

Factors Controlling Dissolution

Progress in formulation design, establishment of useful *in vitro* dissolution tests, and the ability to anticipate absorption

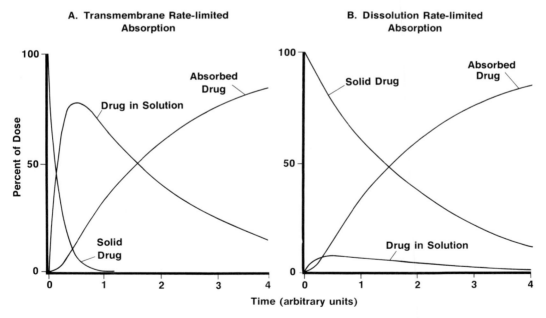

Figure 3-6. *When absorption is transmembrane rate-limited most of the drug has dissolved before an appreciable fraction has been absorbed. In contrast, when dissolution rate-limits absorption, very little drug is in solution at the absorption site; drug is absorbed as soon as it dissolves. Notice that the majority of drug not absorbed is always found at the rate-limiting step: in solution in case A and as a solid in case B.*

problems with certain drugs, come with an understanding of the factors controlling dissolution. These factors are embodied in the relationship:

$$\begin{array}{l}\text{Rate} \\ \text{of} \\ \text{dissolution}\end{array} = K \cdot A \cdot \left[\begin{array}{l}\text{Saturated} \\ \text{solution} \\ \text{at solid} \\ \text{surface}\end{array} - \begin{array}{l}\text{Concentration} \\ \text{in} \\ \text{bulk of} \\ \text{solution}\end{array}\right] \quad 5$$

where K is a constant and A is the surface area of the dissolving solid. Let us examine each of these factors separately.

Surface Area. Expanding the surface exposed to the solvent hastens dissolution. Reducing the size of the solid particles is the most common means of achieving this goal. Yet, for convenience, the opposite is done. For example, fine particles of drugs are compressed or compacted into tablets and capsules. Clearly, this manufacturing process must be reversed if the surface area is to be enlarged sufficiently to ensure adequate dissolution. To this effect, materials (disintegrants) are incorporated into tablets that cause them to swell, upon contact with water, then to disintegrate into granules that finally deaggregate into the original fine drug particles.

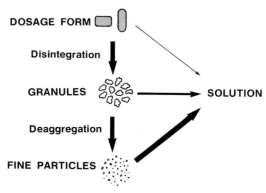

Well-formulated products intended for rapid absorption disintegrate and deaggregate within minutes of administration. Failure to do so may be the cause of poor absorption.

Solubility. It should be recalled that the concentration of drug in solution at the absorption site is kept low in dissolution rate-limited absorption, because dissolved drug rapidly enters the body. The driving force for dissolution is then directly related to the solubility of the drug at the surface of the dissolving solid. This explains why tablets, capsules, and even suspensions of sparingly soluble drugs are prone to absorption problems. Even if dissolution were not the rate-limiting step and a saturated solution at the absorption site could be maintained, the rate of absorption of these drugs would still be low owing to the low aqueous solubility. Among such drugs are digoxin, griseofulvin, and spironolactone. All have low aqueous solubilities, 10 mg/liter or less, as do phenylbutazone, tolbutamide, and warfarin. The last three drugs, however, are weak acids whose dissolution can be markedly increased by using a salt. For example, sodium tolbutamide is absorbed much more rapidly than the free acid. The explanation lies in the different concentration at the surface of the dissolving solid. For tolbutamide, this concentration is the low aqueous solubility of the free acid, whereas for sodium tolbutamide the corresponding concentration is the saturated solution of the salt. Since the salt is much more soluble than the free acid, dissolution of the former is much the faster. Likewise, the hydrochloride or sulfate salt of a base dissolves more rapidly than does the corresponding free base.

Other means of promoting dissolution have been employed. When a drug exists in more than one crystalline (polymorphic) state, the more rapidly dissolving polymorph or amorphous solid is used.

pH. The rate of dissolution depends upon the concentration gradient of dissolving drug that exists between the surface of the solid and the bulk of the solution. Any means of increasing this gradient promotes dissolution. For acids and bases, adjusting the pH of the medium is one way of affecting removal. As an example, consider the dissolution of a base in water and in an acidic solution. In water, as the base dissolves, it produces a saturated solution in the immediate vicinity of the dissolving particle. Further away the concentration falls off as drug diffuses into the body of the solution. Build-up of drug in the water around the solid lowers the concentration gradient and hinders further dissolution. If, however, hydrogen ions are available to consume the dissolved free base by converting it to the soluble cation, the gradient of free base is maintained and dissolution is more rapid. Thus, bases dissolve more rapidly in an acid medium, whereas for analogous reasons, acids dissolve more rapidly in an alkaline medium.

Two methods of increasing the dissolution rate of a base have been considered: use of a salt and use of an acidic environment. Of these, using a salt generally results in faster dissolution. The manyfold increase in solubility of the salt over that of the free base more than compensates for the continual removal of the base in an acidic solution. This is also true for acids. Thus the sodium salt of an acid generally dissolves more rapidly than does the free acid (Table 3-5).

Stirring. Consider now a common situation, the ingestion of a solid formulation of the sodium salt of a sparingly soluble acid. The salt rapidly dissolves at the surface upon contact with the gastric fluid, forming a saturated solution. However, as the salt diffuses away from the surface it is neutralized by hydrogen ions. The free acid formed is at a concentration in excess of its solubility, so the drug precipitates in a finely divided state. Subsequent events depend largely upon the stirring rate around the dissolving particle. With rapid stirring, the precipitate is swept away into the bulk of the solution, creating fresh surface for neutralization and further dissolution. The result is rapid dissolution of the sodium salt and the formation of finely divided precipitate of the acid, of large surface area, dispersed in a saturated solution of the acid. These are excellent conditions for rapid absorption. If, on the other hand, stirring is slow, then the less soluble precipitated acid can form a crust around the dissolving particle of the salt. Further dissolution is thereby hindered, especially if the freshly precipitated acid grows to moderately sized crystals, with an associated small surface area. Now, dissolution and absorption may be even slower than from a well-formulated preparation of finely divided free acid. In practice, both situations probably occur.

Peristaltic movements in the stomach are

Table 3-5. Dissolution of Acids and Their Sodium Salts into Acidic and Neutral Solutions[a]

	Dissolution Rate (mg/100 min/cm² of dissolving surface)	
	pH 1.5	pH 6.8
Phenobarbital	0.24	1.2
Sodium salt	200	820
Salicylic acid	1.7	27
Sodium salt	1870	2500
Sulfathiazole	Less than 0.1	0.5
Sodium salt	550	810

[a] Taken from the data of Nelson, E.: Comparative Dissolution Rates of Weak Acids and Their Sodium Salts. J. Am. Pharm. Assoc., (Sci. Ed.) *47:* 297–299, 1958.

generally feeble but variable. Mixing in the antrum can be quite vigorous. The disintegration rate, deaggregation rate, location of the dosage form in the stomach, and the state of the patient each influence the stirring rate around the dissolving particle. Stirring is generally sufficient to ensure complete and rapid drug absorption from solid dosage forms containing the salts of acids and bases. There are exceptions, however. Thus, the slower absorption of warfarin from some tablets of sodium warfarin, than from some tablets of the acid, is probably explained by poor formulation and by slow stirring, with the resultant precipitation of this insoluble acid around the larger particles of the salt.

As previously mentioned, little drug is generally absorbed from the stomach. Nonetheless, dissolution in the gastric fluid is a prerequisite to the absorption of some drugs. This point is well illustrated by a study of the absorption of various marketed products of tetracycline hydrochloride. Only those which rapidly dissolve in an acidic solution are well absorbed. This amphoteric antibiotic, freely soluble in both strongly acidic and alkaline solutions, is poorly soluble at pH 5.8, the pH of the intestinal fluid. Only that which dissolves in the stomach is apparently absorbed. Perhaps, the sparingly soluble tetracycline precipitates onto undissolved particles entering the intestine, thereby limiting further dissolution.

Gastric Emptying and Intestinal Motility. The possible role of gastric emptying in the absorption of drugs given as tablets or capsules can be understood by considering the following situations.

First, there is the situation in which the drug dissolves before much has entered the intestine. Here, gastric emptying clearly influences the rate of drug absorption. Hastening stomach emptying, for example, hastens drug absorption from solution.

Next, there is the situation in which a drug does not dissolve in the stomach,

whereas, in the intestine, it can both rapidly dissolve and pass across the intestinal wall. Gastric emptying then dramatically affects the time and perhaps the rate of drug absorption. An enteric-coated product is an extreme example of this situation. Erythromycin and penicillin G are rapidly hydrolyzed to inactive products in the acidic environment of the stomach. Salicylic acid is a gastric irritant. A solution to both types of problems has been to coat these drugs with a material resistant to acid, but not to the intestinal fluids. Many such enteric-coated products are single tablets, and the time taken for an intact tablet to pass from the stomach into the intestine varies unpredictably from 20 min to several hours. Accordingly, such enteric-coated products are not to be used when rapid absorption is required. A product composed of enteric-coated granules is an improvement, because the rate of delivery of the granules to the intestine is more reliable, being less dependent on a single event.

Lastly, there is the situation of a drug, such as griseofulvin, that is sparingly soluble in both gastric and intestinal fluids. There may already be insufficient time for dissolution and absorption when this drug is administered as a tablet. Retaining such a drug in the stomach, by increasing the total time for dissolution, should favor increased availability. The time available for dissolution within the intestine is probably limited to between 4 and 10 hours. Subsequently, as the intestinal fluid and contents move into the large intestine and water is reabsorbed, the resulting compaction of the solid contents limits further dissolution of drug. An additional 2 to 4 hours in the stomach, where dissolution can occur, would significantly extend the time for dissolution. Fats, in particular, delay stomach emptying, and this delay may be one of the explanations for the observed increase in the availability of griseofulvin when taken with a fatty meal or with fats.

Changes in intestinal motility affect both mixing within the intestinal fluids and the intestinal transit time. Mixing may be important if substantial dissolution of drug occurs within the intestine. Rapid mixing favors dissolution and drug absorption. A shorter transit time reduces the likelihood of complete absorption especially if insufficient time for absorption is already a problem. When there is both vigorous intestinal movement and a shortened transit time, as might occur in certain types of diarrhea, predicting the outcome of drug absorption is difficult. It is even more difficult if gastric emptying changes simultaneously.

Precipitation and Redissolution

Absorption is normally complete within 1 or 2 hours of administering an aqueous solution of a drug intramuscularly or subcutaneously. There are exceptions, however, particularly when injecting a solution of a salt of either a sparingly soluble acid or base. For example, chlordiazepoxide hydrochloride, in solution, is commonly given intramuscularly when rapid sedation is desired. However, large doses sometimes appear to be poorly effective or ineffective. Although it is eventually completely available, absorption of this sedative has been shown to be slow from the intramuscular site. Indeed, it is even slower than from the gastrointestinal tract, when capsules of chlordiazepoxide hydrochloride are administered (Fig. 3-7). The explanation involves consideration of pH, solubility, perfusion, and stirring.

In the study referenced in the figure, the same dose, 50 mg chlordiazepoxide hydrochloride, was administered by both routes. The intramuscular dose was dissolved in 1 ml of an aqueous vehicle. Chlordiazepoxide is sparingly soluble; its aqueous solubility is approximately 2 mg/ml. To achieve this high concentration of 50 mg chlordiazepoxide hydrochloride/ml, the vehicle contains 20 percent propylene glycol and 4 percent polysorbate 80, both water-miscible materials that permit a greater solubility of the drug. Being the salt of a strong acid and

a weak base (pKa 4.5), the final pH is low, approximately 3. Upon injection, the buffer capacity of both the tissue and the blood perfusing it gradually restores the pH at the injection site to 7.4. This rise in pH and the absorption of the injected water and water-miscible materials cause chlordiazepoxide base to precipitate out of solution. As movement and hence spreading is minimal, a large mass of drug is deposited around the injection site. The rate of absorption now becomes limited by dissolution of the precipitated drug. However, the small surface area, the low solubility, the limited perfusion, and the minimal stirring tend to keep the rate of dissolution down. The result is protracted absorption over many hours or even days. In contrast, absorption following oral administration is relatively rapid. For reasons already discussed, the greater degree of agitation, the larger volume of fluid at the site, and the higher rate of blood flow to the gastrointestinal tract promote more rapid dissolution and absorption following the ingestion of chlordiazepoxide hydrochloride.

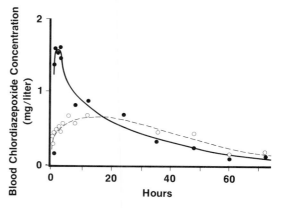

Figure 3-7. *A delayed and lower peak blood concentration of chlordiazepoxide, when given intramuscularly (○--○) as compared to when given orally (●—●), indicates slower absorption from the intramuscular site. On both occasions, 50 mg chlordiazepoxide hydrochloride were administered. (Redrawn from Greenblatt, D.J., Shader, R.I., and Koch-Weser, J.: Slow absorption of intramuscular chlordiazepoxide. N. Engl. J. Med., 291:1116–1118, 1974. Reprinted by permission.)*

Diazepam is sparingly soluble and slowly absorbed when injected intramuscularly. This essentially neutral drug is kept in solution with the aid of propylene glycol. Precipitation at the injection site occurs with the dilution and absorption of this aqueous-miscible solvent.

Dissolution and Drug Delivery Systems

Utilizing the concept that release from a dosage form can rate-limit absorption, various devices have been developed to control the rate of entry of drug into the body. A common approach has been to control the surface area exposed to the dissolving fluid. As drug dissolves, its surface area and, therefore, its rate of release usually decrease. If, however, the surface area is fixed, drug is released at a constant rate. Incorporating the drug into an insoluble matrix is one approach toward achieving this goal. The drug is delivered to the absorption site at a rate dependent on the effective surface area of the matrix, which is under the control of the designer. The duration of release depends upon both the release rate and the amount of drug in the matrix.

Study Problems

(Answers to Study Problems can be found in Appendix G.)

Listed in Table 3-6 are four drugs together with some of their physical properties.

Table 3-6.

Property or Characteristic	Drug A	Drug B	Drug C	Drug D
Molecular weight	327	273	315	378
pKa	8.4 (Acid)	9.8 (Amine)	Neutral	Quaternary Ammonium Compound
Polarity of un-ionized form	Nonpolar	Nonpolar	Polar	—
Solubility of un-ionized form (mg/liter)	1.3	150	—	—

1. Choose the drug(s) (A,B,C,D) that most appropriately completes each of the following statements:
   (a) The gastrointestinal absorption of drug _____, when given in solution, is the most sensitive to changes in intestinal pH.
   (b) The greatest diffusion limitation in crossing the intestinal epithelium is likely to be seen with drug(s) _____ .
   (c) Delayed gastric emptying slows the absorption of drug(s) _____ when given orally in solution. (Assume passive diffusion and drug stability in the gastro-intestinal tract.)
   (d) Muscle blood flow is likely to be a major determinant in the absorption of drug(s) _____, when injected intramuscularly as an aqueous solution, pH 7.4.
   (e) The gastrointestinal absorption of drug(s) _____, when taken as a tablet, is unlikely to be rate-limited by dissolution.

2. Assuming that the conventional single dose of both drugs A and B is 100 mg and that both drugs are stable in the gastrointestinal fluids, circle the most appropriate drug, word, or phrase (in italics) that completes the following statements.
   (a) The sodium salt of drug A dissolves *much faster, much slower, at essentially the same rate,* in a solution of pH 3 than (as) does the free acid in a solution of pH 8. (Assume that all other factors, such as surface area, and stirring, are the same.)
   (b) The hydrochloride salt of drug B should dissolve *much faster, much slower, at essentially the same rate,* in the stomach of a patient with achlorhydria (no gastric acid secretion) than (as) in a patient with normal gastric function.
   (c) Drug A is poorly available when taken orally as the free acid with 100 ml of water. The availability of this drug should be significantly increased by taking the drug *with 200 ml of water, in divided doses during the day, on an empty stomach.*
   (d) Absorption problems are likely to be greater with drug *A, B,* when administered intramuscularly as an aqueous solution of the salt.

4

distribution

Objectives:

The reader will be able to:

1. Define the following terms:
   a. Apparent volume of distribution
   b. Plasma protein binding
   c. Perfusion limitation in distribution
   d. Diffusion limitation in distribution
   e. Tissue to blood equilibrium distribution ratio
   f. Fraction unbound (and bound) in plasma.

2. State the fraction of body volume of an average adult that is assignable to plasma, blood, and to intracellular, extracellular, and total body water.

3. Given the volume of distribution and the fraction unbound in plasma, calculate the fraction of drug in the body that is
   a. In the plasma
   b. Bound to plasma proteins
   c. Outside the plasma
   d. Unbound.

4. Determine the plasma concentration, the amount of drug in the body, and the apparent volume of distribution when any two of these values are known.

5. Describe the effects of perfusion limitation, diffusion limitation, protein binding, and the tissue/blood equilibrium distribution ratio on the distribution of drugs to the tissues.

DISTRIBUTION refers to the reversible transfer of drug from one location to another within the body. Definitive information on the distribution of a drug requires its measurement in various tissues. This kind of information has been obtained in animals, but is lacking in human pharmacology. Useful information on the distribution of drugs in man can be derived, however, solely from observations of blood or plasma drug concentrations. This chapter explores the concepts of distribution useful in clinical pharmacokinetics.

Aspects of Rate of Distribution

The distribution of drugs to the body tissues occurs at various rates and to various extents. Several factors determine the distribution pattern of a drug, including the delivery of drug to a tissue, the ability of a drug to pass through tissue membranes, and the binding of drug to plasma proteins and to tissue components.

Perfusion-Rate Limitation

The rate of distribution of a drug between blood and a tissue, like rate of absorption (see Chap. 3) can be limited either by perfusion or by diffusion. A *perfusion rate-limitation* prevails when the tissue membranes present no barrier to distribution, a condition likely to be met with both small and highly lipophilic drugs diffusing across almost all tissue membranes, and with most drugs diffusing across such loosely knit membranes as muscle capillary walls (see Chap. 3).

Perfusion is usually expressed in units of ml per min per volume of tissue. As seen in Table 4-1, the perfusion rate of tissues varies from approximately 10 ml per min per ml of lung, down to values of only 0.025 ml per min per ml of resting muscle or of fat. All other factors remaining equal, well-perfused tissues take up a drug much more rapidly than do poorly perfused tissues. Moreover, as the subsequent analysis shows, there is a direct correlation between tissue perfusion rate and the time required to distribute a drug to a tissue. The rate of presentation of a drug to a tissue is the product of blood flow, Q, and the arterial blood concentration, C_A, that is,

$$\text{Rate of presentation} = Q \cdot C_A \qquad 1$$

The net uptake into the tissue is the difference between the rate of presentation and the rate of leaving the tissue, $Q \cdot C_V$, where C_V is the emergent venous concentration. Therefore,

$$\text{Net rate of uptake} = Q \cdot (C_A - C_V) \qquad 2$$

If the arterial concentration is constant with time, the amount in the tissue at equilibrium when the net uptake is zero, is:

$$\begin{matrix}\text{Amount in tissue} \\ \text{at equilibrium}\end{matrix} = K_p \cdot V_T \cdot C_A \qquad 3$$

where K_p is the *equilibrium distribution ratio* of concentration in tissue to concentration in blood and V_T is the volume of tissue.

To demonstrate the consequence of a perfusion-rate limitation, consider how long it would take at a constant blood concentration simply to convey to a tissue the amount that is there when equilibrium is achieved. This time can be calculated by dividing the amount in the tissue at equilibrium, Equation 3, by the rate of presentation to the tissue, Equation 1. Therefore,

Time to convey to tissue the amount contained at equilibrium

$$= \frac{K_p \cdot V_T \cdot C_A}{Q \cdot C_A} = \frac{K_p \cdot V_T}{Q} = \frac{K_p}{Q/V_T} \qquad 4$$

From this relationship it is seen that the two factors, equilibrium distribution ratio, K_p, and the perfusion rate, Q/V_T, determine the time.

As examples, consider the distribution of a drug to kidney, muscle, and fat. The perfusion rates and the equilibrium distribution ratios for this drug in these tissues are given in Table 4-2.

Using the kidney as the first example, the time required to deliver the amount that is present when equilibrium is reached with a constantly maintained blood concentration is $[K_p/(Q/V_T)]$ 0.25 min. The time for muscle would be 40 min, and for fat it would be as long as 4800 min or 3.3 days. In practice it would take even longer, than the times calculated above, to approach equilibrium. Constant tissue uptake has been assumed in the calculation but, as seen from Equation 2, net uptake of the drug decreases as the tissue level rises.

These simple examples illustrate two basic principles, namely, equilibrium takes longer to achieve the poorer the perfusion and the greater the partitioning into the tissue. The latter is contrary to what one might intuitively anticipate. However, the greater the tendency to concentrate in a tissue the longer it takes to deliver to that tissue the amount needed to reach distribu-

Table 4-1. Blood Flow Under Basal Conditions and the Relative Size and Water Content of Different Organs and Tissues[a]

Organ	Percent of Body Volume	Percent Water	Blood Flow (ml/min)	Percent of Cardiac Output	Perfusion Rate (ml/min/ml of tissue)	Relative Perfusion Rate[b]
1. Adrenal glands	0.03	—	25	0.2	1.2	17
2. Blood	7	83	(5000)[c]	(100)	—	—
3. Bone	16	22	250	5	0.02	0.3
4. Brain	2	75	700	14	0.5	7
5. Fat	10	10	200	4	0.03	0.4
6. Heart	0.5	79	200	4	0.6	8
7. Kidneys	0.4	83	1100	22	4	55
8. Liver	2.3	68	1350	27	0.8	11
Portal			(1050)	(21)		
Arterial			(300)	(6)		
9. Lungs	0.7	79	(5000)	(100)	10	140
10. Muscle	42	76	750	15	0.025	0.35
11. Skin	18	72	300	6	0.024	0.35
(Cool weather)						
12. Thyroid gland	0.03	—	50	1	2.4	34
TOTAL BODY	100	60	5000	100	0.071	1.0

[a] Compiled from data of Guyton, A.C.: *Textbook of Medical Physiology*, 5th ed. W.B. Saunders, Philadelphia, 1976, p. 251; and Skelton, H.: The storage of water by various tissues of the body. Arch. Intern. Med., *40*: 140–152, 1927. Copyright 1927. American Medical Association.
[b] Perfusion rate relative to the average perfusion rate of the whole body.
[c] Values in parentheses given for comparison.

Table 4-2. Tissue Perfusion Rates and Equilibrium
Distribution Ratios of a Drug

Tissue	Equilibrium Distribution Ratio (tissue/blood) (K_p)	Perfusion Rate (ml/min/ml of tissue) (Q/V_T)
Kidney	1	4
Muscle	1	0.025
Fat	120	0.03

tion equilibrium. Stated differently the affinity of a drug for a tissue accentuates an existing limitation imposed by perfusion.

Diffusion-Rate Limitation.

This situation probably arises for polar drugs diffusing across tightly knit lipoid membranes.

Figure 4-1 demonstrates the diffusion-rate limitation in the passage of compounds into the cerebrospinal fluid. In these studies, the concentration of each drug was measured in the cerebrospinal fluid, relative to that in plasma water with time following the attainment and maintenance of a constant plasma concentration. Because the vascular perfusion of the central nervous system was the same for each of the drugs studied, the widely differing rates of passage into the cerebrospinal fluid must result from a limitation in the diffusion through a lipoid barrier, a *diffusion limitation.* These differences in rate of entry are a function of both the lipid to water partition coefficient and the degree of ionization (Table 4-3), suggesting that only the un-ionized drug penetrates into the brain. For example, the partition coefficients of salicylic acid and pentobarbital are similar, yet the time required to reach distribution equilibrium is far shorter for pentobarbital because, being the weaker acid, a greater fraction is un-ionized in plasma, pH 7.4.

With large differences in perfusion of and diffusion into various tissues it would appear to be impossible to predict tissue distribution of a drug. However, either of these two factors may limit the rate of distribution, thereby simplifying the situation and

allowing some conclusion to be drawn. Consider, for example, the following question: Why, on measuring total tissue concentration, does the general anesthetic thiopental enter the brain much more rapidly than it does muscle tissue? Yet, for penicillin the opposite is true. The explanation lies in the properties of these drugs and tissue membranes.

Thiopental is nonpolar, lipophilic, and being a much weaker acid (pKa 7.6), it is only partially ionized at the pH of plasma. As such, thiopental readily diffuses into both the brain and muscle; entry into both tissues is perfusion rate-limited. Since the perfusion of the brain, particularly gray matter, is one to two orders of magnitude greater than that of muscle (Table 4-1), entry of thiopental into the brain is the more rapid process at plasma pH.

Penicillin, a more polar compound, does not readily pass membranes. The faster rate of entry of penicillin into muscle than into brain is a result of the more porous nature of the muscle capillaries. For many tissues, e.g., kidney and muscle, the capillary membranes appear to be very porous and have little influence on the entry of drugs of usual molecular weight (100–400) into the interstitial fluids, regardless of the drug's physicochemical properties. There may be diffusion limitations at the tissue cell membrane, but in terms of measurement of drug in the *whole* tissue, there would appear to be only a partial impedance to the entry of either ionized or polar compounds, or both. Other tissues, for example much of the central nervous system, anatomically have diffusion limitations at the level of the capil-

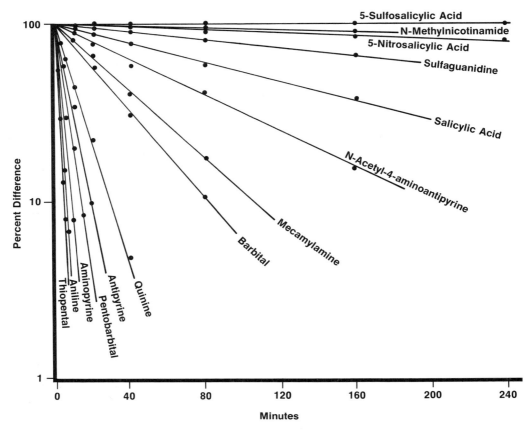

Figure 4-1. *The equilibration of drug in the cerebrospinal fluid with that in plasma is often diffusion-rate limited. The ratio of drug concentrations (cerebrospinal fluid/unbound in plasma) is shown for various drugs in the dog. The plasma concentration was kept relatively constant throughout the study. (Redrawn from the data of Brodie, B.B., Kurz, H., and Schanker, L.S.: The importance of dissociation constant and lipid solubility in influencing the passage of drugs into the cerebrospinal fluid. J. Pharmacol. Exp. Ther., 130: 20-25, 1960. Copyright 1960, The Williams and Wilkins Co., Baltimore.)*

laries that impede movement of drug into the tissue as a whole, as observed with penicillin.

The effect of a high equilibrium distribution ratio on the time to achieve distribution equilibrium, discussed previously for a perfusion-rate limitation, applies equally well to a diffusion rate-limitation. A diffusion-rate limitation simply decreases the rate of entering the tissue from that limited by perfusion. Where the equilibrium lies is independent of which process rate-limits the approach to equilibrium.

All drugs should reach distribution equilibrium when the unbound concentrations in tissue and plasma are equal, if the concentration of drug in blood is maintained long enough. Sometimes, however, this is not observed. Several alternative mechanisms exist for drugs to leave a tissue besides diffusing directly to the blood. Alternatives include excretion, metabolism, active transport out of the tissue and bulk flow of the interstitial fluids to both lymphatic channels and ducts. All these mechanisms tend to result in a lower unbound concentration of drug in the tissue than in the plasma. Active transport into the tissue cells could, of course, have the opposite effect.

Table 4-3. Physicochemical Properties and Time for Cerebrospinal Fluid Concentration to Reach 50 Percent of Equilibrium Value for Selected Acidic Drugs[a] of Figure 4-1[b].

Drug	pKa	Fraction Un-ionized at pH 7.4	Partition Coefficient of Un-ionized Form (n-heptane/water)	Effective Partition Coefficient at pH 7.4[c]	Time to Reach 50 Percent of Equilibrium Value (min)
Thiopental	7.6	0.6	3.3	2.0	1.4[d]
Pentobarbital	8.1	0.8	0.05	0.042	4
Barbital	7.5	0.6	0.002	0.0012	27
Salicylic acid	3.0	0.004	0.12	0.0005	115
Sulfaguanidine	> 10	1.0	0.001	<0.001	231

[a]Similar correlation is observed for basic drugs.
[b]Data from reference in Fig. 4-1 and Hogben, C.A.M., Tocco, D.J., Brodie, B.B., and Schanker, L.S.: On the mechanism of intestinal absorption of drugs. J. Pharmacol. Exp. Ther., *125;* 275-286, 1959.
[c]Fraction un-ionized at pH 7.4 times partition coefficient of un-ionized form.
[d]Probably perfusion rate-limited.

Binding to Plasma Proteins.

A third factor that may influence the rate of distribution is that of binding of drug to plasma proteins. Acidic drugs commonly bind to albumin, an abundant plasma protein. Basic drugs often bind to α_1-acid glycoprotein and lipoproteins. Many endogenous substances, vitamins and metal ions, are bound predominantly to globulins.

Binding is a reversible phenomenon. The rates of association and dissociation are usually rapid (milliseconds). Consequently, the associated, bound, and dissociated, unbound, forms of the drug can be assumed to be at equilibrium at all times and under virtually all circumstances. Only the unbound drug is thought to be capable of diffusing into a tissue. In the absence of a diffusion limitation as with lipophilic compounds, the initial rate of uptake is equal to the rate of presentation, regardless of the extent of protein binding, within limits of course. Thus, the more extensively bound such a drug is to plasma protein, the more quickly is drug distributed. This more rapid distribution is an explanation for the role of plasma proteins in distributing the highly bound corticosteroids formed in the adrenal glands. On the other hand, for polar compounds, diffusion is rate-limiting and dependent on the unbound concentration. As will be shown later in this chapter, the unbound concentration is negligibly affected by changes in plasma binding, and accordingly for such polar compounds plasma binding has little effect on the rate of distribution.

Equilibrium Considerations

Apparent Volume of Distribution

The amount of drug in the body can never be directly measured in humans. Observations are made of the concentration of drug in plasma or sometimes in blood.

The concentration in the plasma with time following the administration of a single dose depends on the rate and extent of distribution to the tissues and on how rapidly the drug is eliminated. For most drugs distribution occurs more rapidly than does elimination. The concentration achieved after distribution is complete is a result of the dose and the extent of distribution into the tissues. This extent of distribution can be determined by relating the concentration obtained with a known amount of drug in the body. This is analogous to the determination of the volume of a reservoir by dividing the amount of dye added to it by the resultant concentration, after thorough mixing. The volume measured is, in effect, a dilution space.

The apparent volume into which a drug distributes in the body at equilibrium is called the *(apparent) volume of distribution.* Plasma, rather than blood, is usually measured. Consequently, the volume of distribution, V, is the volume of plasma at the drug concentration, C, required to account for all the drug in the body, Ab.

$$V = Ab/C \qquad\qquad 5$$

$$\frac{\text{Volume of}}{\text{distribution}} = \frac{\text{Amount in body}}{\text{Plasma drug concentration}}$$

The volume of distribution is useful in estimating the plasma concentration when a known amount of drug is in the body or, conversely, in estimating the dose required to achieve a given plasma drug concentration. How the volume of distribution is measured is presented in Chapter 7.

The volume of distribution is a direct measure of the extent of distribution. It rarely, however, corresponds to a real volume. Drug distribution may be to any one or a combination of the tissues and fluids of the body. Furthermore, the binding to tissue components may be so great that the volume of distribution is many times the total body size.

To appreciate the effect of tissue binding, consider the distribution of 100 mg of a drug in a 1-liter system composed of water and 10 grams of activated charcoal and where 99 percent of the drug is adsorbed onto the charcoal. When the charcoal has settled, the concentration of drug in the water phase would be 1 mg/liter; thus, 100 liters of the aqueous phase would be required to account for all the drug in the system, a volume much greater than that of the total system. Similarly, a drug that binds to tissue components may have a volume of distribution that greatly exceeds the body size. Values of the volumes of

distribution for selected drugs are shown in Figure 4-2.

A few compounds do distribute into real body volumes; they may even be used to measure them. Table 4-4 lists such compounds together with the physiologic volumes into which they are known to distrib-

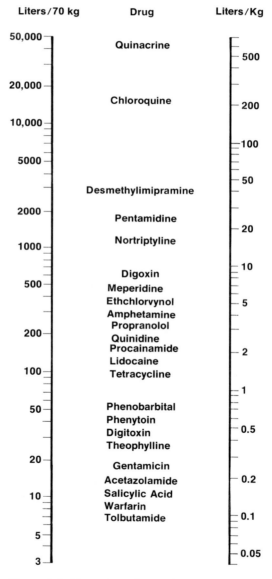

Figure 4-2. *The volume into which drugs apparently distribute varies widely.*

Table 4-4. Body Fluids and Substances that Distribute Within and Define These Fluids

Fluid	Volume (liters)[a]	Percent of Body weight	Substances Primarily Distributed in Fluid
Extracellular water	13–16	18–22	Inulin, Na^+, Br^-, I^-
Plasma	3	4	Evans blue
Interstitial fluids	10–13	14–18	—
Intracellular water	25–28	35–40	—
Transcellular water[b]	0.7–2	1–3	—
Total body water	40–46	55–65	Antipyrine Caffeine Ethanol

[a] Estimates for standard 70-kg man
[b] Includes gastrointestinal secretions, lacrimal fluids, nasal secretions, and so on.

ute approximately. Such examples are rare, however. Even if the volume of distribution of a drug corresponds to the value of a physiologic volume, one cannot conclude unambiguously that the drug only distributes into that volume. The binding of drugs in plasma and in tissues complicates the situation and often prevents making any conclusion about the actual volume into which the drug distributes. An exception is where the drug is restricted to the plasma; the volumes of distribution, apparent and real, are then the same, about 3 liters in an adult. This last situation only occurs when the drug is highly bound to plasma proteins and is not bound in the tissues. Even here, the apparent volume cannot be an equilibrium value, because plasma proteins slowly equilibrate between plasma and other extracellular fluids. The apparent volume of plasma proteins, about 7 liters for albumin, is perhaps a better estimate of the minimum value for any drug. For drugs that are neither tissue nor plasma protein bound, the volume of distribution varies between the extracellular fluid volume (16 liters) and the total body water (42 liters), depending upon the degree to which the drug gains access to the intracellular fluids.

Knowing the plasma volume V_p and the volume of distribution, V, the fraction of drug in the body in plasma and the fraction outside plasma can be estimated. The amount in plasma is $V_p \cdot C$; the amount in the body is $V \cdot C$. Therefore

$$\text{Fraction of drug in body in plasma} = \frac{V_P}{V} \qquad 6$$

It is evident that the larger the volume of distribution, the smaller is the fraction in plasma. For example, for a drug with a volume of distribution of 100 liters, only 3 percent resides in plasma.

The remaining fraction given by

$$\text{Fraction of drug in body outside plasma} = \frac{(V - V_P)}{V} \qquad 7$$

includes that in the blood cells. For the example considered above, 97 percent is outside of plasma. Although this fraction can be readily determined, the actual distribution of drug outside plasma cannot.

Plasma Protein Binding

One of the primary goals of measuring plasma concentrations is to relate pharmacologic response and toxicity to concentration. For practical reasons, plasma (or serum) has become the reference fluid for measuring drug concentration. In many respects this choice is unfortunate. The unbound drug concentration is undoubtedly more closely related to the activity of the drug, yet it is only occasionally measured, primarily because the methods available for doing so are often tedious and lack accuracy. Whole-blood concentration is preferred over the plasma concentration for assessing the distribution of drug into and its elimination from tissues, because it is drug in whole blood, not that just in plasma, which is delivered to the tissues.

The principal concern with plasma-protein binding is related to its variability within and between patients in various therapeutic settings. The degree of drug binding to plasma proteins is frequently expressed as the ratio of the bound concentration to the total concentration. This ratio, fb, has limiting values of 0 and 1.0. Drugs with a value of fb greater than 0.9 are said to be highly bound, and those with a value of fb less than 0.2 are said to show little or no plasma protein binding.

As stated previously, the unbound concentration, rather than the bound concentration, is frequently more important in therapeutics. Therefore, the value of the fraction of drug in plasma that is unbound to plasma proteins, fu, is of greater utility than that of fb. This fraction is simply related to fb by

$$fu = 1 - fb \qquad 8$$

Approximate values of fu for representative drugs in the concentration range usually associated with therapy and at normal serum protein concentrations are shown in Figure 4-3.

Binding is a function of the affinity of the protein for the drug. Because of a limited number of binding sites on the protein, binding also depends on the concentrations of both drug and protein. Assuming a single binding site on the protein, P, the association is simply summarized by the following reaction:

$$D \;+\; P \;\rightleftharpoons\; DP \qquad 9$$
$$\text{Drug}\quad\text{Protein}\quad\text{Drug-protein}$$
$$\text{complex}$$

Equilibrium may lie either to the right or to the left. High affinity, of course, implies that equilibrium lies far to the right. This is a relative statement, however, since the greater the protein concentration for a given drug concentration, the greater the bound drug concentration and the converse. From mass law considerations, the equilibrium is expressed in terms of the concentrations of unbound drug, (D), unbound protein, (P), and drug-protein complex, (DP).

$$K = \frac{(DP)}{(D)\cdot(P)} \qquad 10$$

The association constant, K, is a direct measure of the affinity of the protein for the drug.

Using the fraction of the total concentration that is unbound, fu, the unbound concentration is $fu \cdot C$ and the bound concentration is $(1 - fu)C$. It therefore follows that

$$K \cdot (P) = \frac{(1 - fu)}{fu} \qquad 11$$

or

$$fu = \frac{1}{1 + K \cdot (P)} \qquad 12$$

From this relationship the value of fu is seen to depend upon the unbound protein concentration as well as upon the affinity of the protein for the drug. The unbound protein concentration, in turn, depends upon the total concentration of protein, (P_t), and the concentration of the drug-protein complex, since $(P_t) = (P) + (DP)$. Usually only a small fraction of the available binding sites is occupied at therapeutic drug concentrations; therefore, the fraction unbound is relatively constant and independent of the drug concentration. Under conditions in which most of the available sites are occupied, (DP) approaches (P_t), the binding varies with the drug concentration, and the binding is said to show concentration dependence. At all concentrations the degree of binding depends upon both the affinity constant and the protein concentration. Differences in these last two factors are primarily responsible for the variability observed in plasma-protein binding. Decrease in apparent affinity is often observed in uremia and in the presence of other drugs. The plasma concentration of a binding protein can be decreased, e.g., albumin in chronic liver disease, or increased e.g., α_1-acid glycoprotein in stress conditions.

Tissue Binding

The fraction of drug in the body located in the plasma is also dependent on binding to tissue components as shown schematically in Figure 4-4. A drug may have a great affinity for plasma proteins, but still be primarily in the tissue. This situation would occur if the tissue has an even higher affinity for the drug. The affinity of a tissue for a drug may be for any of several reasons, including binding to tissue proteins (such as albumin) or to nucleic acids or, in the case of adipose tissue, dissolution in fat.

Unlike plasma binding, tissue binding of a drug cannot be measured directly. Handling of a tissue results in its disruption and loss of integrity. Even so, tissue binding is important in drug distribution, and its effect may be appreciated by considering the model shown in Figure 4-5. In this model, drug in the body is accounted for in the plasma, volume V_P, and in two tissue compartments, one of volume V_{T_1}, and the other of volume V_{T_2}. At distribution equilibrium the tissue/plasma ratio of drug concentrations is K_{P_1} and K_{P_2} in the respective tissues. The amount of drug in each location can then be expressed in terms of the plasma concentration, C, the volumes of the tissues, and the distribution ratios as follows:

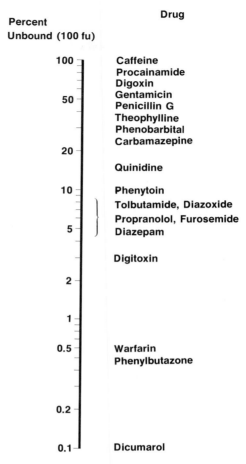

Figure 4-3. *The fraction of drug in plasma not bound to proteins varies widely among drugs.*

$$Ab = \underset{\substack{\text{Amount} \\ \text{in plasma}}}{V_P \cdot C} + \underset{\substack{\text{Amount in} \\ \text{tissue 1}}}{V_{T_1} \cdot K_{p_1} \cdot C} + \underset{\substack{\text{Amount in} \\ \text{tissue 2}}}{V_{T_2} \cdot K_{p_2} \cdot C} \quad 13$$

The volume of distribution of the drug, V, is simply the parameter which, when multiplied by the plasma drug concentration (Eq. 5), accounts for all the drug in the body. From this it follows that,

$$V = V_P + V_{T_1} \cdot K_{p_1} + V_{T_2} \cdot K_{p_2} \quad 14$$

Thus, the volume of distribution is the volume of plasma plus the sum of the products of each tissue volume and the respective equilibrium distribution ratio. For drugs

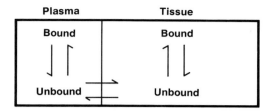

Figure 4-4. *At equilibrium the distribution of a drug within the body depends upon the binding to both plasma proteins and tissue components. Only the unbound drug is capable of entering and leaving the tissues.*

that bind strongly to tissue components, the values of the distribution ratios, (K_{p_1}, K_{p_2}), may be much greater than unity. Consequently, the apparent tissue volumes may be much greater than the real volumes, and the apparent volume of distribution much greater than the total body volume.

Tissue binding may be inferred from measurement of drug binding in the plasma. Consider, for example, the following mass balance relationship.

$$V \cdot C = V_P \cdot C + V_T \cdot C_T \qquad 15$$

Amount in body	Amount in plasma	Amount in tissues

in which V_T is the physical volume of distribution outside the plasma into which the drug distributes and C_T is the average total drug concentration throughout this volume.

Dividing by C,

$$V = V_P + V_T \cdot \frac{C_T}{C} \qquad 16$$

Apparent volume of distribution	Volume of plasma	Apparent volume of tissue

Recall that the fraction of drug in plasma unbound to plasma proteins is given by

$$fu = \frac{Cu}{C} \qquad 17$$

Similarly, the fraction unbound to tissue components, fu_T, is

$$fu_T = \frac{Cu_T}{C_T} \qquad 18$$

Assuming that distribution equilibrium is achieved when the unbound concentrations in plasma, Cu, and in tissues, Cu_T, are equal, then the ratio of Equations 17 and 18 becomes

$$\frac{C_T}{C} = \frac{fu}{fu_T} \qquad 19$$

which on substituting into Equation 16 yields

$$V = V_P + V_T \cdot \frac{fu}{fu_T} \qquad 20$$

From this relationship it is seen that the apparent volume of distribution increases when fu is increased, and decreases when fu_T is increased, as might occur by displacement from plasma proteins or tissue binding sites, respectively.

Since the plasma volume, V_P, is known and the values of fu and V are measurable, the value of V_T/fu_T can be determined.

$$\frac{V_T}{fu_T} = \frac{(V - V_P)}{fu} \qquad 21$$

Taking phenylbutazone as an example, V is about 10 liters, V_P, is 3 liters, and fu is 0.005; therefore V_T/fu_T is 1400 liters. Clearly this

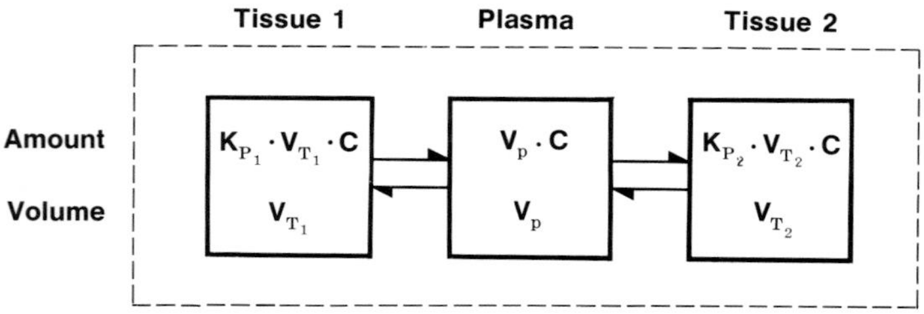

Figure 4-5. *The effect of tissue binding on drug distribution is illustrated by a drug that distributes between plasma and two tissues. The physiologic volumes are V_P, V_{T_1}, and V_{T_2}, respectively. At equilibrium the amount of drug in the tissue depends on the equilibrium distribution (partition) ratio, the tissue volume, and the plasma concentration.*

	Tissue 1	Plasma	Tissue 2
Amount	$K_{P_1} \cdot V_{T_1} \cdot C$	$V_P \cdot C$	$K_{P_2} \cdot V_{T_2} \cdot C$
Volume	V_{T_1}	V_P	V_{T_2}

drug must be bound to the tissues somewhere. To say how much is tissue bound requires an assumption about the physical volume into which the drug distributes. If a drug does not traverse membranes, drug in the tissue would be restricted to extracellular fluids outside the central nervous system. If it does pass readily through membranes, total body water minus the plasma volume might be a better estimate of V_T. In general, V_T should be between these limits, that is, 12 and 39 liters. Assuming that phenylbutazone passes membranes readily, then V_T equals 39 liters, and the value of fu_T is about 0.03. In other words, 97 percent of phenylbutazone in the tissues is bound, despite a small volume of distribution. The small volume of distribution is a consequence of the plasma protein binding being greater than the tissue binding, $fu/fu_T = 0.18$.

Defining V_b as the proportionality constant between the amount in the body and the blood drug concentration, relationships similar to Equations 20 and 21 can be derived that relate V_b to the blood volume, V_B, the fraction unbound in blood, fu_b, the fraction outside blood that is unbound, fu_T', and the physiologic volume outside blood into which the drug distributes, V_T'. The relationships are

$$V_b = V_B + V_T' \cdot \frac{fu_b}{fu_T'} \qquad 22$$

and

$$\frac{V_T'}{fu_T'} = \frac{(V_b - V_B)}{fu_b} \qquad 23$$

The relationship between the volume of distribution (blood) and the binding of a drug is demonstrated by (+)-propranolol as shown in Figure 4-6. The linear relationship indicates that V_T'/fu_T' is a constant. Furthermore, using Equation 23, a usual blood volume of 5 liters, and a limiting value of V_T' of 37 liters (total body water minus the blood volume), the fraction unbound in the tissues is about 0.02. In contrast to phenylbutazone, this drug is more tightly bound in the tissue than in the blood. Also, it is apparent that differences in the binding of propranolol in blood account for most of the variation observed in its volume of distribution (blood).

Total and Unbound Plasma Drug Concentrations Relative to a Given Amount of Drug in the Body

Variations in both plasma and tissue binding give rise to differences in the volume of distribution. Under these conditions the plasma concentration poorly reflects the amount of drug in the body. Whether or not the unbound plasma concentration of drug is a better reflector of the amount in the body depends upon the source of the variability in drug distribution. To appreciate this point, Equations 5 and 20 may be combined to give

$$Ab = \left(V_P \cdot C + \frac{V_T \cdot Cu}{fu_T} \right) \qquad 24$$

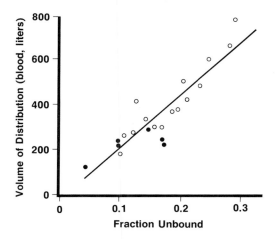

Figure 4-6. *The volume of distribution (blood) of (+)-propranolol varies with the fraction unbound. The observation was made in 6 control subjects (●) and in 15 patients (○) with chronic liver disease, after an intravenous bolus (40 mg) of (+)-propranolol. (Data from Branch, R.A., Jones, J., and Read, A.E.: A study of factors influencing drug disposition in chronic liver disease, using the model drug (+)-propranolol. Br. J. Clin. Pharmacol., 3: 243–249, 1976.)*

For most drugs the volume of distribution is much greater than the plasma volume; therefore, from Equation 6, the amount in the plasma can be ignored. Approximately then,

$$Ab = \frac{V_T}{fu_T} \cdot Cu \qquad 25$$

Thus, the unbound concentration, Cu, is insensitive to a change in plasma protein binding. For example, if plasma binding is diminished (fu increased), Cu would remain unaltered but the total concentration ($C = Cu/fu$) would fall. Differences in tissue binding, seen as changes in fu_T, cause both C and Cu to change relative to a given amount of drug in the body.

Another view of the effect of binding on drug distribution is gained from the volume of distribution based on the unbound plasma concentration, V_u. This parameter relates the unbound concentration, Cu, to the amount in the body; therefore,

$$Ab = V_u \cdot Cu = V \cdot C \qquad 26$$

For a drug that does not bind either in plasma or in the tissues, the volumes of distribution, based on unbound and total drug in plasma, are the same and are equal to the body water (42 liters). When there is binding, the unbound volume term will be greater than total body water. From Equation 26, it follows that

$$\begin{array}{l} \text{Percent} \\ \text{unbound} \\ \text{in body} \end{array} = \frac{\text{Total body water} \cdot 100}{V_u} \qquad 27$$

The percent unbound in body for three drugs is shown in Table 4-5.

Clearly, for antipyrine, both the unbound and total plasma concentrations reflect drug in the body. For phenylbutazone only 2 percent is unbound, and so the possibility exists of appreciably affecting the unbound concentrations, particularly if both plasma and tissue binding are altered simultaneously. This situation can arise because phenylbutazone is predominantly bound to albumin, a protein located in both plasma and tissues. Although it has the same volume of distribution as phenylbutazone, the unbound concentration of salicylic acid is less sensitive to a change in binding since only 58 percent of drug in the body is bound.

Table 4-5. Percent Unbound in Body of Some Drugs

Drug	Volume of Distribution (liters)	Fraction Unbound in Plasma (fu)	Unbound Volume of Distribution (V_u) (liters)	Percent Unbound in body
Antipyrine	37	0.88	42	100
Phenylbutazone	10	0.005	2000	2
Salicylic acid	10[a]	0.1	100	42

[a]At doses of 600 mg or less.

Study Problems

(Answers to Study Problems can be found in Appendix G.)

1. Using the information in Table 4-6, rank the lungs, kidneys, heart, liver, and skin in

increasing *affinity* (equilibrium distribution ratio = tissue concentration/blood concentration at equilibrium) for a drug whose tissue distribution is perfusion rate-limited.

Table 4-6.

Organ	Time to Deliver the Amount Contained in the Tissue at Distribution Equilibrium (min)	Perfusion Rate (ml/min/ml tissue)
Lung	10	14
Kidney	20	4
Heart	32	0.8
Liver	100	0.4
Skin	420	0.02

2. The volume of distribution of quinacrine is about 40,000 liters.
   (a) The plasma concentration when 1 gram of drug is in the body would therefore be _____ mg/liter.
   (b) The amount of drug in the body when the plasma concentration is 0.015 mg/liter is _____ mg.
   (c) The percentage of drug in the body that is outside the plasma is _____.

3. The volume of distribution of a drug in man is observed to be 13 liters. Indicate which one (or more) of the following statements is (are) consistent with this observation: The drug is:
   (a) Highly bound to plasma proteins and is concentrated in the liver and the kidney.
   (b) Bound to tissue components throughout the body and is highly bound to plasma proteins.
   (c) Not bound to plasma proteins.

4. Briefly comment on the validity of each of the following statements:
   (a) The volume of distribution of salicylic acid is 9–12 liters in man in the usual antipyretic dose (600 mg). Therefore, the extracellular fluids contain virtually all the drug in the body.
   (b) The equilibrium distribution ratio for a drug between liver and plasma is 50; therefore its volume of distribution must be at least 75 liters.
   (c) A drug that reaches distribution equilibrium within 30 minutes, yet whose volume of distribution is 200 liters, must distribute primarily into highly perfused organs.

5. (a) Digitoxin has a volume of distribution of about 40 liters and that in plasma is 97 percent bound. What fraction of drug in the tissues is bound to tissue components? Assume that the unbound drug distributes evenly throughout total body water.
   (b) Digoxin has a volume of distribution of about 600 liters and that in plasma is 23 percent bound. Making the same assumption as above, is digoxin more or less extensively tissue bound than digitoxin?

5

clearance and renal excretion

Objectives

The reader will be able to:

1. **Define, in both words and equations, clearance, blood clearance, total clearance, and renal clearance.**

2. **Calculate the extraction ratio from blood clearance and organ blood flow.**

3. **Ascertain from the value of its extraction ratio whether the clearance of a drug will be perfusion rate-limited.**

4. **Ascertain the relative contribution of the renal and extrarenal routes to total elimination from their respective clearance values.**

5. **Given renal clearance and binding data, determine if a drug is predominately reabsorbed from or secreted into the renal tubule.**

6. **Describe where filtration, secretion, and reabsorption of drugs occur within the nephron.**

7. **State the average value of glomerular filtration rate and renal blood flow.**

8. **Ascertain from the value of the renal extraction ratio whether the renal clearance of a drug is dependent on its binding to plasma proteins.**

9. **Anticipate those drugs for which a change in either urine pH or urine flow will alter the value of their renal clearance.**

THIS chapter is concerned with the concept of clearance, particularly with reference to the renal excretion of drugs. The practical applications of the clearance concept will become evident in subsequent chapters.

Concept of Clearance

Of the concepts in pharmacokinetics, *clearance* has the greatest potential for clin-

ical applications. It is also the most useful parameter for the evaluation of an elimination mechanism.

Proportionality Constant: Rate and Concentration

Just as the parameter, volume of distribution, is needed to relate the concentration to the amount of drug in the body, so there is a need to have a parameter to relate the concentration to the rate of drug elimination. Clearance, denoted by *Cl*, is that proportionality factor. Thus,

Rate of elimination = Clearance × Concentration   1

For a given rate of elimination, the value of clearance obviously depends on the site of measurement, blood, plasma, or plasma water.

The units of clearance, like those of flow, are volume per unit time. For example, if the clearance value is l liter/hour, then at a concentration of l mg/liter, the rate of drug elimination is l mg/hour. Ordinarily, as the concentration of a drug in blood increases, so does its rate of elimination; clearance remains the same.

Loss Across an Organ of Elimination

Clearance may be viewed in another way, namely, from the loss of drug across an organ of elimination. This physiologic approach has a number of advantages, particularly in predicting and in evaluating the effects of changes in blood flow, plasma protein binding, enzyme activity, or secretory activity on the clearance of a drug. Figure 5-1 is a summary of the various ways of viewing mass balance across an eliminating organ.

The rate of presentation of a drug to an organ of elimination is the product of blood flow, Q, and the concentration in blood entering the arterial side, C_A, that is, $Q \cdot C_A$. Similarly, the rate at which the drug leaves on the venous side is $Q \cdot C_V$, where C_V is the concentration in the returning venous blood. The difference between these rates is the rate of drug extraction by the organ,

$$\text{Rate of extraction} = Q(C_A - C_V) \quad 2$$

Thus, the drug at the eliminating organ has been accounted for by mass balance.

If the rate of drug extraction is related to the rate at which it is presented to the organ, a useful parameter, the extraction ratio, E, is derived:

$$E = \frac{\text{Rate of extraction}}{\text{Rate of presentation}} = \frac{(C_A - C_V)}{C_A} \quad 3$$

The value of the extraction ratio can lie anywhere between zero, when no drug is eliminated, and one, when no drug escapes past the organ.

If, instead, the rate of drug extraction is related to the incoming concentration, one obtains by definition (Equation 1),

$$\text{Clearance} = \frac{Q(C_A - C_V)}{C_A} \quad 4$$

1. Mass Balance

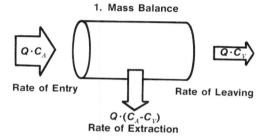

Rate of Entry   Rate of Leaving

$Q \cdot (C_A - C_V)$
Rate of Extraction

2. Mass Balance Normalized to Rate of Entry

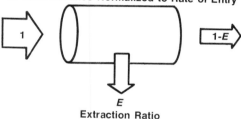

E
Extraction Ratio

3. Mass Balance Normalized to Entering Concentration

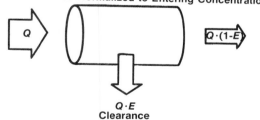

$Q \cdot E$
Clearance

Figure 5-1. *The extraction of a drug by an eliminating organ may be considered from the fundamental concepts of mass balance: 1, The extraction of drug may be accounted for from its rates in and out of the organ. 2, Normalizing to the rate of entry provides a means of determining the fraction extracted, the extraction ratio. 3, Normalizing to the entering concentration allows one to account for the drug in terms of clearance and blood flow. The symbols are defined in Equations 2 through 5.*

in this instance blood clearance, since the concentration in blood is measured. On substituting Equation 3 into Equation 4, the following is obtained:

$$\text{Blood clearance} = \frac{\text{Blood}}{\text{flow}} \times \text{Extraction ratio} \qquad 5$$

Clearance is then simply the product of the extraction ratio of a drug and blood flow, that is, the volume of blood from which all the drug would appear to be removed per unit time. For example, if the extraction of a drug across an organ is 0.5, and organ blood flow is 1 liter/min, then 500 ml of the incoming blood is effectively completely removed of drug each minute as it passes through the organ.

Extraction Ratio and Dependence of Clearance on Blood Flow

There are basic principles that can be explained by the organ model depicted in Figure 5-1. Consider the relationship between clearance and blood flow. For a drug that is virtually all removed as it passes through the eliminating organ, the extraction ratio approaches 1 and clearance approaches its maximum value, organ blood flow. Changes in blood flow produce corresponding changes in clearance and, from Equation 2, changes in rate of extraction, but *not* in the extraction ratio. Clearance is then said to be *perfusion rate-limited*. At the other extreme, that is, where the extraction

ratio approaches zero, the values of the arterial and venous concentrations of drug are almost identical. This is seen from Equation 3. The rate of extraction is dependent on the drug concentration in the blood in the organ; its value is virtually identical to the arterial concentration. In this last situation, since a change in flow produces no change in drug concentration within the organ, neither rate of drug elimination nor clearance change; it follows from Equation 5, however, that the extraction ratio will vary inversely with a change in flow. These relationships are summarized in Table 5-1. Examples of drugs with extraction ratios that are low (less than 0.3), intermediate (0.3–0.7), and high (greater than 0.7) are listed in Table 5-2.

Description of Clearance by Organ, Process, or Site of Measurement

Clearance can be described in terms of the eliminating organ, e.g., hepatic clearance, renal clearance, or pulmonary clearance. It can also be described by the difference between renal excretion and elimination by all other processes, e.g., renal clearance and extrarenal clearance. How an organ clears the blood of drug may also be described by the nature of the elimination process, e.g., metabolic clearance or excretory clearance. Furthermore, the value of the clearance term depends on the reference fluid. Thus, to be specific, the clear-

Table 5-1. Changes in Clearance and Extraction Ratio with Changes in Blood Flow[a]

Drug with	Blood Flow	Extraction Ratio	Clearance
High extraction ratio	↑	↔	↑
	↓	↔	↓
Low extraction ratio	↑	↓	↔
	↓	↑	↔

[a]Symbols: ↑—increase; ↔—little or no change; ↓—decrease.

Table 5-2. Hepatic and Renal Extraction Ratios of Representative Drugs and Metabolites

	Extraction Ratio		
	Low	Intermediate	High
Hepatic[a] extraction	Amobarbital Diazepam Digitoxin Isoniazid Phenobarbital Phenylbutazone Phenytoin Procainamide Salicylic Acid Theophylline Tolbutamide Warfarin	Aspirin Quinidine Codeine Nortriptyline	Alprenolol Arabinosyl-cytosine Desipramine Isoproterenol Lidocaine Meperidine Morphine Nitroglycerin Pentazocine Propoxyphene Propranolol Salicylamide
Renal[a] extraction	Acetazolamide Chlorpropamide Diazoxide Digoxin Furosemide Gentamicin Phenobarbital Sulfisoxazole Tetracycline Tobramycin	Procainamide (Some) Penicillins Quaternary ammonium compounds	(Many) Glucuronides (Some) Penicillins (Many) Sulfates

[a]At least 30 percent of the drug is eliminated by this route.

ance of a drug eliminated, e.g., by metabolism in the liver, using plasma concentration measurements would then be hepatic metabolic plasma clearance. In practice, however, the term plasma is dropped; it is assumed that plasma is the site of measurement unless stated otherwise. For example, the renal clearance of a drug refers to its renal plasma clearance.

Additivity of Clearance

The anatomy of the human body dictates that the clearance of a drug by one organ adds to the clearance of another. This is a consequence of the circulation. Consider, for example, a drug that is eliminated by renal excretion and by hepatic metabolism. Then

$$\text{Rate of elimination} = \text{Rate of renal excretion} + \text{Rate of hepatic metabolism} \qquad 6$$

Dividing the rate of removal associated with each process by the incoming drug concentration, which for all organs is the same (C_A), gives the clearance associated with that process:

$$\frac{\text{Rate of elimination}}{C_A} = \frac{\text{Rate of renal excretion}}{C_A} + \frac{\text{Rate of hepatic metabolism}}{C_A}$$

or   7

$$\text{Total Clearance} = \text{Renal Clearance} + \text{Hepatic Clearance}$$

Thus, total clearance is the sum of the

clearances by each of the eliminating organs. Total clearance, subsequently often simply called clearance, is one of the most common terms used in pharmacokinetics.

Because of the additivity of clearance, the relative contribution of any organ to drug elimination is readily calculated. For example, the fraction of drug excreted unchanged (designated *fe*), being the fraction of total elimination that occurs via renal excretion, is just the fraction that renal clearance is of total clearance.

One exception to the additivity of clearance is pulmonary clearance. This is a consequence of the blood supply to the lungs being in series, rather than in parallel, with other organs of elimination and a consequence of the total cardiac output passing through the lungs before reaching the site of measurement, usually blood in a peripheral vein. The concentration measured is that leaving, rather than entering, the lungs. The use of this concentration to calculate clearance is inconsistent with its definition (see Eq. 4). Indeed, clearance values calculated in this manner may greatly exceed cardiac output, making interpretation difficult.

Plasma Versus Blood Clearance

For many applications in pharmacokinetics, it matters little whether clearance measurements are based on drug in plasma or in blood. The exception is when a clearance value is used to estimate the extraction ratio of the drug. Then the blood clearance value must be used, because it is this parameter that is directly related to organ blood flow and the extraction ratio (see Eq. 5). Measurement of drug in plasma does not take into account drug in or bound to blood cells, which may be available for elimination. For example, the renal (plasma) clearance of mecamylamine can exceed renal plasma flow, which on first glance might appear impossible. This antihypertensive agent concentrates on or in the erythrocytes, yet this source of drug is

evidently still available for excretion into the urine.

The plasma rather than the blood clearance value of a drug is the one more frequently reported. Thus, if one wishes to estimate the extraction ratio, one needs to convert this clearance value based on plasma to one based on blood. This conversion is accomplished by experimentally determining the blood to plasma concentration ratio, because it follows from Equation 1 that

$$\frac{\text{Plasma clearance}}{\text{Blood clearance}} = \frac{\text{Blood concentration}}{\text{Plasma concentration}} \quad 8$$

The concentration ratio is a function of the hematocrit and of the binding of drug to both plasma proteins and blood cell components. The relationship is derived in Appendix A. Strong binding to plasma proteins produces a ratio less than 1.0. A high affinity for blood cells gives a ratio greater than 1.0.

Renal Excretion

Renal excretion of a drug depends upon its physicochemical properties, upon its binding to plasma proteins, and upon the physiology of the kidney. The salient features of the renal handling of drugs follow.

Physiologic Mechanisms

The Nephron—Anatomy and Function. The basic anatomic unit of renal function is the nephron, shown in Figure 5-2. The basic components of the nephron are the glomerulus, the proximal tubule, the loop of Henle, the distal tubule, and the collecting tubule. The glomerulus receives the blood first and filters some plasma water. The filtrate passes down the tubule. Most of the water is reabsorbed; only 1 to 2 ml/min leave the kidney as urine. On leaving the glomerulus the same blood perfuses the proximal and distal portions of the tubule, through a series of interconnecting channels. Only a fraction of the total blood sup-

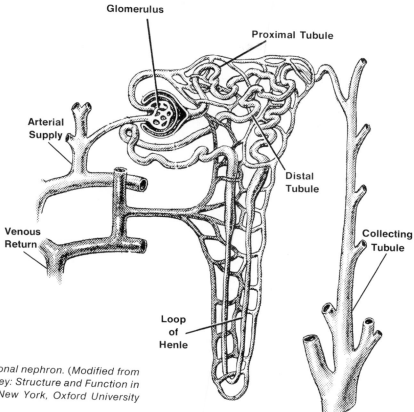

Glomerulus

Proximal Tubule

Arterial
Supply

Distal
Tubule

Venous
Return

Collecting
Tubule

Loop
of
Henle

Figure 5-2. *The functional nephron. (Modified from Smith, H.W.: The Kidney: Structure and Function in Health and Disease, New York, Oxford University Press, 1951.)*

ply to the nephron, however, reaches the terminal end of the distal tubule and the collecting duct.

The appearance of drug in the urine is the net result of filtration, secretion, and reabsorption. The first two processes add drug to the lumen of the nephron; the last process involves the movement of drug from the lumen back into the body. The excretion rate of a drug is, therefore,

$$\text{Rate of excretion} = \text{Rate of filtration} + \text{Rate of secretion} - \text{Rate of reabsorption} \quad 9$$

Let us look at each process in turn.

Glomerular Filtration. Approximately 25 percent of the cardiac output, 1.2 to 1.5 liters of blood per min, goes to the kidneys. Of this volume, about 10 percent is filtered at the glomerulus. Only drug in plasma

water is filtered; drug bound to macromolecules or blood cells is unable to pass across the glomerular membranes. The filtrate contains the drug at a concentration identical to that in plasma water, namely, Cu.

The rate at which plasma water is filtered, 125 ml/min, is conventionally called the glomerular filtration rate, GFR. It follows that

$$\text{Rate of filtration} = GFR \cdot Cu \quad 10$$

Recall that the fraction unbound, fu, is the ratio of the unbound to total plasma drug concentration; therefore,

$$\text{Rate of filtration} = fu \cdot GFR \cdot C \quad 11$$

If a drug is only filtered and all filtered drug is excreted into the urine then the rate of excretion is the rate of filtration. Since renal clearance, Cl_R, by definition, is,

$$Cl_R = \frac{\text{Rate of excretion}}{\text{Plasma concentration}} \qquad 12$$

it follows that for such a drug its renal clearance (by filtration) is $fu \cdot GFR$.

Creatinine, an endogenous substance, and inulin, an exogenous polysaccharide, are not bound to plasma protein nor secreted, and all the filtered load of each substance is excreted into the urine. Accordingly, the renal clearance value of each of these substances is a close measure of GFR.

Active Secretion. Filtration always occurs. Secretion is inferred when the rate of excretion exceeds the rate of filtration of a drug (Eq. 9). Stated differently, since substitution of Equation 10 into Equation 9 and division by the plasma drug concentration gives,

$$Cl_R = fu \cdot GFR + \frac{\left[\begin{array}{c} \text{Rate of} \\ \text{secretion} \end{array} - \begin{array}{c} \text{Rate of} \\ \text{reabsorption} \end{array} \right]}{\text{plasma concentration}} \qquad 13$$

secretion must take place when renal clearance exceeds clearance by filtration. Some reabsorption can occur but it must be less than secretion.

Separate mechanisms exist for secreting acids (anions) and bases (cations), including quaternary ammonium compounds, from the plasma into the tubular lumen. The secretory processes are located predominantly along the proximal tubule. Although active, these acid and base transport systems lack a high degree of specificity, as demonstrated by the wide variety of substances transported by them. As expected, however, substances transported by the same system compete with each other.

Secretion can be so extensive that virtually all the drug in the blood is removed whether or not bound to plasma protein or located in blood cells. Para-aminohippuric acid (PAH), an exogenous organic acid, is handled in this manner; it is also located within blood almost exclusively in the plasma and it is not reabsorbed. The renal clearance of PAH is therefore a measure of

renal plasma flow. Only the unbound drug is capable of crossing the cells lining the tubule; thus, the transport of all the drug out of the blood requires rapid dissociation of the drug-protein complex and movement of drug out of the blood cells. Evidently, this can occur with PAH, and as mentioned previously, with mecamylamine. The findings with these compounds also imply that most of the blood supply is in contact with the proximal tubule, that the transport mechanism(s) is able to remove the unbound drug rapidly, and that the blood must be in the active transport region for a sufficient period of time to allow all drug to be stripped off protein and to be removed from blood cells.

Reabsorption. Reabsorption is the third and perhaps the most important factor controlling the renal handling of drugs. Reabsorption must occur if the renal clearance is less than the calculated clearance by filtration (see Eq. 13). Some secretion may still occur but it must be less than reabsorption. Reabsorption varies from being almost absent to being virtually complete. Active reabsorption occurs for many endogenous compounds, including vitamins, electrolytes, glucose, and amino acids. For the vast majority of drugs, however, which are exogenous compounds, reabsorption is a passive process. The degree of reabsorption depends on the properties of the drug, e.g., its polar-nonpolar nature, its state of ionization, and its molecular weight. The membranes of the cells that form the tubule are lipoidal in nature, a characteristic shared in common with most membranes of the body. They act as a barrier to water-soluble and ionized substances. Thus lipophilic molecules tend to be extensively reabsorbed; polar molecules do not. Reabsorption also depends on physiologic variables such as the rate of urine flow and the pH of the urine.

Reabsorption occurs all along the nephron. To understand why this is so requires an understanding of the fate of the water

filtered at the glomerulus. The events, depicted in Figure 5-3, show that the majority,
80 to 90 percent, of the filtered water is
reabsorbed in the proximal tubule. Most of
the remainder is reabsorbed in the distal
tubule and collecting ducts. Changes in
urine flow are mediated here. If no water is
reabsorbed in the distal tubule, urine flow is
about 15 to 25 ml/min. Normally, however,
water is reabsorbed to the extent that urine
flow is 1 to 2 ml/min and lower.

Consequently, with water reabsorption,
drugs concentrate in the filtrate. In fact, if a
drug is neither reabsorbed (generally polar)
nor secreted, the concentration of drug in
the urine will be about 100 times as great as
that unbound in plasma. This is a result of
the rate of excretion being equal to the rate
of filtration, that is,

$$GFR \cdot Cu = \frac{\text{Urine}}{\text{Flow}} \times \frac{\text{Urine}}{\text{Concentration}} \quad 14$$

| Rate of | Rate of |
| filtration | Excretion |

From which it is readily seen that

$$\frac{\text{Urine concentration}}{Cu} = \frac{GFR}{\text{Urine flow}}$$

When the GFR is 100 times the urine flow
the urine concentration is 100 times that
unbound in plasma. Thus, reabsorption of
water favors the reabsorption of a drug that
diffuses across tubular membranes.

Renal Clearance

When the rate of excretion of a drug is
directly proportional to the plasma concentration,

$$\text{Rate of excretion} = Cl_R \cdot C \quad 15$$

renal clearance is constant. This constancy
is the basis for the use of urine data to
determine the time course of a drug in the
body (Chap. 7). Interpretation of urine data
with regard to levels of drug in the body is
clearly complicated for drugs whose renal
clearance varies. Factors that influence

renal clearance include plasma drug concentration, plasma protein binding, urine
flow, and urine pH.

Plasma Drug Concentration. Both filtration
and reabsorption are usually passive processes, the rates of which are directly related to the plasma drug concentration.
Active secretion and active reabsorption are
saturable processes, that is, they have a
maximum capacity. This is shown in Figure
5-4 for active secretion. The maximum rate
of tubular secretion is often called the T_M
value. The rate of transport increases in
direct proportion to the plasma concentration until the transport approaches its capacity. Further increases in the drug concentration then produce little change in the
rate of transport. Consequently, the clearance by secretion decreases as the plasma
drug concentration increases.

Secretion never occurs alone; filtration is
always a component and passive reabsorption may or may not be. Figure 5-4 also
demonstrates how the rate of excretion of a
drug that undergoes filtration and secretion,
but no reabsorption, always increases with
plasma concentration. While the rate of
secretion approaches a maximum, the rate
of filtration increases in direct proportion to
the plasma concentration. The same events
are shown in curve B in Figure 5-5.

There may be little to no excretion at low
plasma concentrations for a drug that is
actively reabsorbed, for example, glucose
and vitamins. Drug appears in urine when
its rate of filtration (plus secretion, if any)
exceeds the capacity of the active reabsorption process. This condition occurs when the
plasma concentration exceeds what is
sometimes called the threshold concentration.

Renal clearance is the rate of drug excretion divided by its plasma concentration. A
drug that is filtered only, and is not bound
in plasma, has the same renal clearance at
all concentrations, as shown schematically
in curve A of Figure 5-5. Curve B depicts
the events that occur for a drug that is

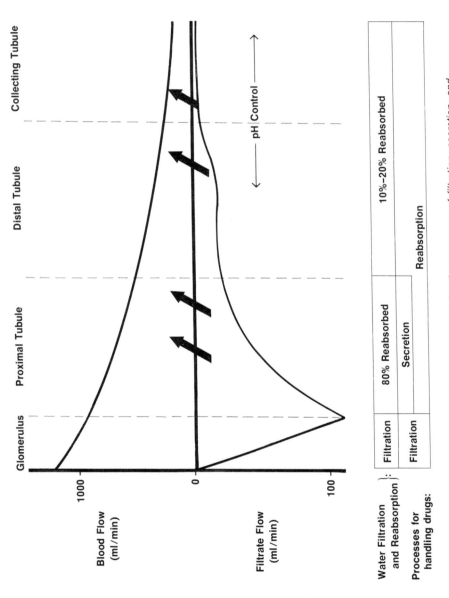

Figure 5-3. The handling of drugs by the nephron includes the processes of filtration, secretion, and reabsorption. Both reabsorption of water and control of urine pH influence the reabsorption process. The schematic diagram shows the approximate locations where the processes for most drugs occur.

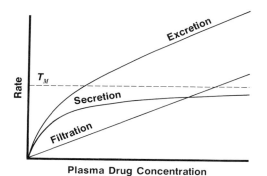

Figure 5-4. *The rate of secretion has a limiting value, the maximum transport rate* T_M*, whereas the rate of filtration increases in direct proportion to the plasma concentration of a drug. Consequently, the rate of excretion of a drug that is both filtered and secreted increases with its plasma concentration, but not in direct proportion. Reabsorption is assumed not to occur.*

actively secreted. In the region of plasma concentrations well below those required to approach saturation, renal clearance is highest and remains essentially constant. The therapeutic concentration of most actively secreted drugs lies within this region. At higher plasma concentrations, renal clearance decreases; the lower limiting value is that contributed by both filtration and passive reabsorption. The same limitation applies to a drug that is actively reabsorbed, curve C. However, at low concentrations the renal clearance of an actively reabsorbed drug is less, not more.

Plasma Protein Binding. The effect of altered binding on renal clearance of a drug depends upon its extraction ratio. If the extraction ratio is high, renal clearance depends upon blood flow and not upon plasma binding. Conversely, if the extraction ratio is low, renal clearance is sensitive to changes in plasma binding. These relationships apply despite the complex nature of the processes governing renal excretion.

To demonstrate these generalizations, first consider a drug that undergoes filtration, but neither secretion nor reabsorption. Because the filtered drug is at the same concentration as that unbound in plasma, there is no tendency for the drug bound to plasma proteins to dissociate to form unbound drug. The renal clearance of such a drug is $fu \cdot GFR$; thus, as the fraction unbound changes so does the renal clearance.

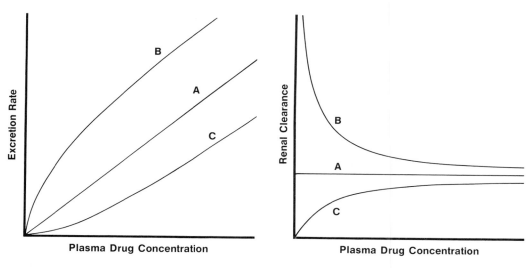

Figure 5-5. *The relationships of the rate of excretion (on left) and of renal clearance (on right) with the plasma concentration depend on whether the drug undergoes filtration only (drug A), filtration and secretion (drug B), or filtration and active reabsorption (drug C).*

The extraction ratio of such a drug is low. For example, even if the drug is totally unbound in blood ($Cu = C_b$), the extraction ratio is still only 0.08. This follows since

Extraction ratio

$$= \frac{\text{Rate of extraction } (GFR \cdot Cu)}{\text{Rate of presentation (renal blood flow} \cdot C_b)}$$

$$= \frac{125 \text{ ml/min}}{1500 \text{ ml/min}} = 0.083$$

Suppose next, that in addition to filtration a drug is secreted, but poorly. Then, the concentration at the secretion site is almost identical to the plasma drug concentration, C. Since the rate of secretion depends on the unbound drug concentration, in this case Cu (or $fu \cdot C$), it follows that the renal clearance, being the sum of the clearance associated with filtration ($fu \cdot GFR$) and secretion, must also be directly proportional to the value of fu. The same relationship holds when a low extraction ratio results from extensive reabsorption.

As seen previously for a drug that is actively secreted to the point that virtually all the drug presented to the kidney is removed, changes in protein binding have little or no effect on the renal clearance. For a drug with an intermediate extraction ratio renal clearance changes with protein binding. However, the closer the extraction ratio is to 1, the smaller the change in clearance. Examples of drugs with various renal extraction ratios are listed in Table 5-2.

Reabsorption and Urine pH. In contrast to that of the blood, the pH of urine varies widely and, therefore, so can the degree of reabsorption of certain weak acids and weak bases. This influence of pH on reabsorption can be thought of in equilibrium terms or in terms of the rate of reabsorption.

Equilibrium Considerations. A drug cannot be completely reabsorbed unless reabsorption is active. Passive reabsorption continues only until the diffusible species

attains the same concentration in both urine and plasma water.

To appreciate the factors influencing renal clearance under equilibrium conditions, first consider the reabsorption of an un-ionized nonpolar drug. If reabsorption were to continue until equilibrium is reached, the concentration in the urine and that unbound to plasma proteins, Cu, would be identical. Consequently,

$$Cl_R = \frac{\text{Urine flow} \times \text{Urine concentration}}{\text{Plasma concentration}} \qquad 16$$

and since $Cu = fu \cdot C$, it follows that

$$\frac{\text{Renal}}{\text{clearance}} = fu \cdot \text{Urine flow} \qquad 17$$

This last relationship is a simple test of how close reabsorption is to equilibrium. An un-ionized nonpolar drug may have a renal clearance below this value only if it is actively reabsorbed. Moreover, the renal clearance of a highly bound drug may be small since the urine flow is normally only 1 to 2 ml/min. Note also that at constant urine flow, its renal clearance is directly proportional to the fraction unbound.

For weak acids and weak bases the pH of the urine is an additional factor that determines reabsorption. Although there is some change in the pH of the filtrate as it passes down the proximal tubule, the major adjustment is at the end of the distal tubule and in the collecting duct. The extremes of urine pH are 4.5 and 7.5 under forced acidification and alkalinization, respectively; on the average, urine pH is 6.3. These extremes contrast with the narrow range of plasma pH, 7.3 to 7.5. Thus, a large pH gradient may exist between plasma and urine.

Urine pH is altered by diet, by drugs, and by the clinical state of a patient. The pH of the urine also varies during the day. Respiratory and metabolic acidosis produces acidification, and respiratory and metabolic alkalosis produces alkalinization. An exception to this is when the metabolic acidosis is of renal origin, for example, renal tubular acidosis, in which case the urine is alkaline. Drugs such as the carbonic anhydrase inhibitor, acetazolamide, produce an alkaline urine.

The renal clearances for several weak acids and bases, listed in Table 5-3, were calculated using the Henderson-Hasselbalch equation (Chap. 3) and Equation 16, assuming that equilibrium is achieved between un-ionized drug in urine and plasma and that the ionized form is not diffusible. From the values in the table it appears that the renal clearance of acids, pKa less than 6.0, can be much less than urine flow, whereas that of bases can be only slightly less because urine pH is never much higher than plasma pH.

An interesting observation may be made with regard to the renal clearance of weak bases. At low urine pH the renal clearance, by calculation, approaches renal blood flow. Such a high clearance value usually suggests active secretion. It is unlikely, however, that such a high clearance value can be obtained by passive diffusion—for three reasons. First, the fraction of renal blood flow that reaches the end of the distal tubule and collecting duct, where the major change in pH occurs, is small. Second, the calculation of renal clearance is based on the ratio of urine concentration to plasma concentration leaving, rather than entering,

the kidney. The venous concentration here is less than that entering the kidney, particularly when the extraction ratio of the drug is high—a perfusion rate-limited condition. Third, the high values of calculated clearance apply to bases, which at blood pH values tend to be almost completely ionized; thus the rate of movement through the membranes, which depends on the concentration of un-ionized drug, is reduced. A similar argument applies to weak acids. Accordingly, a renal clearance value greater than the *GFR* for either acids or bases at normal urine pH probably suggests active secretion.

A Rate Process in Reality. The foregoing discussion was based on equilibrium concepts, but passive reabsorption seldom approaches equilibrium. The primary consideration is how rapidly equilibrium is approached. In reality, then, reabsorption must be considered from a kinetic rather than from an equilibrium point of view, as was absorption of drugs from the gastrointestinal tract (Chap. 3).

The rate at which reabsorption occurs depends on the ability of the un-ionized drug to diffuse across membranes, its polarity, and the fraction of drug in the lumen that is un-ionized. The percent un-ionized for the same drugs listed in Table 5-3 is

Table 5-3. Calculated Renal Clearances (ml/min) of Selected Nonpolar Weak Acids and Weak Bases at Various Values of Urine pH[a]

Drug	Nature	pKa	Urine pH		
			4.4	6.4	7.9
A		2.4	0.001	0.1	3
B	Acid	6.4	0.1	0.2	3
C		10.4	1.0	1.0	1.0
D		2.4	1.0	1.0	1.0
E	Base	6.4	90	2	0.9
F		10.4	1000	10	0.3
G		12.4	1000	10	0.3

[a] No binding of drug to plasma proteins, $fu = 1.0$; urine flow of 1 ml/min; pH of plasma is constant at 7.4.

given in Table 5-4. The calculation is based on the Henderson-Hasselbalch equation (Chap. 3).

Weak Bases. The effect of urine pH on the cumulative amount of unchanged methamphetamine (pKa 10) that is excreted in the urine is shown in Figure 5-6. After 16 hours about 16 percent of the dose is excreted unchanged when the urine pH is not controlled. On alkalinizing the urine by ingesting sodium bicarbonate only 1 to 2 percent of the dose is in the urine, while acidification by ingesting ammonium chloride results in 70 to 80 percent recovery in the urine. Clearly, for this drug, urine pH is important in determining the contribution of the renal route to total elimination.

Even under conditions of no pH control, urine pH varies throughout the day and the excretion of methamphetamine fluctuates accordingly. The excretion rate after a single dose increases during periods of lower pH and decreases during periods of higher pH (Fig. 5-7). The explanation for these observations is contained in Tables 5-3 and 5-4. At low urine pH both equilibrium and kinetic considerations favor high renal clearance of a drug of pKa 10. In particular, the percent un-ionized and hence the un-ionized concentration in the renal tubule are so small that there is little opportunity for reabsorption within the time that the drug resides in the nephron. At high urine

pH with a greater percent of drug un-ionized in the tubule, both equilibrium and rate considerations favor reabsorption. Drugs that show these substantial changes in renal clearance are said to be pH sensitive.

The effect of urine pH on the reabsorption of basic drugs, in general, follows:

1. A basic drug that is polar in its un-ionized form is not reabsorbed, regardless of its degree of ionization in the urine, unless actively transported. The aminoglycoside tobramycin is an example; its renal clearance is independent of urine pH.

2. A very weakly basic nonpolar drug, whose pKa is around 6 or below, such as propoxyphene, is extensively reabsorbed at all values of urine pH because the percent of drug in the diffusible un-ionized form is sufficient to have no limiting effect on the rate of reabsorption, regardless of urine pH. Furthermore, equilibrium favors reabsorption. The renal clearance of such a drug may vary with urine pH but its value is low, especially if the drug is highly bound to plasma proteins.

3. For a strong base, with a pKa value approaching 12 or greater, such as guanethidine, little or no reabsorption is expected throughout the range of urine pH, because ionization is so extensive. Accordingly its renal clearance is independent of urine pH and is generally high.

Table 5-4. Percent Un-ionized of Selected Weak Acids and Weak Bases at Various Values of Urine pH[a]

Drug	Nature	pKa	Urine pH 4.4	6.4	7.9
A		2.4	1.0	0.01	0.0003
B	Acid	6.4	99	50	3
C		10.4	100	100	99.7
D		2.4	99	100	100
E	Base	6.4	1.0	50	97
F		10.4	0.0001	0.01	0.3
G		12.4	10^{-6}	0.0001	0.003

[a]Same drugs as in Table 5-3.

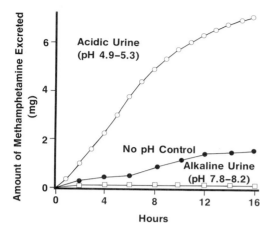

Figure 5-6. *The cumulative urinary excretion of methamphetamine (11 mg orally) in man varies with the urine pH. (Adapted from Beckett, A.H., and Rowland, M.: Urinary excretion kinetics of methylamphetamine in man. Nature, 206: 1260–1261, 1965.)*

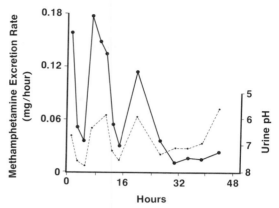

Figure 5-7. *The urinary excretion rate (—) of methamphetamine (11 mg orally) is dramatically influenced by the urine pH (– – –). The urine pH is clearly not controlled. (Adapted from Beckett, A.H., and Rowland, M.: Urinary excretion kinetics of methylamphetamine in man. Nature 206: 1260–1261, 1965.)*

4. For a basic nonpolar drug with a *pKa value between 6 and 12* the extent of reabsorption varies from negligible to almost complete (equilibration) with changes in urine pH. The renal clearance of such a drug varies markedly with urine pH.

Weak Acids. The principles developed for weak bases also apply to weak acids. However, for acids, an increase in pH causes more ionization, not less. Consequently, acids are reabsorbed less and have larger renal clearance values at higher values of urine pH.

Again, the effect of pKa in reabsorption is seen by inspecting Tables 5-3 and 5-4. An acid with a pKa value of 2 or less, chromoglycic acid, is so completely ionized at all urine pH values that it is simply not reabsorbed; its renal clearance is generally high and insensitive to pH. At the other extreme, a very weak acid with a pKa value above 8, such as phenytoin, is mostly un-ionized throughout the range of urine pH; its renal clearance is always low and insensitive to pH. Only for an acid whose *pKa lies between 3.0 and 7.5* is renal clearance pH sensitive. Note in Table 5-3 that for all

nonpolar acids equilibrium favors reabsorption.

The effect of pH on the renal clearance of basic and acidic drugs of various pKa values is summarized in the schematic diagram of Figure 5-8. Curves are shown for both acidic (pH 5) and alkaline (pH 7.5) urine. The scheme is not intended to be accurate. Variations in urine flow and polarity of the un-ionized form of a drug, as well as active secretion and active reabsorption, preclude it from being so.

Effect of Urine Flow. Urine flow can only have a substantial effect on the renal clearance of a drug that is mostly reabsorbed. Certainly, the effect is most dramatic when the reabsorption approaches equilibrium.

Ethyl alcohol and methyl alcohol are examples of compounds that are reabsorbed to the extent that the concentration in the urine is virtually the same as that in the plasma regardless of urine flow. Consequently, from Equations 16 and 17, the renal clearance is approximately equal to urine flow and is, therefore, urine-flow dependent.

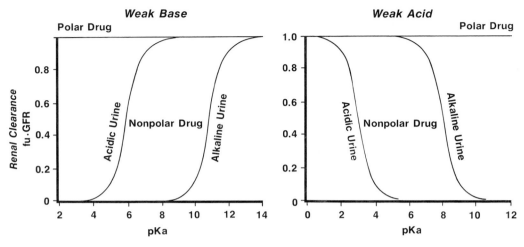

Figure 5-8. *Scheme showing how the renal clearance relative to the clearance by filtration (fu · GFR) of nonpolar weak bases (left) and weak acids (right) depends on both pKa and urine pH; the drugs are assumed to be equally nonpolar. Also shown is how the value for polar compounds (top horizontal lines) is high and independent of ionization. All drugs are assumed to be not secreted.*

Weak acids and bases that show pH-sensitive reabsorption also generally show flow-rate dependence. Again, however, the degree to which the renal clearance is changed by flow depends on the extent of reabsorption. If 50 percent of that filtered and secreted is reabsorbed at normal urine flow, 50 percent is excreted. Increased urine flow decreases reabsorption toward zero, but renal clearance cannot be increased by more than a factor of two. Figure 5-9 shows how the renal clearance of phenobarbital (pKa 7.2) varies with urine flow. As expected the renal clearance of this drug is pH sensitive as well as flow-rate dependent.

For polar substances that are not reabsorbed, e.g., mannitol, gentamicin, penicillin, creatinine, and para-aminohippuric acid, the rate of excretion is the rate of filtration plus the rate of secretion. For a given plasma drug concentration the rate of excretion is constant. An increase in the urine flow only produces a more dilute urine.

Forced Diuresis and Urine pH Control

Increased urine flow by forced intake of fluids and, in some cases, the coadministra-

tion of mannitol or another diuretic, can increase the excretion of some drugs. More rapid elimination is, of course, desirable for the purpose of detoxifying a patient who is overdosed. There are several criteria that must be met for forced diuresis to be of value:

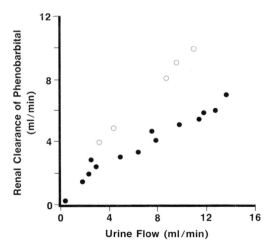

Figure 5-9. *The renal clearance of phenobarbital varies with urine flow in man. It is also a function of urine pH: without alkalinization (●); with alkalinization (○). (Redrawn from Linton, A.L., Luke, R.G., and Briggs, M.D.: Methods of forced diuresis and its application in barbiturate poisoning. Lancet, 2: 377–380, 1967.)*

1. Renal excretion under conditions of forced diuresis must become the major route of drug elimination. Increasing the renal clearance of a drug tenfold, for example, does little to hasten drug elimination from the body, if renal clearance normally is only 1 percent of total clearance.

2. The compound must normally be extensively reabsorbed in the kidney tubule.

3. If the reabsorption is pH sensitive, both forced diuresis and pH control may be of value. This applies if forced diuresis or pH control alone only partially prevents reabsorption.

The last point bears further discussion. Suppose that, on alkalinizing the urine, the reabsorption of a weak acid is decreased from 90 to 10 percent of that filtered and secreted. The addition of forced diuresis will be of little additional value; the excretion rate can only be increased by a further 10 percent. The converse applies to the use of pH control when forced diuresis almost completely prevents reabsorption.

Study Problems

(Answers to Study Problems can be found in Appendix G.)

1. The renal clearances and the fractions unbound to plasma proteins of three drugs are listed below:

	Renal Clearance	Fraction Unbound
Drug A	20	0.50
Drug B	12.5	0.10
Drug C	10	0.02

State the likely contribution of filtration, secretion, and reabsorption to the renal handling of each of these drugs.

2. For each of the following multiple choice questions, indicate the letters of *all* (one or more) of the correct answers. The symbol *fe* refers to the fraction of the drug eliminated that is excreted unchanged.

(a) The renal clearance of a given acidic drug is not sensitive to changes in urine pH because:

(*i*) It is secreted but not reabsorbed.

(*ii*) It has a pKa value of 5.

(*iii*) The fraction of that filtered that is reabsorbed varies with urine pH.

(*iv*) It has a small volume of distribution.

(*v*) All of the drug is renally excreted unchanged, *fe* = 1.

(b) Forced diuresis is likely to significantly enhance the elimination of a drug,

(*i*) Which is both polar and slowly removed from the body.

(*ii*) For which most of the filtered and secreted drug is reabsorbed and *fe* is greater than 0.5.

(*iii*) Which is neutral, polar and which has a value of *fe* greater than 0.9.

(*iv*) Which is not secreted and the ratio of its renal clearance to inulin clearance is one.

(c) A renal clearance of 312 ml/min for oxacillin indicates that:

(*i*) It is secreted into the luminal contents of the nephron.

      (*ii*) Its renal extraction ratio is 0.1.
      (*iii*) The majority of oxacillin entering the body is excreted in the urine unchanged.
      (*iv*) It is not bound to plasma proteins.
  (d) The renal clearance of a drug is constant with time if
      (*i*) Its value exceeds 300 ml/min.
      (*ii*) The concentration in urine is independent of urine flow.
      (*iii*) A constant fraction of filtered and secreted drug is reabsorbed.

3. The relationship between glucose excretion rate and its plasma concentration in a healthy individual is displayed in Table 5-5. Briefly explain this observation and prepare either a table or a graph of glucose renal clearance in ml/min as a function of its plasma concentration.

Table 5-5. Glucose Excretion Rate at Various Plasma Glucose Concentrations

Excretion Rate (mg/min)	5	66	151	256	400	520	631
Plasma Glucose Concentration (mg/100 ml)	200	301	398	503	605	708	799

4. The renal clearance of the acid, probenecid (Benemid), is low and pH sensitive, yet the drug diminishes the renal clearance of penicillin G.
  (a) Briefly explain this observation.
  (b) Will altering the plasma concentration of penicillin G influence its renal clearance in the presence of probenecid?
  (c) Suggest a reason why the renal clearance of penicillin G (pKa 2.9) is insensitive to urine pH changes.

5. Payne et al. (Br. Med. J., *3*:819, 1967) were interested, for legal reasons, in determining if the concentration of alcohol in urine could be related to its blood concentration. Table 5-6 summarizes their findings.
  (a) What explanation(s) can you offer for the very close correlation between concentrations of alcohol in blood and in urine?
  (b) Would you expect the excretion rate of alcohol to correlate with the plasma alcohol concentration? Discuss briefly.

Table 5-6. Frequency Distribution of the Ratio of Alcohol Concentrations, Urine/Blood

Percent of Observations	9	51	32	8
Urine Concentration / Blood Concentration	< 1.2	1.2–1.4	1.4–1.6	> 1.6

From Payne et al.: Br. Med. J., *3:* 819, 1967.

6

hepatic clearance and elimination

Objectives

The reader will be able to:

1. Define, in words and in equations, hepatic clearance and biliary clearance.

2. Ascertain from the value of the hepatic extraction ratio whether the hepatic clearance of a drug is dependent on its binding to plasma proteins or on blood flow.

3. Describe capacity-limited elimination kinetics and discuss the mechanisms responsible for such.

4. Determine the biliary clearance of a drug from its bile to plasma concentration ratio and the bile flow.

5. Describe the role that biliary excretion can play in drug disposition.

6. Explain the statement:
   "The elimination rate constant, or the fractional rate of elimination of a drug, is dependent on the values of both its total clearance and volume of distribution."

Biotransformation

METABOLISM is the major mechanism for elimination of drugs from the body. Some drugs are eliminated almost entirely unchanged by the kidneys, but these drugs are relatively few.

The consequences of drug metabolism are manifold. Biotransformation provides a mechanism for ridding the body of undesirable foreign compounds and drugs; it also provides a means of producing active and toxic compounds. Numerous examples are now recognized where the administered drug is really an inactive prodrug, which is converted into a pharmacologically active metabolite. Often both the drug and its metabolite(s) are active. The duration and intensity of the pharmacologic and toxic responses vary with their time course in the body. The disposition of active metabolites, as well as that of the compound administered, is therefore of therapeutic concern.

Restricting ourselves to the elimination of the compound administered, we can make a few generalizations:

1. Unless metabolized, a nonpolar, un-ionized compound remains in the body for a long time; its renal clearance is low. Not

unexpectedly, this statement also applies to nonpolar acids of pKa greater than 8 and to nonpolar bases of pKa lower than 6, as well as to substances that do not ionize.

2. Since metabolism and renal excretion are parallel processes, the fraction eliminated by each route depends upon the contribution of each to the total clearance.

3. The major routes of biotransformation can be predicted for many compounds based on the functional groups present.

Pathways of Metabolism

The most common routes of drug metabolism are oxidation, reduction, hydrolysis, and conjugation. Frequently, a drug simultaneously undergoes metabolism by several competing pathways. The amount of each metabolite formed depends on the relative rates of each of the parallel pathways.

The metabolites may undergo further metabolism. For example, oxidation, reduction, and hydrolysis are often followed by a conjugation reaction. These reactions occur in series or are said to be *sequential.*

Table 6-1 contains representative drugs whose pathways of biotransformation are classified by chemical alteration and by site of metabolism. Several metabolic transformations occur in the endoplasmic reticulum of the liver and of certain other tissues. On homogenizing these tissues the endoplasmic reticulum is disrupted with the formation of small vesicles called *microsomes.* For this reason, metabolizing enzymes of the endoplasmic reticulum are called microsomal enzymes. Drug metabolism, therefore, may be classified as microsomal and nonmicrosomal.

Hepatic Elimination

Although drug metabolism can take place in many organs, the liver most often has the greatest metabolic capacity and consequently has been the most thoroughly studied. Analogous to the kidney the most direct quantitative measure *in vivo* of the liver's ability to eliminate a drug is hepatic clearance. Hepatic clearance includes biliary excretory clearance, which is subsequently discussed, and hepatic metabolic clearance.

Hepatic Clearance

As with other organs of elimination, the removal of drug by the liver may be considered from mass balance relationships. Figure 6-1 shows schematically the appropriate blood supply to the liver via the portal vein (1050 ml/min) and the hepatic artery (300 ml/min). Using an average entering blood concentration, C_A, the rate of presentation of drug to the liver is $Q_H \cdot C_A$, where Q_H is the combined hepatic blood flow. The rate at which a drug leaves the liver is $Q_H \cdot C_V$, where C_V is the hepatic venous concentration of drug. Therefore,

$$\text{Rate of elimination} = Q_H(C_A - C_V) \quad 1$$

From the definition of clearance,

$$\frac{\text{Hepatic}}{\text{clearance}} = \frac{\text{Rate of elimination}}{C_A} \quad 2$$

it follows that

$$\frac{\text{Hepatic}}{\text{clearance}} = \frac{Q_H(C_A - C_V)}{C_A} \quad 3$$

that is

$$\frac{\text{Hepatic}}{\text{clearance}} = \underset{\substack{\text{Hepatic} \\ \text{blood} \\ \text{flow}}}{Q_H} \cdot \underset{\substack{\text{Hepatic} \\ \text{extraction} \\ \text{ratio}}}{E_H} \quad 4$$

Note that in the last equation, it is the hepatic *blood* clearance that relates the extraction ratio to the blood flow. The effects of altering blood flow and plasma-protein binding on clearance and extraction ratio are questions of fundamental importance.

There are at least five processes that may affect the ability of the liver to extract a drug from the blood. They are shown in Figure 6-2. While the drug is in the liver it has the opportunity to partition out of the blood cell, to dissociate off the plasma proteins, to pass across the hepatic membranes, and to be either transported into the bile or metabolized by an enzyme, or both. For a drug to have a high extraction ratio (approaching unity), none of these processes may be slow or rate limiting. Conversely, a drug with a low extraction ratio (approaching zero) must be rate-limited somewhere in the overall scheme. This rate limitation could be a slow enzymatic reaction, process *e*; poor biliary transport, process *d*; poor diffusion into the hepatic cell, process *c*; slow diffusion out of the blood cell, proc-

Table 6-1. Patterns of Biotransformation[a] of Representative Drugs[b]

Prodrug	Drug	Active Metabolite	Inactive Metabolite[c]
	Acetohexamide —(R)→	Hydroxyhexamide	
Acetylsalicylic Acid[d]	—(H)- - -→	Salicylic Acid →	(C)→ Salicyl (acid) glucuronide; (C)→ Salicyl (phenolic) glucuronide; (C)- - -→ Salicyluric acid; (O)→ Gentisic acid
Chloral Hydrate	- - -(R)- - -→	Trichloroethanol —(C)→	Trichloroethanol glucuronide; (O)→ Trichloroacetic acid; - - -→ Trichloroacetic acid
	Glutethimide —(O)→	Hydroxyglutethimide —(C)→	Hydroxyglutethimide glucuronide
6-Mercaptopurine	- - -(C)- - -→	6-Mercaptopurine ribonucleotide	(O)→ 6-Thiouric acid
Phenacetin —(O)→		Acetaminophen →	(C)→ Acetaminophen glucuronide; (C)- - -→ Acetaminophen sulfate
Phenytoin —(O)→			p-Hydroxyphenytoin
	Succinylcholine —(H)→	Succinylmonocholine —(H)→	Choline
Theophylline			(O)→ 1-Methylxanthine; (O)- - -→ 1,3-Dimethyluric acid
	Tolbutamide —(O)→		Hydroxy-tolbutamide —(O)→ Carboxy-tolbutamide

[a]Classification: microsomal, —→; nonmicrosomal, - - -→; (O), oxidation; (R), reduction; (H), hydrolysis; (C), conjugation.
[b]For each drug only representative metabolic pathways are indicated.
[c]Inactive at concentrations obtained following the therapeutic administration of the parent drug.
[d]Its status as a prodrug or drug for anti-inflammatory activity is not well established.

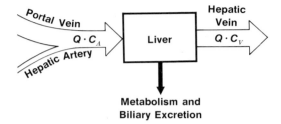

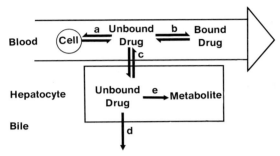

Figure 6-1. *Drug is delivered to the liver via both the portal vein and the hepatic artery and returned to the rest of the body by the hepatic vein. At steady state the difference between the rate of presentation, $Q \cdot C_A$, and the rate of return, $Q \cdot C_V$, is the rate of extraction by metabolism and by biliary excretion.*

Figure 6-2. *Drug in the blood is bound to blood cells (process a) and to plasma proteins (process b); however, it is the unbound drug that diffuses (process c) into the hepatocyte. Within the hepatocyte, the unbound drug is subject to secretion into the bile (process d) or to enzymatic biotransformation (process e). The metabolite leaves the hepatocyte via the blood or the bile or it is subjected to further transformation.*

ess *a*; or a result of tight binding to plasma proteins, process *b*. A combination of these factors could also be involved. One important conclusion can be made, however. The rate of drug elimination in the liver should be directly related to the concentration of drug unbound in the plasma except, perhaps, if process *a* is rate limiting. If processes *d* and *e* are slow and process *c* is rapid, the concentration in the hepatocyte, available for biliary transport or enzymatic reaction, is that unbound in plasma. If processes *d* and *e* are rapid, but process *c* is slow, the concentration that determines elimination is still that unbound to plasma proteins.

The effects of altering blood flow and plasma protein binding on hepatic clearance depend, as expected, on the extraction ratio of the drug. The line of reasoning is analogous to that presented in Chapter 5.

Blood Flow. For a drug with an extraction ratio approaching 1, hepatic clearance is now perfusion rate-limited, and its value approaches that of hepatic blood flow. Changing blood flow alters clearance, but has little or no effect on extraction ratio. There are, of course, practical limits as to how much the flow can be decreased without producing anoxia and affecting the viability of the liver.

For a drug with a low extraction ratio, the arterial and venous concentrations of

the drug across the liver are almost the same. Thus, changing the blood flow has little effect on the unbound concentration to which the liver is exposed. Whether process *c* in Figure 6-2 or processes *d* and *e* are rate limiting, the rate of elimination by the liver would remain the same with blood flow changes. Thus, the clearance remains unaltered, and consequently, the extraction ratio changes inversely with changes in blood flow. These conclusions have been summarized in Chapter 5 (see Table 5-1). Secondary to a decreased blood flow, however, there may be reduced metabolism if the supply of cofactors, e.g., oxygen and sulfate, are rate determining.

Plasma Protein Binding. For a drug with a high extraction ratio, the liver is clearly capable of removing all the drug presented to it in spite of binding to blood cells and to plasma proteins. The rate of elimination depends on the total concentration in the blood. Certainly, a decrease in binding aids in removing a drug; but in this case it is all removed anyway. Therefore, neither the extraction ratio nor the clearance is affected by changes in binding.

For a drug with a low extraction ratio the

opposite is observed. As seen previously, the rate of elimination depends on the unbound concentration.

$$\underset{\substack{\text{Rate of} \\ \text{elimination}}}{} = \underset{\substack{\text{Clearance based} \\ \text{on unbound} \\ \text{concentration}}}{Cl_u} \times \underset{\substack{\text{Unbound} \\ \text{concentration}}}{Cu} \quad 5$$

Here, clearance based upon the unbound concentration, sometimes referred to as the *intrinsic clearance,* is a measure of hepatocellular activity. It is analogous to the glomerular filtration rate, GFR, but is dissimilar in that its value varies with the drug. Expressing the rate of hepatic elimination relative to the plasma concentration, it is apparent that the hepatic (plasma) clearance, varies proportionally with changes in plasma binding:

$$\underset{\substack{\text{Hepatic} \\ \text{clearance}}}{} = \underset{\substack{\text{Clearance} \\ \text{based on} \\ \text{unbound} \\ \text{concentration}}}{Cl_u} \times \underset{\substack{\text{Fraction} \\ \text{in plasma} \\ \text{unbound}}}{fu} \quad 6$$

For example, if the value of *fu* varies twofold so will the hepatic clearance, but the value of the intrinsic clearance remains unchanged. A similar conclusion is drawn for a drug with a low extraction ratio when relating hepatic blood clearance to the fraction in blood unbound. Table 5-2 lists drugs with high and low hepatic extraction ratios.

Drug concentration. A typical characteristic of enzymatic reactions and active transport processes is a limitation in the capacity of the process. There is only so much enzyme present in the liver, and therefore there is a maximum rate at which metabolism can proceed. A limitation in the rate of metabolism can also be a consequence of a limitation in the availability of the cosubstrates and cofactors required in the enzymatic reaction. Similarly, for active biliary excretion there is a maximum rate at which a drug can be excreted into the bile.

Most of our present knowledge of enzyme kinetics is derived from studies *in vitro* in which substrate, enzyme, and cofactor concentrations are controlled. Correlation of such studies with those performed *in vivo* has been difficult. Many factors are involved *in vivo* that cannot be isolated. Nevertheless, the basic principles of enzyme kinetics have application in pharmacokinetics.

The upper curve in Figure 6-3 is characteristic of metabolism by a given enzyme both *in vitro* and *in vivo*. The behavior displayed is typical of Michaelis-Menten kinetics if the approach to the maximum rate, *Vm,* follows the relationship;

$$\text{Rate of metabolism} = \frac{Vm \cdot C}{Km + C} \quad 7$$

in which *Km* is a constant, the Michaelis-Menten constant. In enzyme kinetics the value of *Vm* is directly proportional to the total concentration of enzyme, and *Km* is an inverse function of the affinity between drug and enzyme. Note in Equation 7 that a value of *C* equal to *Km* gives a rate that is one-half the maximum; this is a convenient way of defining the constant. An estimate of the true *Km* requires measurement of the drug concentration at the metabolizing enzyme site. Lacking this capability *in vivo*, the plasma concentration is conventionally used. At plasma concentrations well below *Km*, which fortunately occurs for most drugs used therapeutically, the rate and the concentration vary in direct proportion. At concentrations above *Km*, the rate approaches the value of *Vm*. Since metabolic clearance is defined as the rate of metabolism relative to the plasma concentration,

$$\text{Metabolic clearance} = \frac{Vm}{Km + C} \quad 8$$

its value decreases at drug concentrations approaching and exceeding the value of *Km*. This is shown in the lower part of Figure 6-3. Note that the maximum clearance is the ratio *Vm/Km* unless, of course, this value is so high that elimination becomes perfusion rate-limited, in which case, the limiting value of clearance is hepatic

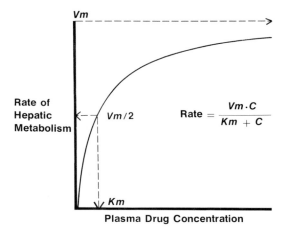

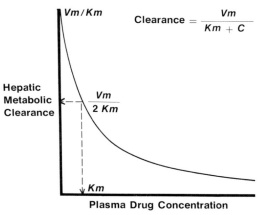

Figure 6-3. *When hepatic metabolism follows Michaelis-Menten kinetics the rate of metabolism increases (top graph), toward a maximum value, Vm, as the plasma drug concentration is increased. The concentration at which the rate is one-half the maximum is the Km value. The metabolic clearance (bottom graph) falls with increasing drug concentration. The concentration at which the clearance is one-half the maximum is also the Km value. The equations for the relationships are shown.*

blood flow. Because of the complexities introduced, the administration of drugs showing saturable metabolism at therapeutic concentrations is difficult.

First-Pass Considerations

To reach the general circulation a drug given orally must pass via the portal system through the liver. The fraction of drug entering the liver that escapes elimination by the organ, F_H, is the upper limit of the oral availability. Its value may be calculated from the hepatic extraction ratio, E_H, since

$$\text{Oral availability} = 1 - \frac{\text{Hepatic extraction ratio}}{\qquad} \qquad 9$$

For example, the antiarrhythmic agent, lidocaine, has an hepatic extraction ratio of 0.7. Accordingly its oral availability is only 30 percent, one reason perhaps why, for this drug, the parenteral route is preferred clinically. Other drugs with a high hepatic extraction ratio (see Table 5-2) likewise have a low oral availability. There may be other factors that limit the drug getting to the portal vein and so further decrease the availability, as described in Chapter 3.

Occasionally drugs with a high hepatic extraction ratio, for example, alprenolol, show increased oral availability when large doses are given. The concentration of drug entering the liver is now sufficiently high to approach or exceed the value of *Km*. The normally high hepatic clearance and extraction ratio is then reduced, and consequently, the availability is increased.

Nonhepatic Metabolism

The liver is often thought of as *the* site of drug metabolism; often it is. However, some metabolizing enzymes are located in other tissues. For example, glucuronide formation occurs in the kidney, in the membranes of the gastrointestinal tract, and in the skin as well as in the liver. The blood contains esterases; these enzymes are also found in many other tissues. The blood clearance, under these circumstances, is theoretically no longer limited by hepatic blood flow. The lung is also rich in some enzymes, and since essentially all the cardiac output passes through this organ, clearance can potentially also be extremely high. The activity of some drug-metabolizing enzymes in the human placenta is high. In some instances the activity is equal to or greater than that in the liver on a weight basis. The therapeutic importance of placental drug metabolism is, however, basically unknown.

Biliary Excretion

All drugs are excreted into the bile. The ability of the liver to do so is expressed by biliary clearance, which is analogous to renal clearance and can be calculated from:

$$\frac{\text{Biliary}}{\text{clearance}} = \frac{\text{(Bile flow)} \times \text{(Concentration in bile)}}{\text{Concentration in plasma}} 10$$

In man, bile flow is a steady 0.5 to 0.8 ml/min. Thus, for a drug with a concentration in the bile equal to or less than that in plasma, the biliary clearance is small. A drug that concentrates in the bile, however, may have a reasonably high biliary clearance. Indeed, the bile to plasma concentration ratio can approach 1000. Therefore biliary clearances of 500 ml/min or higher can be achieved.

Bile does not appear to be a product of filtration, but rather a product of secretion of bile acids and of other solutes. The pH of bile averages about a steady 7.4. The biliary transport of drugs, however, is similar to active secretion in the kidney in that there is a maximum rate of transport. Competitive inhibition of biliary secretion has also been shown.

A few generalizations have been made regarding the characteristics of a drug needed to ensure high biliary clearance. First, the drug must be actively secreted; there appear to be separate secretory mechanisms for acids, for bases, and for un-ionized compounds. Second, it must be polar, and, lastly, its molecular weight must exceed 250. There is little proof, but the latter two requirements may be a consequence of the apparent porous as well as lipophilic nature of both the hepatocyte membranes and bile canniculae. Both nonpolar and small molecules may be reabsorbed. These arguments do not aid in predicting the nature and specificity of the secretory mecha-

nisms, but they do aid in predicting a drug's biliary clearance. For example, glucuronide conjugates of drugs are polar in nature, are ionized, pKa about 3, and have molecular weights exceeding 300. They are usually highly cleared into the bile.

Drug that is excreted in the bile enters the intestine after storage in the gallbladder. In the intestine it may be reabsorbed to complete an enterohepatic cycle. The drug may also be metabolized in the liver, e.g., to a glucuronide. The glucuronide is then excreted into the intestine, where it may undergo hydrolysis by the β-glucuronidase enzymes of the resident flora, back to the drug, which is then reabsorbed. The enterohepatic cycling of drugs directly and indirectly through a metabolite is represented schematically in Figure 6-4.

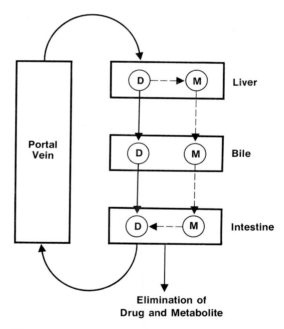

Figure 6-4. *When a drug (D) is absorbed from the intestine, excreted in the bile, and reabsorbed from the intestine (solid line), it has undergone enterohepatic cycling. Similarly, when a drug is converted to a metabolite (M) that is excreted in the bile, converted back to the drug in the intestine, and the drug is reabsorbed (dashed line), the drug has also been enterohepatically cycled, in this case indirectly through a metabolite.*

Dependence of Elimination on Clearance and Distribution

The rate of drug elimination depends on the values of both total clearance, Cl, and plasma drug concentration, C; that is,

$$\text{Rate of elimination} = Cl \cdot C \qquad 11$$

Furthermore, the plasma concentration depends upon the amount of drug in the body, Ab, and the volume into which the drug appears to distribute, V.

$$C = Ab/V \qquad 12$$

Thus,

$$\text{Rate of elimination} = \frac{Cl}{V} \cdot Ab \qquad 13$$

The rate of drug elimination relative to the amount of drug in the body is called the *fractional rate of drug elimination, k*. It is that fraction of the amount in the body that is eliminated per unit time (Fig. 6-5),

$$k = \frac{\text{Rate of elimination}}{Ab} = \frac{Cl}{V} \qquad 14$$

Because clearance is the volume of plasma that is cleared of drug per unit time, from the preceding equation it is apparent that the fractional rate of drug elimination can be thought of in another way, also depicted in Figure 6-5. It is the fraction of the volume of distribution from which the drug is being removed per unit time.

On substituting Equation 14 into Equation 13,

$$\text{Rate of elimination} = k \cdot Ab \qquad 15$$

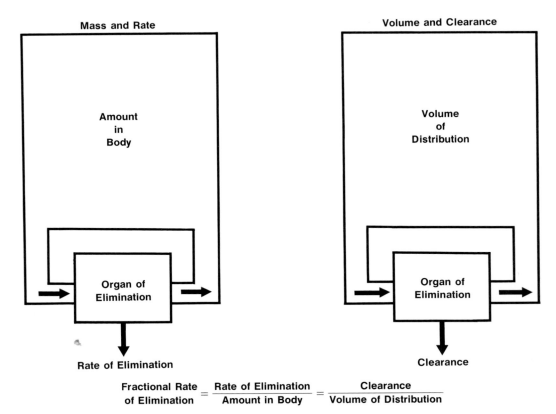

Figure 6-5. *The fractional rate of elimination of a drug can be thought of either as the fraction of the total amount in the body that is eliminated per unit time (left), or as the fraction of the total volume from which the drug is cleared per unit time (right).*

it is apparent that the fractional rate of drug elimination can also be thought of as an elimination rate constant. The value of the rate constant depends upon the values of both clearance and volume of distribution, Equation 14. For this reason a highly cleared drug may be eliminated very slowly. For example, although the clearance of quinacrine is high, about 1500 ml/min, it takes 2 weeks to eliminate 50 percent of the drug from the body. At the other extreme is gentamicin; it has a relatively low clearance of about 120 ml/min and yet it only takes 2 hours to eliminate 50 percent of this drug from the body. This is because the volume of distribution of gentamicin is only about 16 liters; a substantial fraction of the drug in the body is in the blood and is presented to the eliminating organs, in this case primarily the kidneys. The volume of distribution of quinacrine is evidently much larger than that of gentamicin. To estimate its value requires knowledge of the relationship between the time to eliminate one-half the drug in the body, the *elimination half-life* ($t_{1/2}$), and the elimination rate constant. The relationship, derived in Chapter 7, is

$$k = \frac{0.7}{t_{1/2}} \qquad 16$$

Substituting Equation 16 in Equation 14 and rearranging, yields

$$t_{1/2} = \frac{0.7\,V}{Cl} \qquad 17$$

The half-life, too, is therefore a function of volume of distribution and clearance.

Consider the following ideas involving the dependence of half-life on clearance and volume of distribution. A drug that undergoes complete enterohepatic cycling, and yet has a biliary clearance much greater than clearance by other routes of elimination, might be distributed to the bile and subsequently to the intestines in significant amounts, if the intestinal reabsorption is slow. The consequence of biliary obstruction would be a decreased volume of distri-

bution, but no change in clearance, and therefore a shorter half-life. On the other hand, if there is no enterohepatic cycling, the bile and the intestines are not part of the volume of distribution. Then biliary obstruction, by decreasing clearance without affecting distribution, would cause the half-life to increase.

The interrelationships expressed in Equations 14, 16, and 17 are just as readily derived from clearance and volume parameters based on measurements of drug in blood (Cl_b, V_b) or in plasma water (Cl_u, V_u). Thus by definition

Rate of elimination
$$= Cl \cdot C = Cl_b \cdot C_b = Cl_u \cdot Cu \qquad 18$$

and

$$Ab = V \cdot C = V_b \cdot C_b = V_u \cdot Cu \qquad 19$$

Note that each clearance or volume term can be related to another using the definitions $fu = Cu/C$ and $fu_b = Cu/C_b$. For example, $Cl = fu \cdot Cl_u$ and $V_b = fu_b \cdot V_u$. On dividing each term in Equation 18 by the respective term in Equation 19

$$k = \frac{Cl}{V} = \frac{Cl_b}{V_b} = \frac{Cl_u}{V_u} \qquad 20$$

and on substituting Equation 20 into Equation 17, it follows that

$$t_{1/2} = \frac{0.7\,V}{Cl} = \frac{0.7\,V_b}{Cl_b} = \frac{0.7\,V_u}{Cl_u} \qquad 21$$

Thus, the value of the elimination rate constant, k, or the half-life, $t_{1/2}$, is independent of the site of measurement.

Table 6-2 illustrates the half-lives that result from various combinations of clearance and volume of distribution. For a drug that is eliminated by hepatic metabolism and renal excretion, the shortest possible half-life is 1.2 min, a value obtained by substituting the smallest possible volume of distribution, the blood volume, 5 liters, and the largest possible value for clearance, 3 liters/min (the sum of the hepatic and renal

Table 6-2. Half-life of a Drug as Influenced by Clearance and Volume of Distribution[a]

Clearance (ml/min)	Volume of Distribution[a] (liters)				
	5	10	100	1000	10,000
3000	1.16 min	2.3 min	23 min	3.8 hours	38.5 hours
1500	2.3 min	4.6 min	46 min	7.6 hours	77 hours
125	27.7 min	55.4 min	9.2 hours	92 hours	38.5 days
10	5.8 hours	11.6 hours	116 hours	48.1 days	1.25 years
1	58 hours	116 hours	48.1 days	1.25 years	12.5 years
0.1	24 days	48 days	1.25 years	12.5 years	125 years

[a] Based on blood drug concentration. As shown in Equation 21, the table is also applicable to values of clearance and volume of distribution based on either total or unbound plasma drug concentration measurements.

blood flows) into Equation 17. If clearance is low and volume of distribution is large, the half-life can be extremely long.

The volume and clearance parameters based on measurement of drug in blood are useful in considerations of drug extraction in the eliminating organs. The parameters based on the unbound drug concentration are particularly useful in therapeutics, because it is the unbound drug that is thought to relate most closely to the effects of a drug. Both sets of parameters are of value in anticipating and evaluating the pharmacokinetic and therapeutic consequences of alterations in protein binding, blood flow, and other physiologic variables. For convenience of chemical analysis the plasma drug concentration is usually measured, but the volume and clearance parameters so obtained have limitations.

Study Problems

(Answers to Study Problems can be found in Appendix G.)

1. A drug is eliminated almost exclusively by hepatic metabolism; renal and biliary excretion of unchanged drug account for less than 1 percent of total drug elimination. One route of metabolism is glucuronidation, with excretion of all of the glucuronide into the bile (flow rate is 50 ml/hr), at a concentration 110 times that of drug in blood. The excreted glucuronide is neither hydrolyzed in nor reabsorbed from the intestines. The volume of distribution (blood) and the half-life of this drug are 100 liters and 9 hours, respectively.
   (a) Is glucuronidation a major (more than 50 percent) route of elimination of the drug?
   (b) What is the hepatic extraction ratio of this drug? Hepatic blood flow is 1.5 liters/min.
   (c) Is the clearance of this drug more likely to be sensitive to a change in plasma protein binding or to a change in hepatic perfusion?
   (d) Will the half-life of this drug be changed in a patient with biliary obstruction? Briefly comment.

2. (a) Estimate the volume of distribution of quinacrine from the following data: $t_{1/2} = 2$ weeks, clearance = 90 liters/hour.

   (b) Assuming that elimination of quinacrine occurs solely in the liver and that the ratio of blood to plasma drug concentrations is 50 to 1, calculate

   (i)   Its hepatic extraction ratio.

   (ii) The fraction of orally administered drug reaching the liver that escapes hepatic metabolism on the first pass.

   (iii) The volume of distribution based on concentration in blood.

3. What is the shortest half-life that a drug can have if eliminated solely by the liver? Briefly discuss.

4. Prove the following two equalities:

   (a) $Cl_b = fu_b \cdot Cl_u$

   (b) $V = (fu/fu_b) \cdot V_b$

Unifying Problems

(Answers to Unifying Problems can be found in Appendix G.)

Three different drugs A, B, and C are listed in Table 6-3 together with some of their physical properties and disposition characteristics.

1. Indicate the drug(s) (A, B, and C) above for which each of the following statements is probably most applicable:

   (a) The renal clearance of this drug is the most sensitive to changes in urine pH.

   (b) This drug has the highest renal clearance of the three listed.

Table 6-3

Property or Characteristic	Drug A	Drug B	Drug C
Polarity of un-ionized form	Polar	Nonpolar	Nonpolar
pKa	3.0 (weak acid)	9.9 (amine)	Not an acid or a base
Usual dose (mg)	250	100	250
Volume of distribution (liters)	16	300	200
Fraction unbound (fu)	0.4	0.8	*
Half-life	30–40 min	12 hours	18 hours
Fraction excreted unchanged	0.1	0.9	0.05

*Information not given.

(c) This drug most likely shows the greatest diffusion limitation in crossing the placenta to the fetus.

(d) Forced diuresis is most likely to be of value for this drug in a case of drug overdose.

(e) The plasma concentration achieved from a single usual dose of this drug after distribution equilibrium is the lowest.

(f) This drug has the lowest total clearance.

2. Write in the space provided the most appropriate word, term, or value for the following statements:

(a) The clearance of Drug A will _____ if the drug is
      increase, decrease, show little change

significantly displaced from plasma protein binding sites.

(b) Filtration contributes _____ to the renal clearance of Drug B than does secre-
      more, less

tion.

(c) For the drug whose renal clearance is most likely to be sensitive to urinary pH,
      _____ of the urine will *decrease* the clearance and *increase* the
      alkalinization, acidification

half-life of the drug.

3. (a) Drug A is distributed evenly throughout and accounted for within the extracellular fluids. True or false?

(b) Drug C is probably primarily eliminated by _____.
      metabolism, renal excretion

(c) Drug C cannot be highly bound (*fu* less than 0.1) to plasma proteins since it has such a large apparent volume of distribution. True or false?

(d) _____ percent of drug B in the body is located outside the plasma.
      51, 97, 99, 99.9

disposition and absorption kinetics

7

intravenous dose

Objectives

The reader will be able to:

1. **Define the meaning of half-life, elimination rate constant, and first-order process.**

2. **Calculate the values of half-life, elimination rate constant, volume of distribution, and clearance from plasma or blood concentrations of a drug following an intravenous dose.**

3. **Calculate the values of half-life, elimination rate constant, and fraction excreted unchanged from urinary excretion data following an intravenous dose.**

4. **Calculate the value of the renal clearance of a drug from combined plasma and urine data.**

5. **Calculate drug levels in the plasma, in the body, and in the urine with time following an intravenous dose, given the pharmacokinetic parameters.**

ADMINISTERING a drug intravascularly ensures that all of it enters the body. By rapid injection, elevated concentrations of drug in the blood can be promptly achieved; by infusion at a controlled rate a constant concentration can be maintained. With no other route of administration can such promptness and degree of control be as readily achieved. Of the two intravascular routes, the intravenous one is the most frequently employed. Intra-arterial administration, which has greater inherent manipulative dangers, is reserved for situations requiring drug localization in a specific organ or tissue.

The disposition characteristics of a drug are defined by analyzing the temporal changes of drug and metabolites in blood, plasma, and occasionally urine following intravenous administration.

How this information is obtained following a rapid injection of the drug forms the basis of this chapter. The pharmacokinetic information so derived forms a basis for making rational decisions in therapeutics.

Concept of a Bolus

Intravenous administration is most commonly accomplished by infusion. Both rate of infusion and the total amount of drug administered must be considered. For a given dose the shorter the duration of an infusion the earlier and the higher is the maximum concentration in the body fluids. Usually the onset of pharmacologic response(s) is more rapid and the intensity is greater as well. Maximum concentrations are achieved when the dose is placed instantaneously into the blood as a slug or bolus, but the resulting extremely high concentrations may produce adverse effects. These effects may be circumvented by infusing the drug, but then some time may be required for the effect to appear.

Whenever the intent is to administer a drug as rapidly as possible, even though it is infused, it is often said to be given as a bolus dose. A study with procainamide illustrates this point.

Procainamide is usually given orally and in emergencies intramuscularly for the treatment of cardiac arrhythmias. One gram of procainamide hydrochloride, corresponding to 886 mg procainamide base, was injected intravenously to define its disposition kinetics. Injecting this dose within a few seconds would achieve the objective, but the extremely high plasma concentrations seen in these early moments almost certainly would produce a severe lowering of blood pressure. The problem was avoided by infusing procainamide hydrochloride at a constant rate of 100 mg/min for 10 min (Fig. 7-1). Administered in this manner, the peak plasma concentration is

below that which produces significant hypotension, while the amount of drug eliminated during the 10-min infusion is a small fraction of the dose administered. Consequently, from the intent and the lack of elimination, it is said that an intravenous bolus dose of procainamide has been given.

Disposition Viewed from Plasma

Several methods are employed for graphically displaying plasma concentration-time data. One common method, shown with procainamide in Figure 7-1A, is to plot concentration against time on regular or Cartesian graph paper. Depicted in this manner, the plasma concentration is observed to fall rapidly immediately after giving the bolus, in this case from 18 to 6 mg procainamide/liter within 20 min. Thereafter, the rate of decline becomes much slower, taking almost another 3 hours before the concentration falls a further 50 percent to 3 mg/liter. Another method of display that dramatizes these events more vividly is a plot of the same data on semi-

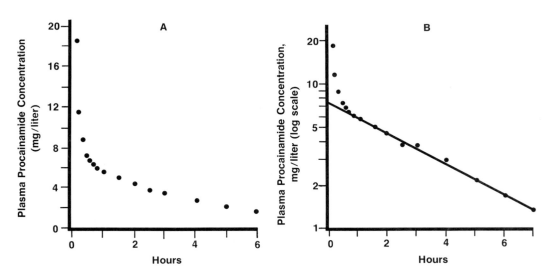

Figure 7-1. A, *Concentration of procainamide, expressed as procainamide hydrochloride, in plasma after an intravenous infusion of 1 gram procainamide hydrochloride at the rate of 100 mg/min for 10 min into a 70-kg volunteer. B, The data shown in A replotted on semilogarithmic graph paper. Note the short distribution phase. (Modified from the data of Koch-Weser, J.: Pharmacokinetics of procainamide in man. Ann. N.Y. Acad. Sci., 179: 370–382, 1971.)*

logarithmic paper (Fig. 7-1B). The time scale is the same as before, but now the ordinate (concentration) scale is logarithmic. Notice the sharp break at about 45 min when the plasma concentration is 6.3 mg/liter. Before this time, the fall is rapid. Thereafter, the decline is slower and, on this semilogarithmic plot, appears to continue linearly. The early phase is commonly known as the *distribution phase* and the latter, the *elimination phase.*

Distribution Phase

The distribution phase is so called because distribution primarily determines the early rapid decline in plasma concentration. For procainamide, distribution is extremely rapid and occurs significantly even over the 10-min period of drug administration. This must be so because the amount of procainamide hydrochloride in plasma at the end of this period is only 48 mg. This value of 48 mg is calculated by multiplying the peak plasma concentration, 16 mg/liter, by the plasma volume, 3 liters. The majority, 952 mg or 95 percent, of the total dose (1 gram) must have already left the plasma and been distributed into other tissues. The rapidity of this process implies that drug uptake must have been primarily into the well-perfused organs, including the liver and the kidney. Some of the drug entering these elimination organs is also cleared from the body, but for procainamide and for many other drugs, the fraction of the administered dose lost during the distribution phase is small.

Elimination Phase

During the distribution phase, changes in the concentration of drug in plasma reflect primarily movement of drug within, rather than loss from, the body. However, with time, distribution equilibrium is established with more and more tissues, and eventually, changes in plasma concentration reflect a proportional change in the concentration of drug in all other tissues and, hence, in the amount of drug in the body. During this proportionality phase, the body acts kinetically as a single container or compartment. Because the decline of the plasma concentration now reflects elimination of drug from the body, this phase is often called the elimination phase.

Elimination Half-Life. The elimination phase is characterized by two parameters, the *elimination half-life* ($t_{1/2}$) and the apparent volume of distribution (V). The elimination half-life is the time taken for the plasma concentration, as well as the amount of the drug in the body, to fall by one-half. The half-life of procainamide, determined by the time taken to fall from 6 to 3 mg/liter, is 2.7 hours (Fig. 7-1B). This is the same time that it takes for the concentration to fall from 4 to 2 mg/liter or from 2 to 1 mg/liter. In other words, for procainamide at the dose administered, the elimination half-life is independent of the amount of drug in the body. It follows, therefore, that less drug is eliminated in each succeeding half-life. Initially there is 1 gram in the body. After about 2.7 hours (1 half-life) 500 mg remain. After 5.4 hours (2 half-lives) 250 mg and after 8.1 hours (3 half-lives), 125 mg remain. In practice, all the drug (97 percent) may be regarded as having been eliminated by 5 half-lives (13.5 hours).

Volume of Distribution. The apparent volume of distribution (V) is obtained by dividing the amount of drug in the body by the plasma concentration (Chap. 4). This calculation requires that distribution equilibrium be achieved between drug in tissues and that in plasma. The amount of drug in the body is known immediately after an intravenous bolus; it is the dose administered. However, distribution equilibrium has not yet been achieved. An estimate is needed of the plasma concentration that would have resulted had all the drug spontaneously distributed into its final volume of distribution. To do this, use is made of the linear decline during the elimination phase seen in the semilogarithmic plot (Fig. 7-1B).

The decline in plasma concentration during the elimination phase can be characterized by the linear equation

$$\log_{10}C = \log_{10}C_0 - k_s t \qquad 1$$

where k_s is the slope of the line in Figure 7-1B and C_0 is the concentration one would determine from this equation at zero time. The negative sign arises because the concentration is declining with time. The term C_0 is an extrapolated value and is an estimate of the concentration which when multiplied by the volume term, V, accounts for the dose administered, i.e.,

$$\text{Dose} = V \cdot C_0 \qquad 2$$

In practice, C_0 is estimated by extrapolating the straight line in Figure 7-1B back to zero time. In the example with procainamide, C_0 is 7.7 mg/liter. Since 1 gram was administered to the patient, the volume of distribution of procainamide is 133 liters. Knowing the volume of distribution the amount of drug in the body can now be estimated at any time during the elimination phase. For example, when the concentration of procainamide in plasma is 2 mg/liter, there are 266 mg in the body.

First-Order Elimination. One may ask why the elimination for procainamide (and for most other drugs) is linear when plotted on semilogarithmic paper. The answer to this question requires a number of manipulations. Equation 1 is expressed in logarithms to the base 10. For reasons that will become apparent, it is first necessary to transpose the relationship to the base of the natural logarithm, e. This transposition is effected simply by realizing that for any number x, $2.3 \log_{10}x = \log_e x$. For example, $\log_{10}2 = 0.301$; therefore, $\log_e 2 = 0.693$. Hence, Equation 1 becomes:

$$\log_e C = \log_e C_0 - kt \qquad 3$$

where $k = 2.3k_s$. Taking the antilogarithm of both sides of Equation 3 yields:

$$C = C_0 \cdot e^{-kt} \qquad 4$$

And multiplying both sides by V, gives

$$Ab = \text{Dose} \cdot e^{-kt} \qquad 5$$

since $C \cdot V$ and $C_0 \cdot V$ are the amount of drug in the body and the dose administered, respectively. Equations 4 and 5 enable the concentration and amount of drug in the body at any time to be estimated using a calculator or the table of exponential functions (Appendix FI). When the decline in the plasma concentration or amount of drug in the body can be described by a single exponential term as given by Equations 4 and 5, it is said to be (mono)exponential. Since the elimination half-life ($t_{1/2}$) is the time taken for the concentration and the amount of drug in the body to fall by one-half, e.g., from C_0 to $\frac{1}{2} C_0$, it follows from Equation 4 that:

$$0.5 = e^{-kt_{1/2}} \qquad 6$$

or

$$e^{kt_{1/2}} = 2$$

Taking the antilogarithms,

$$k \cdot t_{1/2} = \log_e 2 = 0.693$$

one obtains the important relationship,

$$t_{1/2} = \frac{0.7}{k} \qquad 7$$

While the constant k is in the exponent in Equation 4 and can be calculated from Equation 7; its meaning may be better understood by differentiating Equation 4,

$$\frac{dC}{dt} = -k \cdot C_0 \cdot e^{-kt} \qquad 8$$

but since $C = C_0 \cdot e^{-kt}$, it follows that

$$\frac{dC}{dt} = -k \cdot C \qquad 9$$

Multiplying both sides by V, Equation 9 becomes

$$V \cdot \frac{dC}{dt} = -k \cdot V \cdot C \qquad 10$$

or

$$\frac{dAb}{dt} = -k \cdot Ab \qquad 11$$

where Ab is the amount of drug in the body, $V \cdot C$.

The term on the left-hand side of Equation 11 is the rate of change of drug in the body. This is also the rate of elimination of drug from the body. Processes such as this, in which the rate of reaction is proportional to the amount present, are known as *first-order processes*. The proportionality constant is known as the *first-order rate constant* with dimensions of time^{-1}. Because k characterizes the elimination process, it is known as the *elimination rate constant*. Since the rate constant can also be defined by rearranging Equation 11 to yield:

$$k = \frac{dAb}{Ab} / dt \qquad 12$$

the elimination rate constant may simply be regarded as the *fractional rate of drug removal*. For example, since the half-life of procainamide is 2.7 hours, the value of its elimination rate constant is 0.25 hours^{-1}. Hence, the speed of the elimination process of procainamide can either be characterized by its half-life, 2.7 hours, or by saying that the fractional rate of elimination is 0.25 (or 25 percent) of the drug in the body per hour.

It is important to realize that k refers to the fractional rate of elimination and not to the actual amount eliminated per unit time. Consider, for example, that the time scale in Figure 7-1B was in days rather than in hours. The half-life would then be expressed as 0.11 days and the corresponding value for k would be 6.3 days^{-1}. Clearly 6.3 times the dose in the body cannot be eliminated in one day. What is meant is that the fractional rate of elimination, at any moment, is 6.3 times the amount of drug in the body per day. However, because levels in the body decline rapidly, the amount eliminated during the day is, of necessity, less than the dose. To avoid confusion a unit of time must be selected so that the value of k is much less than 1.

Fraction of Dose Remaining. Another view of the kinetics of drug elimination may be gained by examining how the fraction of the dose remaining in the body varies with time. The fraction remaining is obtained by dividing the amount in the body by the dose administered, which, upon appropriate substitution, yields the following:

$$\text{Fraction of dose remaining in the body} = \frac{Ab}{\text{Dose}} = \frac{C}{C_0} = e^{-kt}$$

The fraction of the dose remaining is, therefore, also given either by the ratio C/C_0 or by e^{-kt}. Figure 7-2 is a semilogarithmic plot of this fraction against time expressed relative to the half-life, not against actual time. By so doing the plot is made universal. For all drugs, 50 percent of the dose remains after one half-life and 25 percent remains after two half-lives.

The virtue of expressing time relative to the half-life is seen by letting n be the number of half-lives elapsed after the bolus dose ($n = t/t_{1/2}$). Then, as $k = 0.7/t_{1/2}$,

$$\text{Fraction of dose remaining in the body} = e^{-kt} = e^{-0.7n}$$

But since $e^{-0.7} = \frac{1}{2}$, it follows that

$$\text{Fraction of dose remaining in the body} = (\tfrac{1}{2})^n$$

or

$$C = C_0 \cdot (\tfrac{1}{2})^n$$

Appendix F-II is a table containing values of $(\tfrac{1}{2})^n$. To appreciate the meaning of these values, and to learn how to apply them, consider the following problems:

Q. How much drug remains in the body 4 half-lives after a bolus dose?

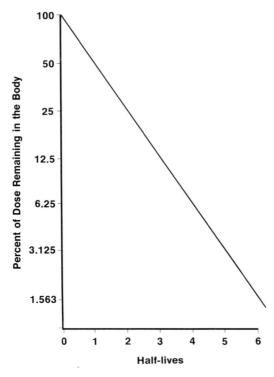

Figure 7-2. *Semilogarithmic plot of the percent dose remaining in the body against time expressed in half-lives. By one half-life, 50 percent of the dose remains in the body, by 3.3 half-lives, 10 percent remains, and by 6 half-lives, only 1.56 percent remains.*

A. $\frac{1}{16}$ or 6.25 percent. The fraction remaining after 4 half-lives ($n = 4$) is $(\frac{1}{2})^4$ or $\frac{1}{2} \times \frac{1}{2} \times \frac{1}{2} \times \frac{1}{2}$.

Q. The half-life of a drug is 6 hours. How much is left in the body 20 hours after a bolus dose?

A. Ten percent. Number of half-lives elapsed since administration (n) = $\frac{20}{6}$ or 3.3. The value of $(\frac{1}{2})^n$ when $n = 3.3$ is 0.1.

Q. Twenty percent of a drug remains in the body 10 hours after a bolus dose. What is the half-life of the drug?

A. 4.3 hours. The value of n which gives a value for $(\frac{1}{2})^n$ of 0.2 is 2.32. Hence the half-life is 10 hours/n or 4.3 hours.

Total Clearance. In Chapter 6 the rate of removal of drug was shown to be the product of its clearance and plasma concentration, that is,

$$\text{Rate of elimination} = \text{Clearance} \cdot C \qquad 13$$

From Equation 10 the rate of elimination is also given by

$$\text{Rate of elimination} = k \cdot V \cdot C$$

which leads to the following important relationship

$$\text{Clearance} = k \cdot V \qquad 14$$

The importance of this equation lies in the fact that from two pharmacokinetic parameters, k and V, one estimates clearance, a physiologic parameter measuring the ability of the eliminating organs to remove drug. Clearance, in turn, may be influenced by such factors as organ blood flow, degree of plasma protein binding, and whether the organ is healthy or diseased. Using Equation 14, the plasma clearance of procainamide is calculated to be 33 liters/hour or 0.5 liters/min.

Clearance and Elimination Half-life. It is more common to refer to the half-life rather than to the elimination rate constant of a drug. Recall that $t_{1/2} = 0.7/k$, so that half-life is related to clearance by:

$$t_{1/2} = \frac{0.7 \times \text{Volume of distribution}}{\text{Clearance}} \qquad 15$$

Equation 15 was purposely arranged in the above manner to stress that half-life and elimination rate constant reflect rather than control volume of distribution and clearance. One can independently alter the volume of distribution or clearance and hence change the half-life but not vice versa. In some instances, the volume of distribution and clearance can change to essentially the same extent, in which case the half-life remains unaltered. To show the application of Equation 15 consider creatinine. It has a clearance of 125 ml/min and is evenly distributed throughout the 42 liters of total body water. As expected by calculation using Equation 15, its half-life is 4 hours. Although inulin has the same clearance as creatinine, it has a half-life of only 1.3 hours because it is restricted to the 16 liters of extracellular water.

Clearance, Area, and Volume of Distribution. Thus far, clearance has been estimated from the half-life and the volume of distribution of a drug. Clearance can be estimated in another way. By rearranging Equation 13, it can be seen that during a small interval of time, dt,

$$\text{Amount eliminated} = \text{Clearance} \cdot C \cdot dt \quad 16$$

where the term $C \cdot dt$ is the corresponding small area under the plasma drug concentration-time curve. For example, if the clearance of a drug is 1 liter/min and the area under the curve between 60 and 61 min is 1 mg × min/liter, then the amount of drug eliminated in that minute is 1 mg. The total amount of drug eventually eliminated, which for an intravenous dose equals the dose administered, is assessed by adding up or integrating the amount eliminated in each time interval from time zero to time infinity, therefore,

$$\text{Dose} = \text{Clearance} \times \text{Area} \quad 17$$

where area is the total area under the concentration-time curve. Thus, once the total area under the plasma concentration-time curve is known (Appendix B), clearance is readily calculated. Note that there is no need to know the half-life or volume of distribution to calculate clearance. Furthermore, this calculation of clearance is independent of the shape of the concentration-time profile.

The volume of distribution (V) is used to relate the plasma concentration to the amount of drug in the body during the elimination phase. Often the value obtained by the method of extrapolation (Eq. 2) is a reasonable estimate of this volume term. Occasionally it is not. The best method of calculating the volume of distribution is to

divide the clearance by the elimination rate constant

$$V = \frac{Cl}{k} = \frac{\text{Dose}}{\text{Area} \cdot k} \quad 18$$

Unlike the method of extrapolation, the present method of estimating V is not restricted to the intravenous bolus situation but can be obtained under a variety of conditions, e.g., long-term intravenous infusions. Consequently, the value of V, estimated using Equation 18, is applied throughout the remainder of this book.

Disposition Viewed from Plasma and Urine

Renal excretion is an important route of elimination for many drugs and their metabolites. Urinary analysis offers a convenient means of estimating some pharmacokinetic parameters. Two factors tend to favor urinary over plasma data analysis. One is the ease of urine collection. The other is the high degree of concentration achieved with many drugs during urine formation, which frequently facilitates chemical analysis.

Much of the interest with urinary analysis in pharmacokinetics stems from the simple relationship that at any instant the rate of drug excretion is the product of its renal clearance and plasma concentration:

$$\text{Excretion rate} = \text{Renal clearance} \times C \quad 19$$

When the renal clearance of a drug is constant the excretion rate is directly proportional to the plasma drug concentration. The excretion rate then mirrors temporal changes of drug in the body.

Constancy of renal clearance is proved when a plot of excretion rate against plasma concentration yields a straight line passing through the origin. In practice, several problems arise in constructing such a plot. Urine is collected over a finite period, e.g., 1 hour or 4 hours, and not instantaneously. Shortening the collection interval, in an attempt to approach an instantaneous excretion rate, tends to increase error owing to incomplete bladder emptying. This is especially true for periods of urine collection of less than 15 min. Lengthening the collection interval, to avoid the problem of incomplete emptying, introduces another problem. Because urine is collected over a time interval, the excretion rate, estimated by dividing the amount excreted in the sample collected by the time interval, is an average value. As such it neither directly reflects the plasma concentration at the beginning nor at the end of the collection time but at some intermediate point. By assuming that the plasma concentration changes linearly with time, the appropriate concentration is that at the midpoint of the collection interval. Because drug levels are in fact changing exponentially with time, this assumption of linear change is reasonable only when drug loss during the interval is small. In practice, the interval should be less than an elimination half-life. Considering these limitations, the data displayed in Figure 7-3 do show that the renal clearance of the antibiotic tetracycline is constant over the therapeutic concentration range and that its value, given by the slope of the line, is 92 ml/min.

Disposition Viewed from Urine Only

Lack of sufficiently sensitive analytic techniques sometimes prevents measurement of the concentration of drug in plasma. In the absence of plasma measurements, neither the volume of distribution nor the renal or total clearance can be determined. Nonetheless, if the drug is in a sufficiently high concentration to be determined in urine, useful information can still be obtained from urine data alone.

Elimination and Excretion Rate Constant

The elimination half-life of the cardiac glycoside, digitoxin, was estimated from urine data before methods were available for measuring the extremely low concentrations in plasma. The approach was to plot the average excretion rate against the midpoint of the collection time on semilogarithmic paper and from the slope of the straight line obtain an estimate of the half-life. Intuitively, the approach is easy to see. Assuming that renal clearance is constant, the urinary excretion rate is proportional to plasma concentration, and plotting urinary excretion rate against time is like plotting

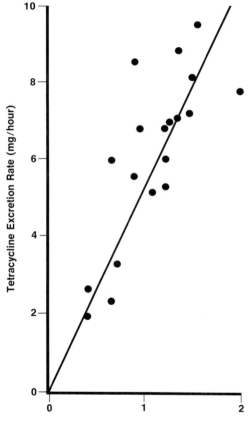

Figure 7-3. *The urinary excretion rate of tetracycline is directly proportional to the serum concentration. (Redrawn from Chulski, T., Johnson, R.H., Schlagel, C.A., and Wagner, J.G.: Direct proportionality of urinary excretion rate and serum level of tetracycline in human subjects. Nature, 198: 450–453, 1963.)*

plasma concentration against time. The half-life is then taken as the time for the urinary excretion rate (or plasma concentration) to fall by one-half. For digitoxin, this is 5 to 6 days in a healthy subject (Fig. 7-4). Conversely, when a straight line is obtained by plotting the urinary excretion rate against the midpoint time, constancy of renal clearance is inferred. The need for using midpoint time follows from the previous discussion; the measured urinary excretion rate reflects the average plasma concentration during the collection interval.

Formal proof of the foregoing discussion is not difficult to derive. Reexpressing Equation 19 in terms of the amount of drug in the body yields:

$$\text{Excretion rate} = \frac{Cl_R}{V} \cdot Ab \qquad 20$$

where Cl_R is renal clearance. As the quotient Cl/V is the rate constant for elimination, so the quotient Cl_R/V is the rate constant for renal excretion, ke. Thus:

$$\text{Excretion rate} = ke \cdot Ab \qquad 21$$

Like k, ke has units of time^{-1} and may be defined as the fractional rate of renal excretion of a drug. At first glance, it would appear that since ke is a proportionality constant, the slope of a semilogarithmic plot of excretion rate against midpoint time should give ke, not k. That this is not the case is evident when Dose $\cdot$ e^{-kt} is substituted for Ab,

$$\text{Excretion rate} = ke \cdot \text{Dose} \cdot e^{-kt} \qquad 22$$

and taking logarithms

$$\log (\text{excretion rate}) = \log (ke \cdot \text{Dose}) - \frac{k \cdot t}{2.3} \qquad 23$$

The intercept at time zero is $ke \cdot$ Dose, and since the bolus dose is known, ke can be calculated. In practice, the uncertainty of complete bladder emptying and the need to collect the urine over short intervals, relative to the elimination half-life of the drug, pose limitations on the quality of excretion rate data. The data often show scatter. When complete urine recovery of drug is assured, estimates of elimination half-life and of elimination and excretion rate constants can be made by analyzing cumulative excretion data (Appendix C). The resultant cumulative excretion plots generally tend to be smoother than the corresponding excretion rate plots.

Renal Excretion as a Fraction of Total Elimination

An important pharmacokinetic parameter is the fraction of the dose entering the systemic circulation that is excreted unchanged, fe. It is a quantitative measure of the contribution of renal excretion to overall drug elimination. Knowing the fraction aids in establishing appropriate modifications in the dosage regimen of a drug for patients with varying degrees of renal function. The value of fe ranges between 0 and 1.0. When the value is low, excretion is a minor pathway of drug elimination. Occasionally, renal excretion is the only route of elimination, in which case the value of fe is

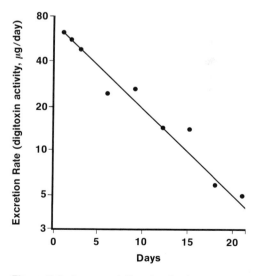

Figure 7-4. Average daily rate of urinary excretion of digitoxin activity for 13 subjects after a single oral dose of 1.2 mg. (Redrawn from Swintosky, J.V.: Excretion equations and interpretation for digitoxin. Nature, 179: 98, 1957.)

one. By definition the difference, $1 - fe$, is the fraction of the dose entering the circulation that is eliminated by nonrenal mechanisms, usually metabolism.

An estimate of fe is most readily obtained from cumulative urinary excretion data, following intravenous administration, since by definition

$$fe = \frac{\text{Total drug excreted unchanged}}{\text{Dose}} \qquad 24$$

In practice, care should always be taken to ensure complete urinary recovery (i.e., collect urine for at least 5 elimination half-lives). In the case of digitoxin the reported value of fe ranges between 0.3 and 0.35 in patients with normal renal function. At any instant, the fraction fe may be defined as the ratio of the rate of excretion to the rate of elimination,

$$fe = \frac{\text{Rate of excretion}}{\text{Rate of elimination}} \qquad 25$$

Appropriately substituting for numerator and denominator, it is seen that

$$fe = \frac{ke \cdot V \cdot C}{k \cdot V \cdot C} = \frac{Cl_R}{Cl} = \frac{ke}{k} \qquad 26$$

Thus, fe may also be defined as the ratio of the renal to total clearance or the ratio of the excretion rate constant to the elimination rate constant. Hence, fe may be calculated by estimating ke/k from the urinary excretion rate data. This is particularly useful in those situations in which total urine collection is not possible. Conversely, having calculated fe from cumulative urinary excretion data (Equation 24) and knowing k, we can estimate the value of ke.

In practice, estimates of Cl, Cl_R, k, and ke are readily obtained whereas those of extrarenal clearance and rate constant for extrarenal elimination are not. These last two parameters are determined by differences. Thus, extrarenal clearance is $(1 - fe) \cdot Cl$ and rate constant for extrarenal elimination is $(1 - fe) \cdot k$.

Estimation of Pharmacokinetic Parameters

Table 7-1 lists pharmacokinetic parameters of some representative drugs in young healthy volunteers. These estimates were made from plasma and urine data obtained following administration of drug by various routes. To appreciate how the pharmacokinetic parameters defining disposition were estimated consider the plasma and urine data in Table 7-2 obtained following an intravenous bolus dose of 50 mg of a drug.

Plasma Data Alone

A plot of plasma concentration versus time indicates that the levels are dropping progressively, but only after the data are plotted on semilogarithmic paper (Fig. 7-5) can the half-life and elimination rate constant be readily determined. The half-life, taken as the time for the concentration to fall in half (e.g., from 1.0 to 0.5 mg/liter, or 0.2 to 0.1 mg/liter), is 2.8 hours, so that k is 0.25 hours^{-1}. Clearance is determined by dividing dose by the area under the curve. The total area under the plasma concentration–time-curve, estimated using the trapezoidal rule (Appendix B), is 10.2 mg-hour/liter and when divided into the dose yields 4.9 liters/hour. The volume of distribution, estimated from Cl/k (Equation 18), is therefore 19.6 liters. This value is virtually identical to that calculated by dividing dose by the intercept concentration at zero time, because no distinct distribution phase is apparent.

Urine Data Alone

The observations are times of urine collection, volumes collected, and concentration of unchanged drug in each sample. These data are treated to derive further information. Especially of interest are the rate and cumulative amount excreted. The amount excreted in each time interval is the product of the volume of urine collected and the concentration, e.g., amount ex-

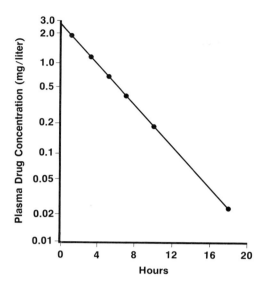

Figure 7-5. Semilogarithmic plot of the plasma concentration-time data given in Table 7-2.

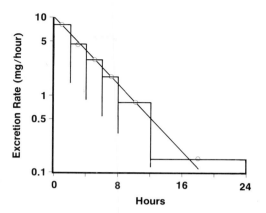

Figure 7-6. Semilogarithmic plot of the rate of excretion against the midpoint time of urine collection. The period over which the average excretion rate was obtained is superimposed. Data from Table 7-2.

creted in Sample 1 is 120 ml × 133 micrograms/ml or 16 mg; the average rate of excretion over the first 2-hour period is therefore 8 mg/hour. The cumulative amount excreted up to any time is the sum of all drug excreted unchanged up to that time. By 24 hours the cumulative amount excreted is 39.1 mg, and since 37.2 mg was excreted in the first 12 hours and only another 1.9 mg was excreted over the next 12 hours, 39.1 mg can reasonably be taken to be the maximum amount of drug that will be excreted.

Excretion rate data are occasionally displayed as a bar histogram but this form of presentation is not as useful as one in which the rate data are plotted against the midpoint of the collection interval on semilogarithmic paper (Fig. 7-6). The time for the excretion rate to fall in half (e.g., from 5 mg/hour to 2.5 mg/hour) is the elimination half-life of the drug (2.8 hours). The intercept at zero time ($ke \cdot Dose$) is 10 mg/hour so that ke, the rate constant for excretion, is 0.2 hours^{-1}. One can arrive at the same answer for k by a different route. The fraction of the dose excreted unchanged, fe, is 39.1 mg/50 mg, or 0.78, so

that ke ($fe \cdot k$) is 0.78 × 0.25, or 0.20 hours^{-1}.

Plasma and Urine Data

Plasma and urine data together are required to estimate the renal clearance of the drug. This parameter is best obtained from the slope of a plot of the excretion rate against the plasma drug concentration at the midpoint time of the urine collection (Fig. 7-7). The straight line implies that the renal clearance is constant and independent of the plasma concentration. The slope of the line indicates that the renal clearance of the drug is 4 liters/hour. Essentially the same value is obtained by multiplying the total clearance (5.0 liters/hour) by fe (0.78) (cf. Eq. 26).

A Question of Precision

Had you, the reader, plotted the same data and calculated the pharmacokinetic parameters, you may have obtained answers that differ from those given. This is not unusual and will occur in many cases when you check your answers to the problems at the end of each chapter against those given in Appendix G. The reason lies in the variability of the system. Sources of

Table 7-1. Average Pharmacokinetic Parameters of Representative Drugs in Young Healthy Adults

Drug	Molecular Weight	pKa	Percent in Plasma Unbound	Clearance (liter/hour/70 kg)
Acetazolamide Acid	222	7.2	4 → 13[d]	2.4
Amphetamine Base	135	9.9	85	9–32[a]
Diazepam Neutral	285	3.4	4	2.7
Digoxin Neutral	781	—	65–80	12
Gentamicin Base	459	—	70–80	7.2
Lidocaine Base	234	7.8	30 → 40[d]	45
Lithium Carbonate Salt	74	—	>90	1.8[b]
Meperidine Base	284	8.7	20–70[c]	66
Phenobarbital Acid	232	7.2	33–71	0.28
Penicillin G Acid	334	2.8	30–50	30
Phenytoin Acid	252	8.3	10	1 ← 2.4[e]
Procainamide Base	235	9.2	80–90	34
Propranolol Base	259	9.5	4–10	49
Sulfisoxazole Acid	267	5.0	6 → 15[d]	1.4
Tetracycline Amphoteric	444	3.3, 7.8, 9.6	70–80	9
Theophylline Acid	180	8.7	36–46	4.3
Tolbutamide Acid	270	5.5	8 → 11[d]	0.80
Warfarin Acid	308	4.8	0.3–1.0	0.16

[a]Depends on urine pH.
[b]Depends on urine flow and sodium output.
[c]Increases with age.
[d]→ denotes increasing value with increasing concentration within the therapeutic range.
[e]← denotes decreasing value with increasing concentration within the therapeutic range.

Table 7-1. Average Pharmacokinetic Parameters of Representative Drugs in Young Healthy Adults (Continued)

Volume of Distribution (liter/70 kg)	Half-life (hours)	Fraction Excreted Unchanged (percent)	Oral Availability (percent)	Drug
14	4.1	66–90	>90	Acetazolamide
290	6–22[a]	5–75[a]	>95	Amphetamine
120	32	<5	>95	Diazepam
760	44	59–80	40–70	Digoxin
21	2	>95	<5	Gentamicin
110	1.5	<5	20–40	Lidocaine
54	21	>95	>95	Lithium Carbonate
320	3.5	2–10[a]	50–70	Meperidine
50	120	20–50	>95	Phenobarbital
23	0.5	60–80	20–40	Penicillin G
50	7 → 40[d]	<5	>90	Phenytoin
140	3	40–55	75–95	Procainamide
180	2.5	<2	15–70	Propranolol
12	6	40–80	>90	Sulfisoxazole
110	8	50–70	50–95	Tetracycline
35	6	<15	>95	Theophylline
8	7	<1	>90	Tolbutamide
8	34	<1	>95	Warfarin

Table 7-2. Plasma and Urine Data Obtained Following an Intravenous Bolus Dose

| | Observation | | | | | Treatment of Urine Data | | |
| | Plasma Data | Urine Data | | | | | | |
Sample	Plasma Concentration[a] (mg/liter)	Time Interval of Collection (hours)	Volume of Urine (ml)	Concentration of Unchanged Drug in Urine (mg/liter)	Amount Excreted in Time Interval (mg)	Excretion Rate (mg/hour)	Cumulative Amount Excreted (mg)	Midpoint Time of Urine Collection (hours)
1	2.0	0–2	120	133	16	8	16.0	1
2	1.13	2–4	180	50	9	4.5	25.0	3
3	0.70	4–6	89	63	5.6	2.8	30.6	5
4	0.43	6–8	340	10	3.4	1.7	34.0	7
5	0.20	8–12	178	18	3.2	0.8	37.2	10
6	0.025	12–24	950	2	1.9	0.15	39.1	18

[a]Plasma sample taken at midpoint time of urine collection.

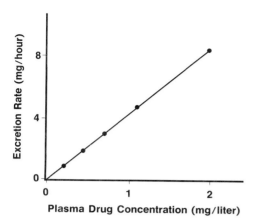

Figure 7-7. *The rate of excretion is directly proportional to plasma drug concentration measured at the midpoint of the urine collection interval. Data from Table 7-2.*

variation include the method of measurement, the conditions of storage and handling of the sample prior to analysis, and the system itself.

Together, at best, they produce an overall variation in the region of 5 to 10 percent in most biologic systems. For example, had the study just considered been repeated subsequently in the same individual the estimated half-life may have been 3.1 hours instead of 2.8 hours. For almost all clinical situations, this degree of variation is acceptable. Variations in the range of 10 to 25 percent are not uncommon. To reflect the acceptable 5 to 10 percent variation, most answers here and throughout the remainder of the book are only given to two significant places, and the value $\log_e 2$, 0.693, has been rounded off to 0.7 (cf. Eq. 7).

Effect of Dose

An adjustment in dose is often necessary to achieve optimal drug therapy. Adjustment is made more readily when the values of the pharmacokinetic parameters of a drug do not vary with dose or with concentration. The possibility for a change with dose exists, however. Recall that binding of

drug within the body depends upon concentration, and that secretory and metabolic processes are saturable. The availability of the drug can also change with dose, for example, when there is a solubility limitation or when an active transport process is involved in absorption. Most drug-induced changes in physiologic function, e.g., cardiac output, vary with drug concentration, which in turn may alter the value of a pharmacokinetic parameter, such as clearance. This type of *dose-dependent* kinetics adds to variability in drug response and makes dose adjustment more difficult.

Evidence of dose dependency is usually assessed by increasing the dose and, after normalizing the resultant plasma concentration or the amount excreted to the dose administered, observing whether such values superimpose at all times. This is referred to as the *principle of superposition*. When the values do not superimpose, dose dependency is inferred. Establishing which pharmacokinetic parameter(s) has changed and identifying the cause of the dose dependency usually require extensive additional experimentation and analysis of the data, aspects that are beyond the scope of this book. Although dose-dependent kinetics is seen within the therapeutic range of doses of such drugs as phenytoin and salicylic acid, this phenomenon is relatively uncommon; the pharmacokinetic parameters are usually independent of dose and the kinetics are often then said to be *linear*. Accordingly, throughout the remainder of the book linear pharmacokinetics is assumed, unless otherwise stated.

Representation of Drug Disposition by a Model

The elimination kinetics of many drugs can be adequately characterized by an elimination rate constant k, or half-life, $t_{1/2}$, and an apparent volume of distribution V (Model A, Fig. 7-8). The total clearance, equal to the sum of clearances by all elimi-

Model A

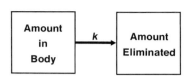

Model B

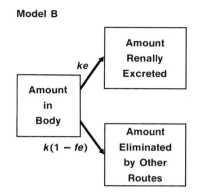

Figure 7-8. Model A, *Simple model depicting disposition occurring from a single compartment of volume V, by an elimination rate constant, k.* Model B, *When excretion is also measured, the elimination rate constant is divided into two components, that associated with excretion (ke) and that associated with loss by other routes [k(1 − fe)].*

nation organs, is given by the product, $k \cdot V$, and has units of volume per unit time. Total clearance can also be obtained by dividing dose administered by the total area under the plasma drug concentration-time profile. When renal excretion of unchanged drug is also measured, the elimination rate con-stant and the total clearance can be divided into two parts, that associated with excretion (ke, Cl_R) and that associated with loss by other routes $(k(1 − fe), \text{ or } Cl(1 − fe))$ as shown in Model B of Figure 7-8. This simple representation of drug disposition is used throughout the remainder of the book.

Study Problems

(*Answers to Study Problems can be found in Appendix G.*)

1. Table 7-3 summarizes plasma data obtained after a bolus dose of a drug.

Table 7-3. Plasma Concentrations of a Drug After Intravenous Administration of a 37.5-mg Dose

Time (hours)	0.8	2.0	4.0	5.0	7.0	10.0
Concentration (mg/liter)	1.60	1.20	0.58	0.32	0.13	0.041

(a) Plot the plasma concentration of drug versus time on three-cycle semilogarithmic paper. Estimate the half-life of the drug.
(b) Estimate the total area under the plasma drug concentration-time curve.
(c) Estimate the total clearance.
(d) Knowing that 37.5 mg of drug was administered, calculate the volume of distribution.

2. Plot on linear and on semilogarithmic graph paper the following plasma concentration-time relationship:

$$C = 0.9e^{-0.347t}$$

where C is in mg/liter and time is in hours.

3. The data given in Table 7-4 are the mean plasma concentrations of lysergic acid diethylamide as a function of time after intravenous administration of 2 micrograms/kg to 5 normal human subjects.

Table 7-4

Time (hours)	0.16	0.33	0.50	1.00	2.00	4.00	8.00
Concentration (μg/liter)	9.5	7.4	6.3	5.3	4.2	2.9	1.2

(a) Prepare a plot of plasma concentration versus time on semilogarithmic paper.
(b) Estimate the half-life and total clearance of the drug.
(c) Given that the mean body weight is 75 kg, calculate the volume of distribution of the drug.

Unifying Problem

(Answers to Unifying Problem can be found in Appendix G.)

1. Swintosky et al. studied the disposition kinetics of sulfaethylthiadiazole. Table 7-5 contains a list of the plasma concentrations and the amounts of drug excreted unchanged with time following an intravenous bolus dose of 2.0 grams sulfaethylthiadiazole to a subject (weight 81 kg).

Table 7-5 [a]

Time (hours)	1	2	4	6	8			
Plasma concentration (mg/liter)	120	102	85	72	58			
Time interval (hours)		0–3	3–6	6–9	9–12	12–15	15–24	24–48
Amount excreted unchanged (mg)		534	436	181	139	110	202	195

[a] From Swintosky, J.V., et. al.: J. Am. Pharm. Assoc. *46*: 403–411, 1957. Reproduced with permission of the copyright owner.

(a) Estimate graphically the volume of distribution, the elimination half-life, and the total clearance of the drug from the plasma data.
(b) Estimate graphically the elimination half-life from a semilogarithmic plot of excretion rate against the midpoint time of urine collection. Compare your answer with that estimated from the plasma data.

(c) Calculate the fraction of the dose excreted unchanged and the renal clearance of the drug.

(d) Given that the average fraction of drug in plasma unbound is 1.6 to 5.7 percent, do the data suggest that sulfaethylthiadiazole is secreted renally?

(e) Estimate the elimination half-life of sulfaethylthiadiazole from cumulative excretion data and compare the answer with that obtained from the plasma and urinary excretion rate data. Before doing so, read the material in Appendix C, which discusses the treatment of cumulative urine data.

8

constant rate intravenous infusion

Objectives

The reader will be able to:

1. **Define plateau level and describe the factors controlling it.**

2. **Describe the relationship between half-life of a drug and time required to approach the plateau level following a constant-rate intravenous infusion with or without a bolus dose.**

3. **Estimate the value of half-life, volume of distribution, and clearance of a drug from data obtained during and following an intravenous infusion.**

4. **Estimate the value of half-life, elimination rate constant, fraction excreted unchanged, and excretion rate constant from urine data obtained during and following an intravenous infusion.**

5. **Estimate the value of the renal clearance of a drug from combined plasma and urine data.**

6. **Use pharmacokinetic parameters to predict drug levels with time during and following a constant intravenous infusion with or without a bolus dose.**

WHILE a single intravenous bolus may rapidly produce the desired therapeutic level of a drug, this mode of administration is unsuitable when the maintenance of plasma or tissue concentrations and, hopefully, of effect is desired. Under these circumstances, it is common practice, in hospital settings, to infuse a drug at a constant rate. This method permits precise and readily controlled drug administration. Usually the solution for injection is infused by gravity from a bottle placed above the patient. The infusion rate is controlled by the flow rate and concentration of drug in the solution. Adjustment in flow is made either by vary-ing the height of the bottle or by regulating the aperture of the tubing connecting the bottle to the needle. When greater precision and control of drug delivery is desired, an infusion pump is used.

Drug Level–Time Relationships

A drug is said to be given as a constant (rate) infusion when the intent is to maintain a stable level (amount or concentration) of drug in the body. In contrast to the short duration of infusion of a bolus dose, the duration of constant infusion is usually much longer than the half-life of the drug.

The essential features of the events following a constant infusion can be appreciated by considering the events depicted in Figure 8-1.

The Plateau Level

At any time during an infusion, the rate of change in the amount of drug in the body (dAB/dt) is the difference between the rate of infusion and the rate of drug elimination;

$$\underset{\substack{\text{Constant rate} \\ \text{of infusion}}}{\frac{dAb}{dt}} = \underset{}{R_{inf}} - \underset{\substack{\text{Rate of} \\ \text{elimination}}}{k \cdot Ab} \qquad 1$$

or expressing the equation in terms of the concentration of drug in plasma,

$$\frac{V \cdot dC}{dt} = R_{inf} - Cl \cdot C \qquad 2$$

On starting a constant infusion the amount of drug in the body is zero; therefore the amount of drug in the body rises and continues to do so until the rate of

elimination matches the rate of infusion. The amount of drug in the body is then said to have reached a *steady-state*, or *plateau*, level, which remains stable as long as the same infusion rate is maintained. Since, at the plateau, the rate of change of amount of drug in the body is zero, it follows that Equations 1 and 2 simplify to:

$$\underset{\substack{\text{Amount at} \\ \text{steady state}}}{Ab_{ss}} = \underset{\substack{\text{Infusion rate} \\ \text{Elimination rate constant}}}{R_{inf}/k} \qquad 3$$

$$\underset{\substack{\text{Concentration} \\ \text{at steady state}}}{C_{ss}} = \underset{\substack{\text{Infusion rate} \\ \text{Clearance}}}{R_{inf}/Cl} \qquad 4$$

Clearly then the only factors governing the amount of drug at the plateau are the rate of infusion and the elimination rate constant. Similarly, only the infusion rate and clearance control the steady-state plasma concentration. Suppose, for example, that a steady-state plasma concentration of procainamide of 4 mg/liter is desired. Since the clearance of this drug is 33 liters/hour,

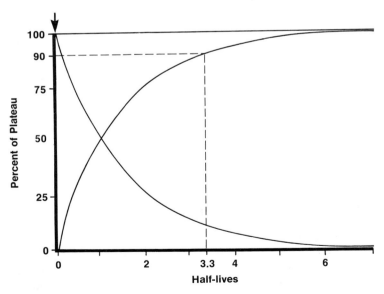

Figure 8-1. *The approach to the plateau is controlled only by the half-life of the drug. Depicted is a situation in which a bolus dose immediately attains and a constant infusion thereafter maintains a constant amount of drug in the body. As the amount of the bolus dose remaining in the body (⌒) falls, there is a complementary rise resulting from the infusion (⌣). By 3.3 half-lives the amount in the body associated with the infusion has reached 90 percent of the plateau level.*

the required infusion rate is 132 mg/hour. Since the elimination rate constant of procainamide is 0.25 hour^{-1}, the corresponding amount of drug in the body at steady state is 528 mg. Alternatively, the amount can be calculated by multiplying the plateau concentration (4 mg/liter) by the volume of distribution of procainamide (133 liters).

To emphasize the factors that control the plateau level consider the following statement: All drugs infused at the same rate and having the same clearance reach the same plateau concentration. This statement is true. The liver and kidney can clear only what they see. These organs are unaware of differences in the tissue distribution of a drug. The rate of elimination depends only on clearance and on the plasma concentration. At the plateau, the rate of elimination is equal to the rate of infusion. The plasma concentration must therefore be the same for all drugs with the same clearance if administered at the same rate. However, the amount of drug in the body differs with differences in volumes of distribution. Only drugs for which clearance and volume of distribution are the same will both the concentration and the amount in the body at the plateau be the same when infused at the same rate. Now consider the next statement: When infused at the same rate, the amount of drug in the body at the plateau is the same for all drugs with the same half-life. This statement is also true. Drugs with the same half-life have the same elimination rate constant. The elimination rate constant is the fractional rate of drug elimination. At the plateau the rate of elimination equals the rate of infusion. It should be recalled that the fractional rate of drug removal is obtained by dividing the rate of elimination by the amount of drug in the · body. Hence the amount of drug in the body at the plateau must be the same for all drugs with the same half-life. Although the amount of drug in the body is the same, the corresponding plateau concentration of a drug varies inversely to its volume of distribution.

A knowledge of the plateau level at a particular infusion rate helps to predict the infusion rate needed to obtain a different plateau level. Thus, provided that clearance is constant, any change in the infusion rate produces a proportional change in the plateau concentration. Returning, for example, to procainamide, since an infusion rate of 132 mg/hour results in a plateau concentration of 4 mg/liter, a rate of 264 mg/hour is needed to produce a plateau concentration of 8 mg/liter.

Time to Reach the Plateau

A delay always exists between the starting of an infusion and the establishment of the plateau level. The sole factor controlling the approach to the plateau is the half-life of the drug. To appreciate this point consider the following situation. Suppose a bolus dose had been given at the start of a constant infusion and that this dose immediately attained the amount at the plateau; clearly the size of the bolus dose must be Ab_{ss}. Thereafter, the amount in the body is maintained at the plateau by the constant infusion. Imagine that a way exists to monitor separately the drug remaining in the body from the bolus and that accumulating due to the infusion. The events are depicted in Figure 8-1. The amount of drug in the body associated with each mode of administration is eliminated as though the other were not present. The level associated with the bolus dose declines exponentially and at any time,

$$\text{Amount of bolus dose remaining in the body} = Ab_{ss} \cdot e^{-kt} \quad 5$$

However, as long as the infusion is maintained, this decline is always exactly matched by the gain resulting from the infusion. This must be so since the sum always equals the plateau level, Ab_{ss}. It therefore follows that the amount of drug in the body associated with a constant infusion (Ab_{inf}) is always the difference between the amount at the plateau (Ab_{ss}) and the amount of the bolus dose remaining, namely,

$$Ab_{inf} = Ab_{ss} - Ab_{ss} \cdot e^{-kt} \qquad 6$$

Or, by dividing through by the volume of distribution,

$$C_{inf} = C_{ss}[1 - e^{-kt}] \qquad 7$$

Thus, both the amount of drug in the body and the plasma concentration (C_{inf}) rise asymptotically toward the plateau following constant drug infusion without a bolus dose.

Practically, it may be more useful to discuss accumulation following a constant infusion in terms of the half-life of a drug. Defining n as the number of half-lives elapsed since the start of the infusion ($t/t_{1/2}$), Equations 6 and 7 can be written as,

$$Ab = Ab_{ss} [1 - (\tfrac{1}{2})^n] \qquad 8$$

and,

$$C = C_{ss} [1 - (\tfrac{1}{2})^n] \qquad 9$$

The amount of drug in the body, or plasma concentration, expressed as a percent of the plateau level, has been calculated at different times after initiation of an infusion and is shown in Table 8-1. In one half-life ($n = 1$), the level in the body is 50

Table 8-1. Percent of the Plateau Level Reached at Various Times Following a Constant Infusion of Drug

Time (in half-lives)	Percent of Plateau
0.5	29
1	50
2	75
3	88
3.3	90
4	94
5	97
6	98
7	99

percent of the plateau. In two half-lives ($n = 2$), it is $1 - (\tfrac{1}{2})^2$ or 75 percent of the plateau. Theoretically, the plateau is only reached when the drug has been infused for an infinite number of half-lives. For practical purposes, however, the plateau may be considered to be reached in 3.3 half-lives (90 percent of the plateau). Thus the shorter the half-life the sooner the plateau is reached. For example, penicillin G (half-life of 30 min) reaches a plateau within minutes (3.3 half-lives is 100 min), whereas it takes 2 to 3 weeks of constant phenobarbital administration (half-life of 5 days) before the plateau is reached (3.3 half-lives is 17 days). The important point to remember is that the approach to the plateau depends *solely* on the half-life of the drug. For example, because the half-life of procainamide is 2.8 hours, it must be infused for 9 hours before a plateau is reached. This is so whether 132 mg/hour is infused to maintain a plateau concentration of 4 mg/liter, or the infusion rate is doubled (264 mg/hour) to maintain a plateau concentration of 8 mg/liter. In the latter case, the procainamide plasma concentration at one half-life is one-half the corresponding plateau value of 8 mg/liter. So, if one wanted to achieve a plateau concentration of 4 mg/liter in 2.7 hours one could infuse at a rate of 264 mg/hour for one half-life and then maintain this concentration by halving the infusion rate to 132 mg/hour.

Levels in the body at times between half-lives can be calculated using the table of $(\tfrac{1}{2})^n$ functions in Appendix F-II. To illustrate the use of this table consider the following questions:

Q. What is the procainamide concentration after 2 hours of constant infusion of 136 mg/hour?

A. 1.6 mg/liter. The value of n is $\tfrac{2}{2.7}$ or 0.74. The value of $1 - (\tfrac{1}{2})^n$ corresponding to an n of 0.74 is 0.4. Since the plateau concentration ultimately achieved is 4 mg/liter, the concentration at 2 hours is 1.6 mg/liter.

Q. What is the half-life of a drug when 30 percent of the plateau is reached at 4 hours?

A. 7.8 hours. The value of n corresponding to 0.3 for $1 - (\frac{1}{2})^n$ is 0.51. The half-life of the drug is therefore $\frac{4}{0.51}$ or 7.8 hours.

Postinfusion

The moment an infusion is stopped, the level falls by one-half each half-life. Indeed, given only the declining levels of a drug, it is impossible to deduce whether a bolus or an infusion had been given. In the example of procainamide, 816 mg are in the body at the plateau following an infusion rate of 204 mg/hour. Approximately 9 hours (3.3 half-lives) after stopping the infusion, only one-tenth of the plateau level or 82 mg remains in the body. The same amount of drug would be found in the body 9 hours after an intravenous bolus dose of 816 mg of procainamide.

Changing Infusion Rates

The rate of infusion of a drug is sometimes changed during therapy. If the object of the change is to effect a new plateau, then the time to go from one plateau to another, whether higher or lower, depends *solely* on the half-life of the drug.

Consider, for example, a patient stabilized on a 136 mg/hour infusion rate of procainamide, which, according to Figure 8-2, should produce a plateau concentration of 4 mg/liter. Suppose the situation now demands a plateau concentration of 8 mg/liter. This new plateau is achieved by doubling the infusion rate to 272 mg/hour. Imagine that instead of increasing the drip rate, the additional 136 mg/hour was administered at a different site and that a way existed of separately monitoring the procainamide in the body from the two infusions. The events, illustrated in Figure 8-2, show that the procainamide concentration associated with the new infusion will rise to 4 mg/liter in exactly the same time as in the first infusion; half the plateau concentration (2 mg/liter) in one elimination half-life (2.7 hours) and so on. Addition of this rising concentration to the preexisting plateau concentration shows that the half-life is the *sole* determinant of the time taken to go from 4 to 8 mg/liter. Needless to say, any readjustment in the infusion rate in less than 3.3 half-lives means that a new plateau concentration will never be established.

The decline from a high plateau to a low one is likewise controlled by the half-life. Consider, for example, the events following the stopping of the supplementary 136 mg/hour infusion rate discussed previously. The procainamide concentration associated with this supplementary infusion will fall to half the existing level in one half-life. In 3.3 half-lives, the total concentration will have almost returned to the preexisting 4 mg/liter concentration. Also, it will take another 3.3 half-lives for most of the procainamide to be removed from the body once the original 136 mg/hour infusion is stopped.

Bolus and Infusion

It takes approximately 9 hours of constant infusion of procainamide before the plateau concentration is reached. It takes even longer for drugs that have half-lives greater than that of procainamide. Situations sometimes demand that the plateau be reached more rapidly. Figure 8-1 suggests a solution. That is, at the start of an infusion, one gives a bolus dose, equal to the amount desired at plateau. Usually the bolus dose is a therapeutic dose and the infusion rate is adjusted to maintain the therapeutic level. When the bolus dose and infusion rate are exactly matched, as in Figure 8-1, the amount of drug in the body associated with the two modes of administration are complimentary, the gain of one always offsetting the loss of the other. By one half-life the amounts of drug in the body associated with bolus and with infusion are equal. By two half-lives 75 percent

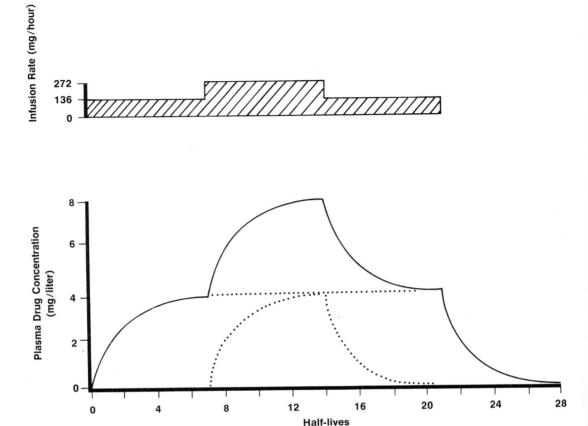

Figure 8-2. *Situation illustrating that the time to reach a new plateau, whether higher or lower than the previous level, depends only on the half-life of a drug. A plateau concentration of 4 mg/liter is reached in approximately 3.3 half-lives after starting a constant infusion of 136 mg/hour of procainamide. Doubling the infusion rate is like maintaining 136 mg/hour and starting another constant infusion of 136 mg/hour. In approximately 3.3 half-lives the procainamide concentration rises from 4 mg/liter to 8 mg/liter. Halving an infusion rate of 272 mg/hour is analogous to stopping the supplementary 136 mg/hour infusion. The plasma concentration of procainamide returns to the 4 mg/liter plateau in approximately 3.3 half-lives.*

of the plateau results from the infusion. Ultimately, as all the bolus dose is eliminated, the plateau level depends *solely* on the infusion rate.

To emphasize this last point, consider two situations. The first, shown in Figure 8-3, is one in which different bolus doses are given at the start of a constant infusion. In case A, drug is infused alone and levels rise, reaching a plateau of 200 mg in approximately 4 half-lives. In case B, the bolus dose of 200 mg immediately attains and the infusion rate thereafter maintains the plateau

level. In case C, the bolus dose of 400 mg is excessive. Now, since the rate of loss from this 400-mg dose is initially greater than the rate of infusion, the level in the body falls. This fall continues until the same plateau as in case B is reached. It should be noticed that the time to reach the plateau depends solely on the half-life of the drug. Thus, in Case C, 300 mg in the body at one half-life, comprised of 200 mg remaining from the bolus and 100 mg from the infusion, lies midway between the bolus dose and the plateau level. By two half-lives, the 225 mg

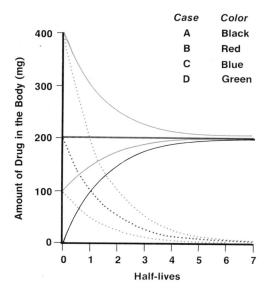

Case	Color
A	Black
B	Red
C	Blue
D	Green

Figure 8-3. *Situations illustrating that the plateau level depends upon the infusion rate and not upon the initial bolus dose. Whether a bolus dose is given (cases B, C, D) or not (case A) at the start of the infusion, the amount of drug in the body at the plateau is the same. The amount of the bolus dose remaining in the body declines exponentially (···) while the level associated with the infusion in all cases rises asymptotically toward the plateau, as portrayed by case A. When not initially achieved it takes approximately 3.3 half-lives to reach the plateau (cases A, C, D).*

in the body lies 75 percent of the way toward the plateau. By approximately 4 half-lives little of the bolus dose remains and the plateau is reached. In case D the bolus dose of 100 mg is below the plateau level. Since the rate of infusion now exceeds the rate of drug elimination, the amount of drug in the body continuously rises until the same plateau as in the previous cases is reached. Once again the time to approach the plateau is controlled solely by the half-life of the drug.

In the second and more common situation, depicted in Figure 8-4, the same bolus dose and infusion rate are administered to three patients, A, B, C, with different half-lives and clearance values. The half-lives in these patients are 3, 6, and 9 hours, respectively. All patients start with the same

amount of drug in the body. In patient B, this amount is maintained because the rate of infusion is exactly matched by the rate of elimination. Since elimination is slower, the level in patient C rises until the rate of elimination equals the infusion rate. The time to reach this higher plateau level is governed solely by the half-life of the drug in this patient. Thus, by one half-life (9 hours), the amount of drug in patient C is midway between the bolus dose and the plateau. By the time the plateau is reached all the bolus dose has been eliminated. Also, it follows from Equation 3 that for a given infusion rate, the amount at the plateau is proportional to the half-life. This is seen in Figure 8-4, where the amount in patient C at the plateau is 50 percent higher than that in patient B. Patient A eliminates the drug more rapidly than does patient B. Accordingly, the amount of drug in patient A falls until a new plateau level, one-half that of patient B, is reached. As always, the approach to the plateau is governed solely by the half-life, which in patient A is only 3 hours. Thus, by 3 hours (one half-life) the level has fallen 50 percent of the way toward the plateau and by 10 hours the plateau is reached.

Assessment of Pharmacokinetic Parameters

Pharmacokinetic parameters are determined just as readily from infusion as from intravenous bolus data. How some of these estimates are made is seen by considering the plasma concentration data in Table 8-2, obtained during and after an infusion of a drug.

Plasma Data Alone

Consider, for the moment, that measurements only during the infusion were available. What can be estimated?

First, dividing the infusion rate of 40 mg/hour by the plateau concentration of 9.5 mg/liter gives the clearance, in this case

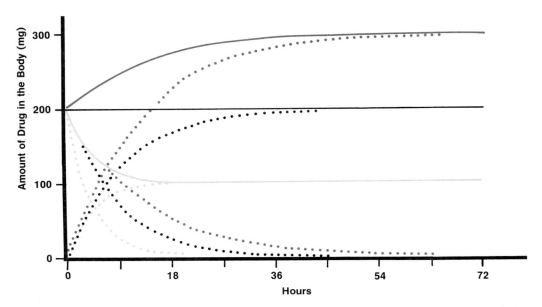

Figure 8-4. *Situations illustrating that the plateau level depends on the half-life. The same bolus dose and constant infusion are given to three patients A, B and C, with half-lives of 3, 6, and 9 hours, respectively. Although the amount of drug in the initial bolus is the same in all three patients, the amount in the body at the plateau differs in direct proportion to their respective half-lives. The percent of the bolus dose remaining with time depends on the individual's half-life, as does the rise in the amount in the body associated with the constant infusion (· · · ·). Only when the rate of loss is immediately matched by the rate of the infusion is the plateau immediately attained and maintained (patient B). Otherwise, the level in the body changes, until after approximately 3.3 half-lives a plateau is reached (patients A and C).*

4.2 liters/hour. Indeed, this is the preferred method for estimating clearance since the plateau concentration can be determined with great precision by averaging those concentrations that clearly lie at the plateau.

Second, the half-life is easily ascertained, being the time taken to reach half the plateau concentration. However, in this example and in most cases, no sample was taken at this time, and so one must interpolate between the observed data. The half-life, estimated in this manner (Fig. 8-5), is approximately 1.5 hours. A more accurate method of estimating the half-life uses all the data obtained during the infusion.

Upon rearranging Equation 7, one obtains

$$C_{ss} - C = C_{ss} \cdot e^{-kt} \qquad 10$$

which upon taking logarithms yields

$$\log (C_{ss} - C) = \log C_{ss} - \frac{k}{2.3} t \qquad 11$$

Thus, the decline obtained by plotting the difference, between the plateau concentration and that at earlier times, against the corresponding time on semilogarithmic paper, should be a straight line. The intercept at time zero is the plateau concentration (C_{ss}) and the slope is $-k/2.3$. These differences in concentration, shown by vertical lines in Figure 8-5, are presented in

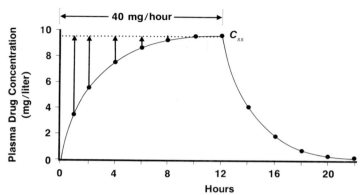

Figure 8-5. *Estimation of pharmacokinetic parameters from plasma data during and after a constant infusion. The vertical arrows represent the differences between the plateau concentration and the concentration observed during the infusion.*

Table 8-2, and have been plotted in Figure 8-6. The data indicate a half-life of 1.65 hours. It should be noted that the longer the time, the closer the concentration approaches the plateau concentration and the greater the error in the difference measurement. Generally, difference values calculated from concentrations beyond 90 percent of the plateau are of little value.

Last, the volume of distribution is calculated knowing clearance and half-life; in this case it is 10 liters.

Consider now the concentration data at and after the end of the infusion. Plotting these data on semilogarithmic paper also gives a straight line, from which the half-life can be determined, since after stopping the infusion

$$C = C_{ss} \cdot e^{-kt} \qquad 12$$

When these data are so plotted, they are observed to superimpose on the previous difference data (Fig. 8-6). In the particular example studied, the half-lives determined

Table 8-2. Plasma Concentration of a Drug During and After a Constant Infusion (40 mg/hour) for 12 Hours

Time (hours)	Observation Plasma Concentration (C, mg/liter)	Treatment of Data $C_{ss}^a - C$ (mg/liter)
During infusion		
1	3.3	6.2
2	5.4	4.1
4	7.6	1.9
6	8.7	0.8
8	9.3	0.2
10	9.6	−0.1
12	9.5	0.0
Postinfusion		
2	4.1	
4	1.8	
6	0.76	
8	0.33	
10	0.14	

[a] The concentration at the 12th hour of infusion.

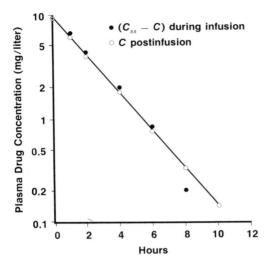

Figure 8-6. *Semilogarithmic plot of the difference (●) between the plateau drug concentration and that observed during the infusion against time. Also plotted are the declining values of the plasma drug concentration (○) against time after stopping the infusion.*

from the rising and declining curves are equal. Occasionally they differ, thereby indicating that drug disposition has changed over the period of study.

Urine Data Alone

Assume that only urine data had been obtained during and after the infusion. What can be estimated? If the renal clearance is constant, the rate of excretion is proportional to the plasma concentration. Then excretion rate data can be treated in a manner analogous to that of plasma data, and estimates can be made of elimination half-life, excretion rate constant, and fraction excreted unchanged (fe). An estimate of fe is obtained at plateau from

$$fe = \frac{\text{Rate of excretion at plateau}}{\text{Rate of infusion}} \qquad 13$$

because the rate of infusion is equal to the rate of elimination. For example, when the infusion rate is 40 mg/hour, the excretion rate at plateau for the drug is 12 mg/hour, so fe is 0.3.

Plasma and Urine Data

Without plasma data one cannot estimate a value for volume of distribution or clearance. When both plasma and urine data are available, renal clearance can be estimated in addition to all the other pharmacokinetic parameters. Moreover, a steady-state experiment, achieved with constant infusion, is the preferred method for estimating renal clearance. At plateau, accurate measurements can be made of both plasma concentration and urine excretion rate. In the preceding example renal clearance, obtained by dividing excretion rate at plateau by C_{ss}, is 1.26 liters/hour.

Study Problems

(Answers to Study Problems can be found in Appendix G.)

1. For prolonged surgical procedures succinylcholine has been given by intravenous drip infusion in order to obtain sustained muscle relaxation. The usual initial dose is 20 mg followed by continuous infusion of 0.5 mg/min. The infusion must be individualized because of great variation in the metabolism. Estimate the elimination half-lives of succinylcholine in patients requiring 0.5 mg/min and 5.0 mg/min respectively to maintain 20 mg in the body.

2. A drug is administered by constant-rate intravenous infusion ($R_{inf} = 3$ mg/min) for 60 min. Table 8-3 gives the plasma concentration of the drug at different times until the end of the infusion period.

Table 8-3

Time (min)	10	20	30	40	50	60
Plasma drug concentration (mg/liter)	2.3	3.5	4.2	4.8	5.0	5.2

Assuming that the plasma concentration of drug has reached a plateau at the end of the infusion,
(a) Calculate the elimination rate constant and the volume of distribution of the drug.
(b) What is the concentration expected 20 min after the end of the infusion?
(c) If the infusion rate is 6 mg/min, what are the expected plasma concentrations of the drug at 20, 40, and 60 min during the infusion?
(d) What is the loading dose required to attain immediately a concentration of 7 mg/liter and what is the infusion rate necessary to maintain it?
(e) If the concentration of 7 mg/liter fails to produce the desired response, what should the new infusion rate be and how long does it take to go from 7 mg/liter to a new plateau concentration of 12 mg/liter?

3. Estimate the values of volume of distribution, half-life, and clearance from the data in Table 8-4. The drug was administered as an intravenous bolus of 250 mg followed immediately by a constant infusion of 10 mg/hour. Assume that the drug instantly distributes.

Table 8-4

Time (hours)	0.3	5.0	20	50
Plasma drug concentration (mg/liter)	9.8	7.6	4.8	4.0

4. Estimate the values of volume of distribution, elimination rate constant, half-life, and clearance from data (Table 8-5) obtained on infusing a drug at the rate of 50 mg/hour for 7.5 hours.

Table 8-5

Time (hours)	0	2	4	6	7.5	9	12	15
Plasma drug concentration (mg/liter)	0	3.4	5.4	6.5	7.0	4.6	2.0	0.9

5. Listed in Table 8-6 are the amounts excreted unchanged during and after a constant infusion of 40 mg/hour for 12 hours of the drug whose corresponding plasma data are given in Table 8-2.

Table 8-6

During infusion	Time interval (hours)	0–1	1–2	2–4	4–6	6–9	9–12
	Amount excreted (mg)	1.9	5.6	14.4	20.8	33	36
Post-infusion	Time interval (hours)	0–1	1–2	2–4	4–6	6–9	9–12
	Amount excreted (mg)	9.7	6.7	6.2	3.4	1.5	0.63

(a) By appropriate treatment of the urinary excretion rate data verify that the half-lives during and after infusion are equal and the same as that estimated from the plasma data.

(b) Confirm that the value for fe, estimated from the cumulative urine data, agrees with the value estimated at the plateau.

9

extravascular dose

Objectives

The reader will be able to:

1. **Describe why absorption is often a first-order process and occasionally a zero-order process.**

2. **Determine whether absorption or disposition rate-limits drug elimination.**

3. **Anticipate the effect of altering rate of absorption, extent of absorption, clearance, or volume of distribution on the level of drug in the body following extravascular administration.**

4. **Estimate the availability of a drug, given plasma concentration or urinary excretion data following both extravascular and intravascular drug administration.**

5. **Estimate the relative availability of a drug, given plasma concentration or urinary excretion data following administration of different dosage forms by the same or by different extravascular routes.**

6. **Estimate the renal clearance of a drug from combined plasma concentration and urinary excretion data following extravascular administration.**

7. **Knowing the availability, estimate clearance, volume of distribution, and elimination half-life from plasma concentration data following extravascular administration.**

FOR systemically acting drugs, absorption is a prerequisite for therapeutic activity when they are administered extravascularly. The factors that influence drug absorption were considered in Chapter 3. In this chapter the following aspects are examined: the impact of rate and extent of absorption on both plasma concentration and amount of drug in the body; the effect of alterations in absorption and disposition on body level–time relationships; and the methods used to assess pharmacokinetic parameters from plasma and urinary data following extravascular administration.

Kinetics of Absorption

A First-Order Process

Figure 9-1 contains a semilogarithmic plot of the amount of salicylic acid remaining to be absorbed from the rat stomach and intestine with time. These are the same data that were presented in Figure 3-5.

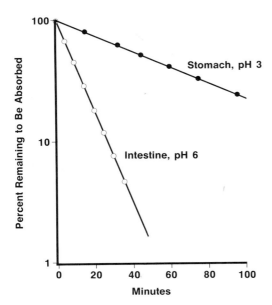

Figure 9-1. *Salicylic acid (pKa 3) is absorbed from both the rat stomach and intestine by first-order kinetics. Despite an environment favoring the un-ionized drug, absorption is slower from the stomach at pH 3 ($t_{1/2}$ = 45 min) than from the intestinal lumen at pH 6 ($t_{1/2}$ = 8 min). (Modified from Doluisio, J.T., Billups, N.F., Dittert, L.W., Sugita, E.G., and Swintosky, J.V. Drug absorption I.: An in situ rat gut technique yielding realistic absorption rates. J. Pharm. Sci., 58: 1196–1199, 1969. Adapted with permission of the copyright owner.)*

Since a straight line on semilogarithmic paper is indicative of a first-order process, these data indicate that salicylic acid in solution is absorbed from the rat stomach and intestine by first-order processes. That is:

$$\text{Rate of absorption} = ka \cdot Aa \qquad 1$$

where ka is the rate constant for absorption and Aa is the amount remaining to be absorbed.

The oral absorption of drugs in man often approximates first-order kinetics. The same holds true for the absorption of drugs from many other extravascular sites including subcutaneous tissue and muscle. A possible explanation for these observations may be gained by recalling from Chapter 3 that the driving force for absorption is the difference between the concentration of the diffusing drug at the absorption site (C_a) and that unbound in the arterial blood perfusing the absorptive membrane (Cu):

$$\text{Rate of absorption} = P \cdot A \cdot (C_a - Cu) \qquad 2$$

where P is the permeability constant and A is the effective surface area. Distribution and elimination of absorbed drug often ensure that the value of Cu is much less than the concentration at the absorption site. It follows therefore that

$$\text{Rate of absorption} = P \cdot A \cdot C_a \qquad 3$$

and assuming that the volume of fluid at the absorption site (Va) remains relatively constant, one obtains upon substitution:

$$\text{Rate of absorption} = \left(\frac{P \cdot A}{Va}\right) \cdot Aa \qquad 4$$

From this last relationship it is seen that absorption is a first-order process and that the permeability constant of the drug, the surface area, and the volume of fluid at the site determine the value of ka.

The preceding analysis is based upon the absorption of drugs from solution. Even when dissolution rate-limits absorption, absorption is still frequently a first-order process. This occurs because the rate of dissolution is a function of the surface area of the dissolving particle, and the surface area often diminishes in an essentially exponential fashion as the drug dissolves.

As with other first-order processes, absorption is characterized by a half-life. The half-life for the absorption of salicylic acid from the rat stomach is 45 min and from the intestine it is only 8 min (Fig. 9-1). The half-life for the absorption of drugs administered in solution usually ranges from 5 min to 1 hour or even longer if the membrane is poorly permeable to the drug or if perfusion is diminished, such as in shock. When absorption is dissolution rate-limited, the half-life can vary from 15 min to many hours. In some instances, especially following oral administration of a sparingly soluble drug, the absorption half-life may be so long that there is insufficient time available at the absorption site for complete absorption. Also, under these circumstances, absorption tends to deviate from first order.

Occasionally a Zero-Order Process

Occasionally a drug is absorbed at essentially a constant (zero-order) rate. The absorption kinetics are called *zero order* here, because the rate of absorption is proportional to the zero power of the amount remaining to be absorbed. This can occur when the concentration of drug in solution at the absorption site remains constant, as it might, for example, when either an excess of dissolving solid maintains a saturated solution of drug or when the surface area of the dissolving material remains constant (see Dissolution and Drug Delivery Systems, 32). A constant rate of absorption can also occur with carrier-mediated transport systems, such as those involved in the gastrointestinal absorption of riboflavin and thiamine, when the concentration of substrate is sufficiently high to occupy most of the carrier.

Differences between zero-order and first-order kinetics are illustrated in Figure 9-2. Zero-order absorption, characterized by a constant rate of absorption, is essentially independent of the amount absorbed. A plot of the amount remaining to be absorbed against time on regular graph paper yields a straight line whose slope is the rate of absorption (Fig. 9-2A). Recall that the amount remaining to be absorbed declines exponentially for a first-order process (Fig. 3-5). Recall also that because the fractional rate of absorption is constant, the decline of a first-order process is linear with time on semilogarithmic paper. In contrast, for a zero-order absorption process, because the rate is constant but the amount remaining is decreasing, the fractional rate of absorption increases with time. This is reflected in an ever-increasing gradient with time in a semilogarithmic plot of the amount remaining to be absorbed (Fig. 9-2B). A method of determining the kinetics of absorption following extravascular administration is given in Appendix D.

Body Level–Time Relationships

Comparison with an Intravenous Dose

Absorption delays and reduces the *magnitude of the peak* compared to that seen

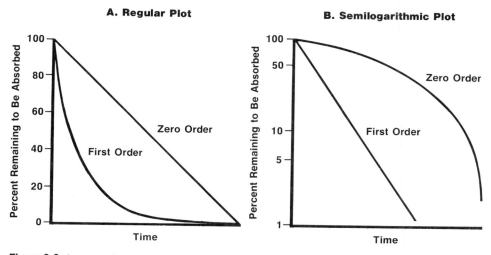

Figure 9-2. *A comparison of zero-order and first-order absorption processes. Depicted are: A, regular; and B, semilogarithmic plots of the amount remaining to be absorbed against time.*

following an equal intravenous bolus dose. These effects are portrayed in Figure 9-3. The rise and fall of the drug concentration in plasma are best understood by remembering that at any time

$$\frac{dAb}{dt} = \frac{dAa}{dt} - k \cdot Ab \qquad 5$$

| Rate of change of drug in body | Rate of absorption | Rate of elimination |

Initially, all the drug is at the absorption site and none is in the body, and so the rate of absorption is then maximal and the rate of elimination is zero. Thereafter, as drug is absorbed, its rate of absorption decreases, whereas its rate of elimination increases. Consequently, the difference between the two rates diminishes. However, as long as the rate of absorption exceeds the rate of elimination the level of drug in the body continues to rise. Eventually, a time is reached when the rate of elimination matches the rate of absorption; the level of drug in the body is then at a maximum. Subsequently, the rate of elimination exceeds the rate of absorption and the amount of drug in the body declines.

The peak level is always lower following extravascular administration than the initial level following an equal intravenous bolus dose. In the former case, at the peak time some drug remains at the absorption site and some has been eliminated, while the entire dose is in the body immediately following the intravenous dose. Beyond the peak time the plasma concentration on extravascular administration exceeds that following the intravenous dose because of the delayed entry of the drug into the body.

Frequently, the rising portion of the plasma concentration-time curve is called the absorption phase and the declining portion the elimination phase. As will be seen, this description may be misleading. Also, if drug is not fully available its concentration may remain lower at all times than that observed after intravenous administration.

Lag time is the delay between drug administration and the beginning of absorption. The lag time can be anywhere from a few minutes to many hours. Long lag times have most commonly been observed following ingestion of enteric-coated tablets. Contributing factors are the delay in stomach emptying and the time taken for the protective coating to dissolve or to swell

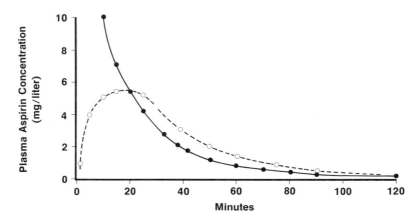

Figure 9-3. *Aspirin (650 mg) was administered as an intravenous bolus (●) and as an oral solution (○) on separate occasions to the same individual. Absorption causes a delay and a lowering of the peak concentration. (Modified from the data of Rowland, M., Riegelman, S., Harris, P.A., and Sholkoff, S.D.: Absorption kinetics of aspirin in man following oral administration of an aqueous solution. J. Pharm. Sci., 61:379-385, 1972. Adapted with permission of the copyright owner.)*

and release the inner contents into the intestinal fluids. Once absorption begins, however, it may be as rapid as from uncoated tablets. Clearly, enteric-coated products should not be used when a prompt and predictable response is desired. A method for estimating the lag time is discussed in Appendix D.

Availability and *area* are also important factors. As mentioned in Chapter 3, and discussed more fully in Chapter 13, the completeness of absorption is of primary importance in therapeutic situations. The availability, *F*, is proportional to the total area under the plasma concentration-time curve, irrespective of its shape. This must be so. Recall from Chapter 7 that:

$$\frac{\text{Total amount}}{\text{eliminated}} = \text{Clearance} \times \text{Area} \qquad 6$$

but the total amount eliminated is the amount absorbed, $F \cdot \text{Dose}$, therefore:

$$\underset{\substack{\text{Amount} \\ \text{absorbed}}}{F \cdot \text{Dose}} = \underset{\substack{\text{Total amount} \\ \text{eliminated}}}{\text{Clearance} \times \text{Area}} \qquad 7$$

Thus, knowing dose, clearance, and area, availability may be determined.

Changing Dose

Increasing the dose, unless this alters the absorption half-life or the availability, produces a proportional increase in the plasma concentration at all times. Hence, the time for the peak remains unchanged but its magnitude increases proportionally with the dose. The explanation is readily apparent. Suppose, for example, that the dose is doubled. Then, at any given time the amount absorbed is doubled and with twice as much entering the body, twice as much is eliminated. Being the difference between the amount absorbed and that eliminated, the amount of drug in the body at any time is, therefore, also doubled. And so too is the total area under the curve. One arrives at the same conclusion by examining Equation 7.

Changing Absorption Kinetics

Alterations in either absorption or disposition produce changes in the amount of drug in the body and in the plasma drug concentration-time profile. This point can be illustrated if one considers the three situations depicted in Figure 9-4 involving changes only in the absorption half-life. All other factors (availability, clearance, and volume of distribution, and hence elimination half-life) remain constant. Notice that the data are presented in semilogarithmic plots.

In case A, the absorption half-life is much shorter than the elimination half-life. In this case, by the time the peak is reached, most of the drug has been absorbed and little has been eliminated. Thereafter, decline of drug from the body is determined primarily by the disposition of the drug, that is, *disposition is the rate-limiting step.* The half-life estimated from the decline phase is, therefore, the elimination half-life.

In case B, the absorption half-life is longer than in case A but still shorter than the elimination half-life. This is observed for a more slowly dissolving dosage form, or when perfusion at the absorption site is diminished. It should be noted that the time to reach the peak is later, because it takes longer for the amount in the body to reach the point where the rate of elimination matches the rate of absorption; the peak concentration is lower, because less drug has been absorbed by that time. Even so, absorption is still essentially complete before the majority of the drug has been eliminated. Consequently, disposition remains the rate-limiting step.

Absorption Rate-Limited Elimination

Occasionally, the absorption half-life is much longer than the elimination half-life and case C prevails. The peak occurs later and is lower than in the two previous cases. The half-life of the decline of drug in the body now corresponds to the absorption half-life. Let us examine the reason for this.

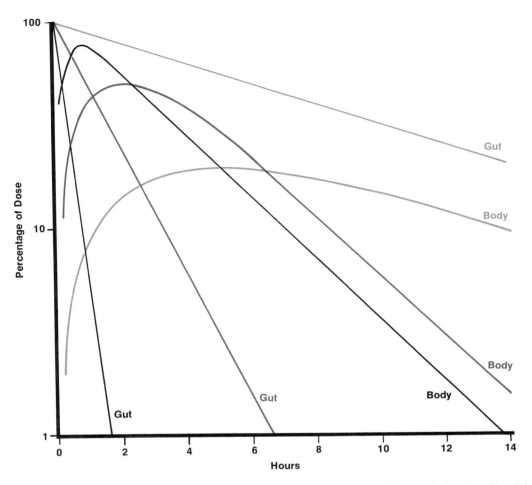

Figure 9-4. *A slowing of absorption delays and decreases the magnitude of the peak. The half-life of the decay phase is that of the slower process. In cases A (black) and B (red), absorption is faster than disposition and the half-life of the decay phase is the elimination half-life of the drug (2 hours). In case C (blue), absorption rate-limits drug elimination; the terminal phase now parallels the loss of drug from the absorption site. In all three cases, availability, clearance, and therefore area, are equal.*

During the rise to the peak, the rate of elimination increases and eventually, at the peak, equals the rate of absorption. However, in contrast to the previous situations, absorption is so slow that much of the drug remains to be absorbed well beyond the peak time. The drug is either at the absorption site or has been eliminated; little is in the body. In fact, during the decline phase, drug cannot be eliminated any faster than it is absorbed. *Absorption is now the rate-limiting step.* Under these circumstances, since the rate of elimination essentially matches the rate of absorption, the following approximation can be written

$$k \cdot Ab \quad = \quad ka \cdot Aa \qquad 8$$
Rate of elimination   Rate of absorption

that is,

$$\text{Amount in body} = \left(\frac{ka}{k}\right) \times \text{Amount at absorption site} \qquad 9$$

Accordingly, the amount of drug in the body (and the plasma concentration) during the decline phase is directly proportional to the amount of drug at the absorption site. For example, when the amount of drug at the absorption site falls by one-half, so does the amount in the body. However, the time for this to occur is the absorption half-life.

Absorption influences the kinetics of drug in the body; but what of the area under the plasma concentration-time curve? Because availability and clearance were held constant, it follows from Equation 7 that the area must be the same for cases A, B, and C.

Distinguishing Absorption from Disposition Rate-Limited Elimination

Although disposition generally is rate-limiting, the preceding discussion suggests that caution may need to be exercised in interpreting the meaning of the half-life determined from the decline phase following extravascular administration. Confusion is avoided if the drug is given intravenously. In practice, however, intravenous dosage forms of many drugs do not exist. An alternative solution to the problem of distinguishing between absorption and disposition rate-limitations is to alter the absorption kinetics of the drug. This is most readily accomplished by giving different dosage forms or by giving the drug by different routes. Two drugs are considered, theophylline and penicillin G.

Food and water influence the absorption kinetics of theophylline, but not the half-life of the decline phase (Fig. 9-5). Here then, disposition is rate-limiting. In contrast, for penicillin, absorption can become rate-limiting by formulation of a sparingly soluble salt (Fig. 9-6).

Changing Disposition Kinetics

What happens to the plasma concentration-time profile of a drug when the absorption kinetics remain constant, but modifications in disposition occur? When

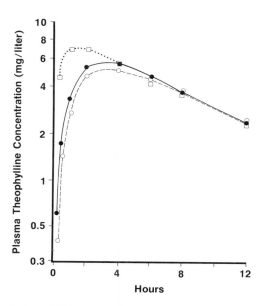

Figure 9-5. *Two tablets, each containing 130 mg theophylline, were taken by 6 healthy volunteers under various conditions. Absorption of the theophylline was most rapid when the tablets were dissolved in 500 ml water and taken on an empty stomach (□). Taking the tablets with 20 ml water on an empty stomach (○) resulted in slower absorption than taking them with the same volume of water immediately following a standardized high carbohydrate meal (●). Despite differences in rates of absorption, however, the terminal half-life (6.3 hours) was the same and, therefore, it is the elimination half-life of theophylline. (Modified from Welling, P.G., Lyons, L.L., Craig, W.A., and Trochta, G.A.: Influence of diet and fluid on bioavailability of theophylline. Clin. Pharmacol. Ther., 7:475-480, 1975.)*

clearance is reduced, but availability remains constant, the area under the plasma concentration-time curve must increase; so must both the time and magnitude of the peak concentration. These events are depicted in Figure 9-7. With a reduction in clearance and, hence, elimination rate constant, a greater amount of drug must be absorbed, and the plasma concentration must be greater prior to the time when the rate of elimination equals the rate of absorption.

As shown in Figure 9-8 the events are different when an increased volume of distribution is responsible for a longer elimi-

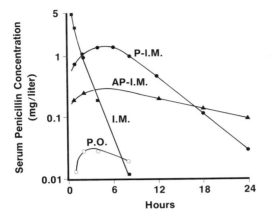

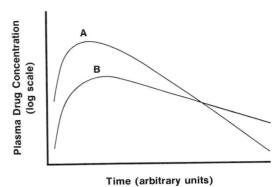

Figure 9-6. *Penicillin G (3 mg/kg) was administered to the same individual on different occasions. An aqueous solution was given intramuscularly (I.M.) and orally (P.O.); procaine penicillin was injected intramuscularly in oil (P-I.M.) and in oil with aluminum monostearate (AP-I.M.). The differing rates of decline of the plasma concentration of penicillin G point to an absorption rate-limitation when this antibiotic is given orally in aqueous solution and intramuscularly as the procaine salt in oil. Distinction between rate-limited absorption and rate-limited disposition following intramuscular administration of the aqueous solution can only be made by giving penicillin G intravenously. (Modified from Marsh, D.F.: Outline of Fundamental Pharmacology. Charles C Thomas, Springfield, Illinois, 1951.)*

Figure 9-8. *Curves A and B depict the plasma drug concentration following extravascular administration before and after a twofold increase in the volume of distribution, without a change in clearance. With the prolongation in the elimination half-life, the time for the peak is delayed and, since the area under the curves must be the same, the peak concentration is reduced.*

nation half-life. Under these circumstances, if availability and clearance remain constant, so does the area under the curve. The peak occurs later and is lower, however. To appreciate why this is so, one should recall that the rate of elimination is the product of clearance and plasma concentration. With a larger volume of distribution more drug must therefore be absorbed before the plasma concentration reaches a value at which the rate of elimination equals the rate of absorption; the absorption rate is lower then and so is the plasma concentration.

Assessment of Pharmacokinetic Parameters

How some of these estimates are made following extravascular administration can be appreciated by considering both the blood concentration-time curves in Figure 9-9, obtained following intramuscular and oral administration of 500 mg of a drug, and the additional information in Table 9-1.

Plasma Data Alone

Availability. Intravenous administration allows calculation of the availability, *F*. The

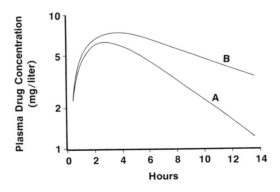

Figure 9-7. *Reducing clearance increases the area under the curve. Curves A and B depict the plasma drug concentration following extravascular administration before and after a twofold reduction in clearance. Area under the curve is increased, and when the elimination half-life is prolonged so too are the magnitude and time of the peak.*

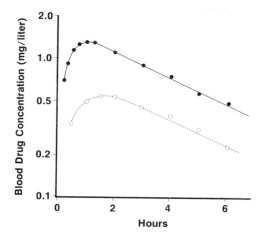

Figure 9-9. *A 500-mg dose was given intramuscularly* (●—●) *and orally* (○. . .○) *to the same subject on separate occasions. The drug is less available and is absorbed more slowly from the gastrointestinal tract. A parallel decline, however, implies that in both instances disposition is rate limiting.*

total area under the concentration-time curve following extravascular administration is divided by the area following an intravenous bolus, appropriately correcting for dose. The basis for this calculation, which assumes that *clearance remains constant,* is as follows:

Intravenous dose

$$\text{Dose}_{I.V.} = \text{Clearance} \times \text{Area}_{I.V.} \quad 10$$

Extravascular (e.g., oral or *per os,* P.O.) dose

$$F_{PO} \cdot \text{Dose}_{PO} = \text{Clearance} \times \text{Area}_{P.O.} \quad 11$$

which upon division yields

$$F_{P.O.} = \left(\frac{\text{Area}_{P.O.}}{\text{Area}_{I.V.}}\right)\left(\frac{\text{Dose}_{I.V.}}{\text{Dose}_{P.O.}}\right) \quad 12$$

For example, appropriately substituting the area measurements in Table 9-1 into Equation 12 indicates that the intramuscular availability of the drug is 97 percent. This value is sufficiently close to 100 percent to conclude that all drug injected into muscle is absorbed. In contrast, only 46 percent is absorbed when it is given orally in solution.

An alternative method of estimating the availability, which gives the same answer, is to substitute the value for clearance directly

into Equation 11. Clearance can be estimated from blood (or plasma) data following either an intravenous bolus dose or a constant infusion.

Relative availability is determined when there are no intravenous data. This is the case for many drugs introduced prior to the realization of the importance of pharmacokinetics that have no intravenous therapeutic use. Cost, stability, solubility limitations, and potential hazards are other major reasons for the lack of an intravenous preparation. Relative availability is determined by comparing different dosage forms, different routes of administration, or different conditions (e.g., diet, disease state). As with the calculation of availability, clearance is assumed to be constant.

Thus, taking the general case:

Dosage form A

$$\underset{\substack{\text{Amount} \\ \text{absorbed}}}{F_A \cdot \text{Dose}_A} = \underset{\substack{\text{Total amount} \\ \text{eliminated}}}{\text{Clearance} \times \text{Area}_A} \quad 13$$

Dosage form B

$$F_B \cdot \text{Dose}_B = \text{Clearance} \times \text{Area}_B \quad 14$$

So that,

$$\underset{\text{availability}}{\text{Relative}} = \frac{F_A}{F_B} = \left(\frac{\text{Area}_A}{\text{Area}_B}\right)\left(\frac{\text{Dose}_B}{\text{Dose}_A}\right) \quad 15$$

The reference dosage form is usually the one that is most available, that is, the one having the highest area-to-dose ratio. In the example considered, this would be the intramuscular dose; the relative availability of the oral dose would be 47 percent. If two oral doses only had been compared, they may have been equally, albeit poorly, available. It should be noted that all the preceding relationships hold, irrespective of route of administration, rate of absorption, or shape of the curve. Constancy of clearance is the only requirement.

Other Pharmacokinetic Parameters. Given only extravascular data, it is sometimes difficult to estimate pharmacokinetic parameters. Indeed, it may be stated that no phar-

Table 9-1. Data Obtained Following Administration of 500 mg of a Drug in Solution by Different Routes

| Route | Blood Data | | Urine Data |
	Area (mg-hour/ liter)	Half-life; Decay Phase (min)	Cumulative Amount Excreted Unchanged (mg)
Intravenous	7.6	190	152
Intramuscular	7.4	185	147
Oral	3.5	193	70

macokinetic parameter can be determined from observations following only a single oral dose. Consider: Area can be calculated without knowing availability, but clearance cannot. Similarly, although a half-life can be ascribed to the decay phase (by preparing a semilogarithmic plot of the blood or plasma concentration-time data), without knowing whether absorption or disposition is rate-limiting, the value cannot be assigned as the absorption or the elimination half-life. Without knowing any of the foregoing parameters, the volume of distribution clearly cannot be calculated.

Fortunately, there is a sufficient body of data to at least determine the elimination half-life of most drugs. Failure of food, dosage form, and, in the example in Figure 9-8, route of administration, to affect the terminal half-life indicates that this must be the elimination half-life of the drug. Also, a drug is nearly always fully available ($F = 1$) from the intramuscular or the subcutaneous site. Hence, clearance can be calculated knowing area (Eq. 7), and the volume of distribution can be estimated once the elimination half-life is known. Consider, for example, just the intramuscular data in Table 9-1. Clearance, obtained by dividing dose (500 mg) by area (7.4 mg-hour/liter), is 1.1 liters/min. Dividing clearance by the elimination rate constant (0.7/185 min) gives the volume of distribution, in this case 300 liters.

Earlier, a range of likely absorption half-lives was quoted. The values were esti-

mated indirectly from the plasma concentration-time profile. Direct measurements of absorption kinetics are impossible because plasma is the site of measurement for both absorption and disposition. To calculate the kinetics of absorption, a method must therefore be devised to separate these two processes. One simple, graphic method for achieving this separation is discussed in Appendix D.

Urine Data Alone

Given only urine data neither clearance nor volume of distribution can be calculated. If the renal clearance of the drug is constant, the rate of drug excretion is proportional to its plasma concentration, and under these circumstances, theoretically, excretion rate data can be treated in a similar manner to the plasma data. In practice, during the first collection of urine, usually 1 or 2 hours after drug administration, absorption of many well-absorbed drugs is complete. Urinary excretion rate data are then of little use in estimating the absorption kinetics of the drug.

Cumulative urine data can be used to estimate availability. The method assumes that the value of fe remains constant. Recall from Chapter 7 that fe is the ratio of the total amount excreted unchanged (Ae_∞) to the total amount absorbed.

$$fe = \frac{Ae_\infty}{F \cdot \text{Dose}} \qquad 15$$

Then, using the subscripts A and B to denote two treatments, it follows that

$$F_A \cdot \text{Dose}_A = Ae_{\infty,A}/fe \qquad 16$$

$$F_B \cdot \text{Dose}_B = Ae_{\infty,B}/fe \qquad 17$$

Amount   Total amount
absorbed   eliminated

which upon division gives:

$$\frac{F_A}{F_B} = \left(\frac{Ae_{\infty,A}}{Ae_{\infty,B}}\right) \cdot \left(\frac{\text{Dose}_B}{\text{Dose}_A}\right) \qquad 18$$

The ratio of the cumulative amount excreted unchanged is therefore the ratio of the availabilities. When one dose is given intravenously, the ratio is the availability of the drug. Otherwise the ratio gives the relative availability. For example, from the cumulative urinary excretion data in Table 9-1, it is apparent that the intramuscular dose is almost completely available; the corresponding value for the oral dose is only 46 percent [(70 mg/152 mg) × 100]. Notice that these values are the same as those estimated from plasma data. This is often the case, and under these circumstances, the need for only a single measurement and the ease and noninvasive nature of the technique make urine analysis the more convenient method for estimating availability.

Plasma and Urine Data

When both plasma and urine data are available, in addition to the other pharmacokinetic parameters, the renal clearance of a drug can be estimated. The approach taken is identical to that discussed following an intravenous dose (Chap. 7). Namely, the rate of excretion is plotted against the plasma drug concentration obtained at the midpoint time of urine collection. Since no knowledge of availability is required, the estimate of renal clearance from combined plasma and urine data following extravascular administration is as accurate as that obtained following intravenous drug administration.

The reason for the low oral availability of the drug ($F = 0.47$) remains to be determined. Poor dissolution can be discounted; the drug was given in solution. The high total clearance (1.1 liter/min) suggests that a significant first-pass hepatic elimination could be the explanation. Let us examine this hypothesis.

As shown previously,

Total blood clearance (Cl_b)	Renal = blood clearance	Extrarenal + blood clearance

From the intravenous data,

Renal blood clearance

$$= fe \cdot Cl_b = \frac{152 \text{ mg}}{500 \text{ mg}} \times 1.1 \text{ liters/min}$$

$$= 0.33 \text{ liter/min}$$

Assuming that all extrarenal clearance is due to hepatic metabolism:

Hepatic
blood $= 1.1 - 0.33 = 0.77$ liter/min
clearance

Recall that the hepatic extraction ratio (E_H) is given by:

$$E_H = \frac{\text{Hepatic blood clearance}}{\text{Hepatic blood flow}}$$

which when appropriately substituting 0.77 liter/min for hepatic clearance and 1.50 liters/min for hepatic blood flow (Table 4-1) gives a value for E_H of 0.51.

The maximum anticipated oral availability is one minus the hepatic extraction ratio or

$$\text{Oral availability} = 1 - 0.51 = 0.49$$

The closeness between prediction and observation suggests that hepatic extraction is a likely explanation for the poor oral availability. Being physiologically determined, no amount of pharmaceutical formulation will improve the situation.

Study Problems

(*Answers to Study Problems can be found in Appendix G.*)

1. Depicted in Figure 9-10 are curves of the plasma drug concentration and of the amount of drug in the body with time following the oral ingestion of a single dose of drug. Draw another curve on each figure that shows the effect of each (A through E) of the following alterations in pharmacokinetic parameters.
   (a) V increased, k decreased
   (b) ka increased
   (c) Cl increased, k increased
   (d) Cl decreased, k decreased
   (e) F decreased
   In each case, assume that the dose administered and all other parameters (among F, ka, V, Cl, and k) remain unchanged.

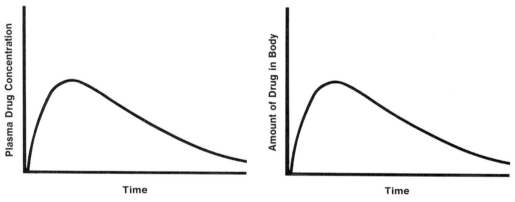

Figure 9-10

2. Rowland et al. (Rowland, M., Epstein, W., and Riegelman, S.: Absorption kinetics of griseofulvin in man. J. Pharm. Sci., *57*:984, 1968) gave griseofulvin orally, 0.5 gram of micronized drug, and, on another occasion intravenously, 100 mg, to human volunteers. The plasma concentration-time data obtained in one subject is tabulated in Table 9-2 below.

   What can be concluded from these data with respect to:
   (a) Rate of absorption of the drug with time on oral administration in this individual?
   (b) Completeness of absorption?

Table 9-2

Time (hours)		0	1	2	3	4	5	7	8	12	24	28	32	35	48
Plasma Griseofulvin Concentration (mg/liter)	Intravenous	0	1.4	1.1	0.98	0.90	0.80	—	0.68	0.55	0.37	—	0.24	—	0.14
	Oral	0	0.4	0.95	1.15	1.15	1.05	1.2	1.2	0.90	1.05	0.90	0.85	0.80	0.50

3. Penamecillin is the acetoxymethyl ester of benzylpenicillin, structures shown below.

$$H = \text{Benzylpenicillin}$$

$$CH_2O-\underset{\underset{O}{\|}}{C}-CH_3 = \text{Penamecillin}$$

There is considerable evidence that penamecillin never reaches the tissues after oral administration, an observation consistent with its known rapid hydrolysis to benzylpenicillin. The latter is found in the serum. The proposed advantage of penamecillin over benzylpenicillin is a more prolonged blood level. A comparison of the mean serum concentrations with time in 10 dogs following oral administration of 25 mg/kg of each of the penicillins is shown in Table 9-3.

Table 9-3

Time (hours)		1	2	4	6	8	10	12
Serum	Following	5.6	2.5	0.38	0.09	0.016	<0.01	—
Benzylpenicillin	Benzylpenicillin							
Concentration	Following	0.4	0.95	0.90	0.50	0.30	0.15	0.09
(mg/liter)	Penamecillin							

(a) What are the relative amounts of benzylpenicillin entering the body following penamecillin and benzylpenicillin?

(b) Assuming a clearance of 8 ml/min/kg for benzylpenicillin in the dog, estimate the fraction of each drug entering the body as benzylpenicillin. Compare your answers to (a) above.

(c) Prepare a semilogarithmic plot of both sets of data. How would you account for the difference in the terminal slopes? Determining the fast and slow rate constants for the benzylpenicillin data following penamecillin, using the method of residuals (Appendix D), helps clarify the situation.

4. Bates et al. (Bates, T.R., Sequeira, J.A., and Tembo, A.V.: Effect of food on nitrofurantoin absorption. Clin. Pharmacol. Ther., 16:63–68, 1974), studying the influence of food and crystal size on the absorption of the weakly acidic (pKa 7.2) broad-spectrum antibacterial agent, nitrofurantoin, obtained the mean total cumulative excretion (Ae_∞) data shown in Table 9-4.

(a) Estimate the relative availability of macrocrystalline nitrofurantoin in the absence and presence of food. What is the basis of your calculation?

(b) What single additional parameter value is needed to determine the availability of nitrofurantoin?

(c) Propose one explanation for the increased availability of oral nitrofurantoin with food, especially observed with the macrocrystalline drug.

Table 9-4.[a] Nitrofurantoin, 100 mg

	Macrocrystalline Capsule		Microcrystalline Tablet	
	Fasting	Nonfasting	Fasting	Nonfasting
Cumulative amount excreted unchanged (mg)	22	40	36	44

[a]From Bates, T.R., Sequeira, J.A., and Tembo, A.V.: Effect of food on nitrofurantoin absorption. Clin. Pharmacol. Ther. *16*: 63–68, 1974.

Unifying Problems

(Answers to Unifying Problems can be found in Appendix G.)

1. Complete Table 9-5 by checking off the pharmacokinetic parameters that can be obtained from the data in Figures 9-11 and 9-12 for each of the drugs.

Table 9-5

Figure	Elimination Half-life	Volume of Distribution	Clearance	Renal Clearance	Availability
Dapsone					
Penicillins					

2. (a) Prove that, independent of the route of administration, and provided that renal clearance is constant, the following relationship holds:

$$\text{Renal clearance} = Ae_\infty/\text{Area}$$

   (b) From the data in Table 9-1 confirm that the renal clearance of the drug is 0.33 liter/min.

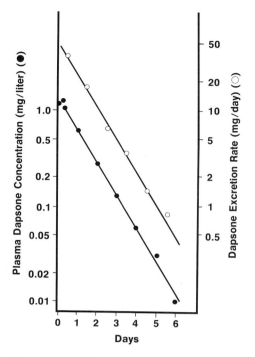

Figure 9-11. *Plasma concentration and excretion rate of dapsone following a 100-mg oral dose.*

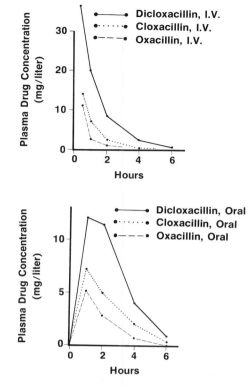

Figure 9-12. *Average serum concentration of three semisynthetic penicillins following 500 mg of each administered intravenously and orally on separate occasions.*

10

metabolite kinetics

Objectives

The reader will be able to:

1. **State the factors that influence the plasma metabolite concentration and the amount of metabolite in the body following drug administration.**

2. **Determine whether or not the elimination of a metabolite is rate-limited by its formation.**

3. **Determine whether the total clearance of a metabolite is less than that of the drug, given plasma concentration-time data following drug administration.**

4. **Describe the consequence of hepatic extraction on plasma metabolite concentrations following oral drug administration.**

5. **State the pharmacokinetic parameters that control the plateau level of metabolite following constant drug infusion.**

6. **Describe why the elimination half-life of metabolite is the sole determinant of accrual of metabolite, when a constant amount of drug is maintained in the body.**

7. **Describe why the elimination half-life of the slowest step, drug elimination or metabolite elimination, controls the accrual of metabolite following a constant drug infusion.**

THE reason for our interest and concern with metabolites can be summed up in four words: action, toxicity, inhibition, and displacement. All too often metabolites are thought of as weakly active or inactive waste products. For many this is so, but as seen in Table 10-1, for many others it is not. Some drugs are inert and depend on metabolism for activation. Some metabolites have pharmacologic properties in common with the parent drug and augment its effect. Some have a different pharmacologic profile and may even be the cause of toxicity. Some are inactive but may, by acting as inhibitors, prolong or augment the response to a drug. Still others may affect the disposition of a drug by competing for plasma and tissue binding sites. It is not sufficient, however, to know that a metabolite possesses any or all of these properties. Unless a sufficient concentration exists at the appropriate site, the presence of metabolite is of little therapeutic concern.

This chapter examines the factors that influence the kinetics of metabolites in the body. The utility of metabolite data in estimating pharmacokinetic parameters is also explored.

Table 10-1. Representative Therapeutically Important Metabolites

Compound Administered	Metabolite
Acetohexamide	Hydroxyhexamide
Acetylsalicylic acid	Salicylic acid
Amitriptyline	Nortriptyline
Chloral hydrate	Trichloroethanol
Chlordiazepoxide	Desmethylchlordiazepoxide
Codeine	Morphine
Diazepam	Desmethyldiazepam
Fluazepam	Desethylfluazepam
Glutethimide	4-Hydroxyglutethimide
Imipramine	Desipramine
Lidocaine	Desethyllidocaine
Meperidine	Normeperidine
Phenacetin	Acetaminophen
Phenylbutazone	Oxyphenbutazone
Prednisone	Prednisolone
Primidone	Phenobarbital
Procainamide	N-Acetylprocainamide
Propranolol	4-Hydroxypropranolol

Single Dose of Drug

Rate-Limiting Steps

To appreciate the factors that influence the amount of metabolite in the body with time following a single dose of drug, consider the scheme:

$$Aa \xrightarrow[ka]{\text{Absorption}} Ab \xrightarrow[km]{\text{Metabolism}}$$

Drug at   Drug in
absorption   body
site

$$Ab(m) \xrightarrow[\text{elimination } k(m)]{\text{Metabolite}} Ae(m)$$

Metabolite   Eliminated
in body   metabolite

in which drug is completely absorbed and metabolized to a single species that, in turn, is eliminated unchanged. Each step is characterized by the respective first-order rate constants, ka, km, $k(m)$. Any step can be the rate-limiting one; the corresponding rate constant has the smallest value. Figure 10-1, a series of semilogarithmic plots of the amount at the various sites against time following a single dose of drug, shows the consequence of a rate limitation in each step.

When absorption is the slowest step (and, therefore, has the longest half-life), most of the drug resides at the absorption site and little exists in the body as either drug or metabolite. Since, for reasons similar to those discussed in Chapter 9, drug and metabolite are eliminated essentially at the same rate that drug is absorbed, the half-life for the decline of drug and metabolite in the body must be the absorption half-life. This situation is relatively uncommon.

A rate limitation in drug disposition, the most common situation, has a number of consequences. First, the half-life of the drug disposition step is longer than that of other steps. Second, there is always more drug than metabolite in the body. Last, metabolite elimination is formation rate-limited; that is, the metabolite is cleared so rapidly that during the decline phase whatever is formed is almost immediately eliminated. Approximately, therefore

$$\underset{\substack{\text{Elimination rate} \\ \text{of metabolite}}}{k(m) \cdot Ab(m)} = \underset{\substack{\text{Formation rate} \\ \text{of metabolite}}}{km \cdot Ab} \qquad 1$$

and on rearranging,

$$\underset{\text{metabolite}}{\text{Amount of}} = \left(\frac{km}{k(m)}\right) \cdot \underset{\text{drug}}{\text{Amount of}} \qquad 2$$

In this case, metabolite declines with the same half-life as the drug.

A metabolite substantially builds up in the body only when its elimination is the slowest step. When this occurs, by the time the peak metabolite level is reached, most of the drug has been absorbed and eliminated; decline of the metabolite is then controlled by its elimination half-life.

In the foregoing simplified scheme the rate of metabolite formation is the rate of drug

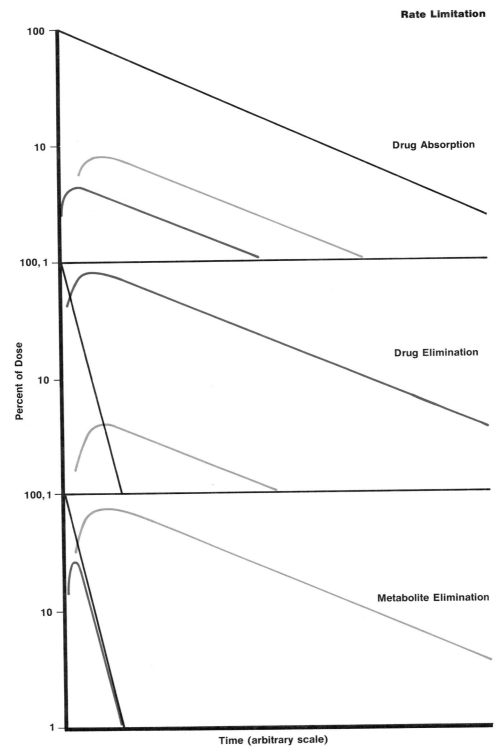

Figure 10-1. *Consequences of a rate limitation. Illustrated are semilogarithmic plots (percent of dose against time) of drug at the absorption site (black), drug in the body (red), and metabolite in the body (blue) when rate limitations occur as indicated. Note that the slowest step controls the half-life for the decay of drug or metabolite in all subsequent compartments.*

elimination. This need not be the case. Equation 1 is valid no matter what fraction of drug is converted to the metabolite. The remainder may be transformed to other metabolites or be excreted unchanged. In Equation 1, $k(m)$ refers to the rate constant for metabolite elimination. Just how many pathways are involved in metabolite elimination is not important. What is important is knowing where the rate-limiting step lies. In any sequence, substances in all compartments beyond the rate-limiting step decline proportionally with the half-life of this slowest step. To emphasize this point consider the following scheme:

$$A \xrightarrow{0.2} B \xrightarrow{1.0} E \xrightarrow{8.2} G \xrightarrow{0.05} H \xrightarrow{0.5} I \xrightarrow{2.0} J$$
with $A \xrightarrow{0.1} C$, $B \xrightarrow{2.2} F$, $A \xrightarrow{0.3} D$

in which A refers to the drug, B through I refer to metabolites, J is the excreted metabolite I, and the number above each arrow is the value of the respective rate constant in hour $^{-1}$.

Q. What is the rate-limiting step in the entire sequence?
A. Elimination of metabolite G, $t_{1/2} = 0.7/0.05 = 13.8$ hours.

Q. What are the half-lives for decay of A, B, E, H, and I from the body following administration of drug?
A. Disposition of A rate-limits B and E, $t_{1/2} = 0.7/(0.1 + 0.2 + 0.3) = 1.2$ hours for A, B, and E. Elimination of G rate-limits H and I, $t_{1/2} = 13.8$ hours.

Plasma Concentration

The preceding discussion, helpful in realizing the importance of rate-limiting steps, dealt with amounts of drug and metabolite in the body. However, plasma concentrations are measured and are of greater interest. Furthermore, in most cases, the volume of distribution of metabolite is not known and, therefore, the amount in the body

cannot be calculated. Our attention therefore turns to clearance, the most important parameter determining plasma concentrations. Several examples are discussed to illustrate the application of the clearance concept to metabolite kinetics.

The first example concerns the potential contribution of a metabolite to drug toxicity. Management of the coma induced by large overdoses of the sedative hypnotic, glutethimide, has been complicated by a poor correlation between the plasma concentration of glutethimide and the clinical course of the patient. The duration of the coma is longer than expected and the depth is greatest long after the plasma concentration of glutethimide has reached a maximum. As illustrated in Figure 10-2 substantial accumulation of a metabolite, 4-hydroxyglutethimide (Table 10-1), seems to be the explanation. Notice that the coma is deepest at the time of the peak metabolite concentration. Although these data do not extend long enough to determine whether the elimination of 4-hydroxyglutethimide is rate-limited by its formation or disposition, they do permit the conclusion to be drawn that the high concentration of this metabolite is due to its clearance being much lower than that of glutethimide. The argument is as follows:

At any time,

$$\text{Rate of change of metabolite in body} = \underbrace{Cl_m \cdot C}_{\substack{\text{Rate of} \\ \text{metabolite} \\ \text{formation}}} - \underbrace{Cl(m) \cdot Cm}_{\substack{\text{Rate of} \\ \text{metabolite} \\ \text{elimination}}} \quad 3$$

where Cl_m is the clearance associated with the oxidation of glutethimide to hydroxyglutethimide, $Cl(m)$ is the total clearance of this metabolite, and C and Cm are the respective plasma concentrations of drug and metabolite.

Integrating the foregoing equation gives the amount of metabolite in the body at any time. However, since no 4-hydroxyglutethimide is present in the body at zero or at infinite time, it follows, upon integrating

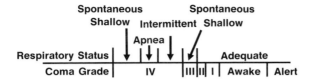

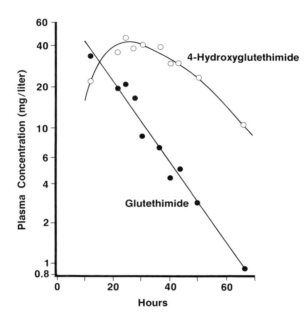

Figure 10-2. *A male patient was admitted to hospital in coma following a 12-gram dose of glutethimide ingested about 11 hours previously. His respiratory status and grade of coma worsened, which correlated with a substantial accumulation of an active metabolite, 4-hydroxyglutethimide. Only when this metabolite declined did the patient's status improve. The accumulation of 4-hydroxyglutethimide is caused by its total clearance being much lower than that of glutethimide. (Modified from Hansen, A.R., Kennedy, K.A., Ambre, J.J., and Fischer, L.J.: Glutethimide poisoning. A metabolite contributes to morbidity and mortality. N. Engl. J. Med., 292: 250–252, 1975. Reprinted by permission.)*

Equation 3 between these time limits, that

$$\frac{\text{Area of metabolite}}{\text{Area of drug}} = \frac{Cl_m}{Cl(m)} \qquad 4$$

where the areas are the total areas under the respective concentration-time profiles. Substituting $fm \cdot Cl$ for Cl_m, where fm is the fraction of drug converted to the metabolite, the following important relationship is obtained:

$$\frac{\text{Area}_{met}}{\text{Area}_{drug}} = fm \cdot \frac{\text{Clearance of drug}}{\text{Clearance of metabolite}} \qquad 5$$

Returning now to Figure 10-2, it is apparent that, even though the plot is semilogarithmic, the area under the metabolite curve is much greater than that under the glutethimide curve. This greater area would be even more apparent were the data plotted on ordinary graph paper. Accordingly, since the value of fm cannot exceed unity,

the clearance of the metabolite must be less than that of glutethimide. If the ratio of areas had been less than 1, then, unless the value of fm is known, the relative total clearance values cannot be assessed. Because no knowledge of the amount of drug in the body is necessary in arriving at the above conclusion, this area method of interpreting metabolite data can be extremely useful, especially in cases of drug poisoning in which the amounts ingested and absorbed are frequently unknown.

The second example deals with propranolol. Based on the data in Figure 10-3, obtained after giving ^{14}C-radiolabeled propranolol intravenously, the drug has the following characteristics: total clearance, 1.5 liters/min; volume of distribution, 500 liters; and elimination half-life, 5 hours. Other data suggest that almost the entire dose is metabolized in the liver. Metabolites of propranolol include one or more glucu-

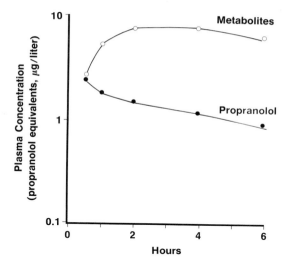

Figure 10-3. *A subject received 1 mg ^{14}C-radio-labeled propranolol intravenously. Plasma concentrations of ^{14}C-propranolol (●) and total radioactivity were measured and the concentration of metabolites (○), expressed in propranolol equivalents, was obtained from the difference in the radioactivities. Note that the elevated metabolite concentration is due to a lower total clearance and smaller volume of distribution of these more polar species. (Modified from Dollery, C.T., Davis, D.S., and Conolly, M.E.: Differences in the metabolism of drugs, depending upon their route of administration. Ann. N.Y. Acad. Sci., 179: 108–112, 1971.)*

ronides and naphthoxylactic acid. These metabolites are measured collectively in plasma as the difference between the total radioactivity and the radioactivity associated with the drug. What can be learned from the data in Figure 10-3?

From considerations of areas of drug and metabolite one can conclude that one or more of the metabolites is cleared more slowly than propranolol. However, the tendency for the decay of metabolites to parallel drug loss suggests that elimination of these metabolites is rate-limited by drug

elimination. Hence, the elimination half-lives of these more polar metabolites must be shorter, and the amount in the body always lower than that of the parent drug. Although the amount is less, the metabolite concentrations are higher because of the much smaller volumes of distribution of these more polar species.

Kinetically, giving an intravenous bolus of drug and measuring the plasma metabolite concentration are the same as giving an oral dose of drug and measuring its plasma concentration. In both situations, one monitors the appearance and disappearance of a species (metabolite in one case, drug in the other) after placing a bolus dose in the preceding compartment, thus,

Absorption

$$Aa \xrightarrow[\text{Absorption}]{ka} Ab \xrightarrow[\text{Elimination of drug}]{k}$$

Drug at absorption site | Drug in body

Metabolism

$$Ab \xrightarrow[\text{Metabolism}]{k} Ab(m) \xrightarrow[\text{Elimination of metabolite}]{k(m)}$$

Drug in body | Metabolite in body

Recall from Chapter 9 that the peak plasma concentration of a drug given extravascularly reflects the balance between drug absorption and elimination. Correspondingly, the 3 hours taken for the metabolites to reach a peak in Figure 10-3 reflects the balance between propranolol elimination and metabolite elimination.

The last example is a comparison of tolbutamide and acetohexamide, two effective hypoglycemic agents. Both are extensively metabolized to the following products,

$$CH_3-\!\!\!\bigcirc\!\!\!-SO_2NHCONHCH_2CH_2CH_2CH_3 \xrightarrow{\text{Oxidation}}$$

Tolbutamide

$$\boxed{HOCH_2}\!\!-\!\!\bigcirc\!\!\!-SO_2NHCONHCH_2CH_2CH_2CH_3$$

Hydroxytolbutamide

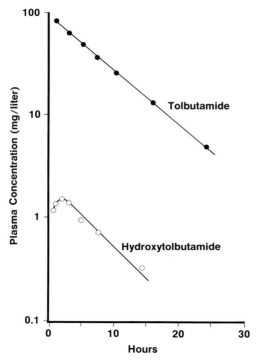

$$CH_3CO-\!\!\!\bigcirc\!\!\!-SO_2NHCONH-\!\!\!\bigcirc \xrightarrow{\text{Reduction}}$$

Acetohexamide

$$CH_3\!\!\mid\!\!\overline{CHOH}\!\!\mid-\!\!\!\bigcirc\!\!\!-SO_2NHCONH-\!\!\!\bigcirc$$

Hydroxyhexamide

Both metabolites are active, but only hydroxyhexamide is therapeutically important. The explanation lies in the differences in their clearances relative to those of their precursors. As seen in Figure 10-4, hy-droxytolbutamide is cleared so much more rapidly than tolbutamide, that concentrations required to augment the effect of the drug are never achieved.

In contrast, hydroxyhexamide, being cleared more slowly than acetohexamide, accumulates substantially and depresses blood glucose long after the majority of acetohexamide has been eliminated (Fig. 10-5).

Tolbutamide elimination clearly rate-limits the elimination of hydroxytolbutamide. Under these circumstances, the ratio of metabolite to drug plasma concentrations is fixed during metabolite decay by the ratio of $fm \cdot Cl$ to $Cl(m)$. Thus, substituting for both clearance and concentration into Equation 1

$$\underset{\substack{\text{Rate of metabolite} \\ \text{elimination}}}{Cl(m) \cdot Cm} = \underset{\substack{\text{Rate of metabolite} \\ \text{formation}}}{fm \cdot Cl \cdot C} \qquad 6$$

and rearranging, yields

$$\frac{\text{Metabolite concentration}}{\text{Drug concentration}} = fm \cdot \frac{Cl}{Cl(m)} \qquad 7$$

In the case of tolbutamide, for example, the value of fm is close to 1 and the 20-fold difference in the total clearance between hydroxytolbutamide and tolbutamide is reflected by the plasma concentration of metabolite being only a small percent of that of tolbutamide.

Impact of Hepatic Extraction on Metabolite Concentration

Ingesting drugs that are cleared by the liver is like taking a mixture of drug and metabolite. The reason, as mentioned in Chapter 3, is that all ingested drug must

Figure 10-4. *A subject received a 1-gram intravenous bolus of tolbutamide. The concentration of tolbutamide in plasma fell with a half-life of 4 hours. Although oxidation to hydroxytolbutamide is almost obligatory for tolbutamide elimination, the plasma concentration of this metabolite is always very low owing to its extremely high clearance value. As a consequence, since the volumes of distribution are similar (0.15–0.30 liter/kg), oxidation of tolbutamide rate-limits hydroxytolbutamide elimination. (Redrawn from Matin, S.B., and Rowland, M.: Determination of tolbutamide and metabolites in biological fluids. Anal. Letters, 6: 865–876, 1973, by courtesy of Marcel Dekker, Inc.)*

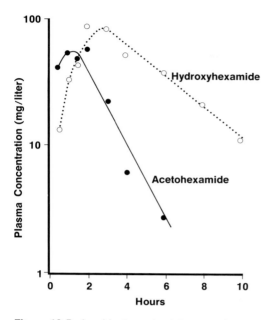

Figure 10-5. *A subject received 1 gram of acetohexamide orally. The lower total clearance of
hydroxyhexamide explains why the plasma concentration of this metabolite of acetohexamide is
soon higher than the parent drug. Furthermore, the
disposition, rather than the formation, of hydroxyhexamide must also be rate-limiting since the concentration of this metabolite declines more slowly
than does that of the drug. (Redrawn from Gallo-
way, J.A., McMahon, R.E., Culp, H.W., Marshall,
F.J., and Young, E.C.: Metabolism, blood levels and
rate of excretion of acetohexamide in human subjects. Diabetes, 16: 118–123, 1967; reproduced
with permission from the American Diabetes Association, Inc.)*

pass through the liver before entering the
general circulation. The composition of the
mixture varies with the hepatic extraction
ratio of the drug. When the extraction of
drug is high, metabolism during absorption
is extensive and the situation comes close to
administering just metabolite.

To appreciate the impact of first passage
of drug through the liver on the plasma
concentration of metabolite, consider the
data in Figure 10-6, obtained following oral
administration of ^{14}C-propranolol. Compared to the situation following an intravenous dose (see Fig. 10-3) the metabolite-
to-drug concentration ratio is much higher

and, paradoxically, the metabolite concentration peaks earlier. These apparently conflicting observations are reconciled by examining the following scheme:

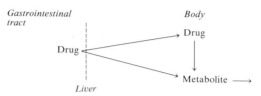

As anticipated from its high hepatic clearance, and confirmed by comparing the
areas under the oral and intravenous propranolol concentration-time curves with
correction for differences in dose, only 30%
of the orally administered dose of propran-

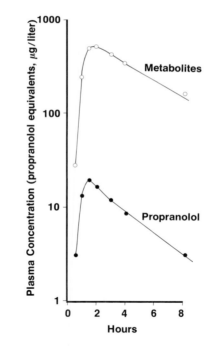

Figure 10-6. *A subject received 40 mg ^{14}C-radio-
labeled propranolol orally. As a consequence of
extensive hepatic clearance, only a small fraction
of the dose is absorbed intact. The remainder appears as metabolite(s), reaching a peak value at
the same time as propranolol. (Modified from
Dollery, C.T., Davis D.S., and Conolly, M.E.: Differences in the metabolism of drugs depending upon
their route of administration. Ann. N.Y. Acad. Sci.,
179: 108–112, 1971.)*

olol filters past the liver. The remainder enters the body directly as metabolite. The small fraction of propranolol absorbed is then handled like an intravenous dose of the drug. Recall that when propranolol is given intravenously, the accrual of metabolites is relatively slow (Fig. 10-3), being dependent on the elimination half-lives of both the drug and the metabolites. In contrast, the concentrations of metabolites peak earlier and are higher after oral propranolol administration, because absorption of this drug (and hence entry of the majority of metabolites) is rapid compared to the elimination of drug or metabolites.

The therapeutic implications of the preceding discussion depend upon the activity of the drug and the metabolite. If the drug is inactive, highly extracted by the liver, and hepatic metabolism is required to generate the active species, a shorter onset and a more intense response may be seen by giving a dose of drug orally than parenterally. On the other hand, if the metabolites are inactive, a larger oral than parenteral dose is required to achieve an equivalent therapeutic response. The situation with propranolol appears to lie somewhere between these two extremes. Following a single dose, the pharmacologic effect is maximal at peak propranolol concentrations, but for a given plasma concentration of propranolol the effect seen orally is greater than that observed following an intravenous dose. The explanation appears to be the presence of a substantial concentration of pharmacologically active metabolites formed on the first pass of propranolol through the liver. These metabolites do not appear to reach detectable concentrations when propranolol is given intravenously.

In Chapter 3 (Table 3-2), the statement was made that chlorpromazine is destroyed, by oxidation to its sulfoxide, within the gastrointestinal tract. Evidence favoring this statement is the failure to detect the sulfoxide when chlorpromazine is given parenterally, yet significant concentrations of the sulfoxide are measured after oral drug administration. Were sulfoxidation to occur primarily within the liver, then the fraction of the dose converted to the sulfoxide should be independent of the route of drug administration. Thus, assuming that ingested drug entirely traverses the gastrointestinal wall and that only hepatic metabolism occurs, drug, whether given orally or parenterally, is equally and fully available to the liver for metabolism. The oral availability of the drug may be low if its hepatic extraction ratio is high, but the fraction of dose converted to a metabolite must be independent of the route of drug administration. The data in Figure 10-7 support this last point. Nortriptyline is highly and almost exclusively cleared by the liver. Using area as a measure of the amount of material in the body, the oral availability of nortriptyline is low, but the amount of the metabolite 10-hydroxynortriptyline entering the systemic circulation is the same, when comparing oral to intramuscular drug administration.

Constant Drug Infusion

In Chapter 8, the kinetics of a constant rate intravenous infusion was examined. Recall that infusion rate and clearance determine the plateau concentration and that half-life alone determines the time to approach the plateau. These observations can be extended to the accumulation of metabolite following constant drug infusion. The essential features can be understood by considering the scheme:

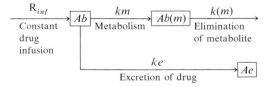

and the events depicted in Figure 10-8.

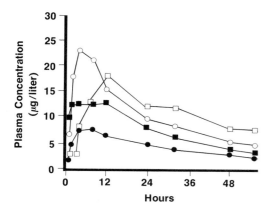

Figure 10-7. *Patients received 40 mg nortriptyline hydrochloride orally and 42.5 mg nortriptyline hydrochloride intramuscularly on separate occasions. Plasma concentration of drug (●-oral, ■-I.M.) and a metabolite, 10-hydroxynortriptyline (○-oral, □-I.M.) were measured; average data in 6 patients are shown. As a consequence of extensive hepatic metabolism, the oral availability of the drug is reduced (F = 0.66). The same amount of metabolite however, enters the systemic circulation. (Redrawn from Alvan, G., Borgå, O., Lind, M., Palmér, L., and Siwers, B.: First pass hydroxylation of nortriptyline: Concentrations of parent drug and major metabolites in plasma. Eur. J. Clin. Pharmacol., 11: 219–224, 1977.)*

The Plateau Level

At any time during drug infusion,

$$\begin{matrix}\text{Rate of change} \\ \text{of metabolite} \\ \text{in body}\end{matrix} = \underset{\substack{\text{Rate of} \\ \text{metabolite} \\ \text{formation}}}{km \cdot Ab} - \underset{\substack{\text{Rate of} \\ \text{metabolite} \\ \text{elimination}}}{k(m) \cdot Ab(m)} \quad 8$$

or expressing the equation in terms of concentration of drug and metabolite in plasma:

$$\begin{matrix}\text{Rate of change} \\ \text{of metabolite} \\ \text{in body}\end{matrix} = Cl_m \cdot C - Cl(m) \cdot Cm \quad 9$$

When the plateau or steady state is reached for both drug and metabolite, the rate of drug elimination matches the rate of infusion and the rate of metabolite elimination matches its rate of formation. Then Equations 8 and 9 simplify to:

$$\begin{matrix}\text{Amount of metabolite} \\ \text{at steady state}\end{matrix} = \frac{km}{k(m)} \cdot Ab_{ss} \quad 10$$

and

$$\begin{matrix}\text{Concentration of} \\ \text{metabolite at} \\ \text{steady state}\end{matrix} = \frac{Cl_m}{Cl(m)} \cdot C_{ss} \quad 11$$

However, since *fm* is the fraction of drug converted to the metabolite, the term $fm \cdot R_{inf}$ must be the rate of metabolite formation at the plateau, so

$$\begin{matrix}\text{Amount of metabolite} \\ \text{at steady state}\end{matrix} = \frac{fm \cdot R_{inf}}{k(m)} \quad 12$$

and

$$\begin{matrix}\text{Concentration of} \\ \text{metabolite at} \\ \text{steady state}\end{matrix} = \frac{fm \cdot R_{inf}}{Cl(m)} \quad 13$$

The only factors controlling the amount of metabolite at the plateau are therefore the rate of drug infusion, the fraction of the drug converted to the metabolite, and the elimination rate constant of the metabolite. Only the first two factors and the total clearance of the metabolite control the plateau plasma concentration of metabolite. Suppose, for example, that one wishes to know the plateau levels of a metabolite when a drug is infused at 5 mg/hour, given that the fraction of drug converted to metabolite, *fm*, is 0.5, that the elimination rate constant of the metabolite, $k(m)$, is 0.1 hour^{-1}, and that the total clearance of metabolite, $Cl(m)$, is 1.0 liter/hour. Then,

Amount of metabolite at plateau

$$= \frac{0.5 \times 5 \text{ mg/hour}}{0.1 \text{ hour}^{-1}} = 25 \text{ mg}$$

Plasma concentration of metabolite at plateau

$$= \frac{0.5 \times 5 \text{ mg/hour}}{1.0 \text{ liter/hour}} = 2.5 \text{ mg/liter}$$

Time to Reach the Plateau

The time required for a metabolite to reach a plateau depends upon whether or

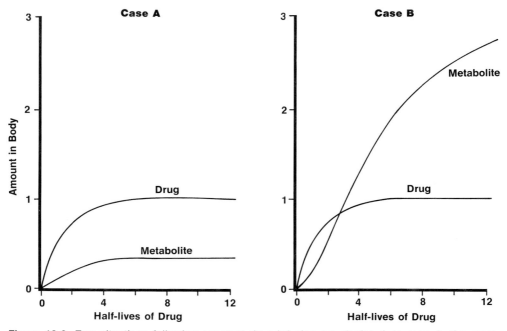

Figure 10-8. *Two situations following constant drug infusion are depicted. In case A, the more usual situation, the metabolite half-life is shorter than that of the drug. Throughout drug accumulation, metabolite levels are virtually at a steady state, and the approach to the metabolite plateau is determined by the half-life of the drug. In the less common situation, case B, the half-life of the drug is less than that of the metabolite. The drug is at steady state well before the metabolite has accumulated appreciably, and the approach of the metabolite to plateau is now determined by the metabolite half-life.*

not a bolus of drug is given at the start of the constant drug infusion. If a dose is given and the infusion maintains that amount of drug in the body, then the approach of the metabolite toward plateau depends only on the metabolite half-life. This point becomes apparent when one realizes that at constant drug concentration, metabolite is formed at a constant rate. As this is analogous to giving a constant infusion of metabolite, it follows (from Chap. 8) that the approach to the plateau is governed *solely* by the metabolite half-life. Thus, one-half the value at the plateau is reached in one metabolite half-life. By approximately 3.3 metabolite half-lives, the plateau is reached. Hence metabolites with short half-lives reach a plateau sooner.

If no bolus is given, the situation is more complicated. The time to reach the plateau is now primarily governed by either the drug or metabolite half-life, whichever is

the longer. To appreciate this point, consider two situations, both shown in Figure 10-8. In the more prevalent situation, case A, the drug has the longer half-life. As expected, the amount of drug in the body reaches a plateau in approximately 3.3 drug half-lives. The metabolite level and hence the rate of metabolite elimination also rises. However, because metabolite elimination is a much faster process than that of the drug, the rate of metabolite elimination soon becomes limited by and approximately equal to its rate of formation. The metabolite is then at virtual steady state with respect to, and cannot rise any faster than, the drug. This follows, since under this condition (Eq. 2)

$$\text{Amount of metabolite} = \left(\frac{k_m}{k(m)}\right) \times \text{Amount of drug}$$

and the metabolite level proportionally reflects the drug level. Therefore the metabolite reaches a plateau in approximately 4 drug half-lives.

In case B, the kinetics of the drug are faster than those of the metabolite. Now the drug reaches steady state before the metabolite level has barely risen. From then on the rate of metabolite formation is constant and, as observed previously, the accumulation of metabolite to the plateau is controlled by the metabolite half-life.

Postinfusion

As should now be anticipated, upon stopping an infusion, the decline of metabolite is governed by the longer half-life, i.e., drug or metabolite. For example, upon stopping a tolbutamide infusion, hydroxytolbutamide declines by one-half each tolbutamide half-life, whereas hydroxyhexamide decline is determined by its half-life after stopping an infusion of acetohexamide.

Assessment of Pharmacokinetic Parameters

Generally, the use of metabolite data to obtain estimates of pharmacokinetic parameters of a drug should be viewed with caution. There are times, however, especially when both drug and metabolite data are available, when insight into a drug's disposition can be gained. When metabolite elimination is rate-limited by drug elimination, urinary excretion of metabolite offers a useful means of monitoring drug elimination.

In summary, a metabolite is of therapeutic importance only when it achieves a sufficiently high concentration to elicit a significant effect. This condition is most likely to occur when a major fraction of the drug is converted to the metabolite, when elimination of the metabolite is the slowest step in the sequence between drug absorption and metabolite elimination, and when the total clearance of the metabolite is less than that of the drug. After constant drug infusion, the plasma concentration of metabolite is governed by the clearance associated with its formation and the total clearance of the metabolite. In the absence of a bolus dose of drug, the approach to the plateau level of a metabolite, following constant drug infusion, is governed either by the elimination half-life of the drug or by that of the metabolite, whichever is the longer.

Study Problems

(Answers to Study Problems can be found in Appendix G.)

1. Elson et al. (Elson, J., Strong, J.M., Lee, W-K., and Atkinson, A.J.): Antiarrhythmic potency of N-acetylprocainamide. Clin. Pharmacol. Ther., *17*: 134–140, 1975) determined the ratio of the plasma concentration of the active metabolite N-acetylprocainamide (see Table 10-1) to that of procainamide in patients on long-term procainamide therapy. The histogram (Fig. 10-9) below shows the results of 33 patients; there is considerable variation. Assuming, as is likely, that these values are reasonable estimates of the ratio at the plateau, comment on which pharmacokinetic parameters of drug and metabolite contribute to the observed variability in the ratio.

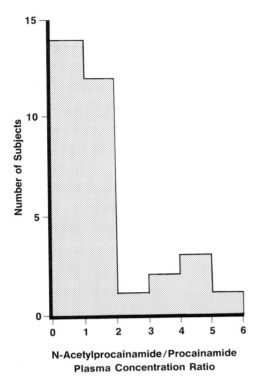

N-Acetylprocainamide/Procainamide
Plasma Concentration Ratio

Figure 10-9.

2. Glycine conjugation, with the formation of salicyluric acid, is one of the major pathways for the elimination of salicylic acid in man. Salicylic acid is cleared slowly from the body, whereas salicyluric acid is cleared so rapidly and completely into the urine that the plasma concentration of this metabolite is very low. Discuss why measuring salicyluric acid in the urine could be successfully used to assess its rate of formation.

3. Listed in Table 10-2 are the plasma concentrations of acetohexamide and its metabolite, hydroxyhexamide, depicted in Figure 10-5.
    Calculate the fraction of acetohexamide converted to hydroxyhexamide and the disposition kinetics of hydroxyhexamide. Assume that oral acetohexamide is fully available, that the absorption of the drug is rapid relative to its elimination, and that the volumes of distribution of drug and metabolite are equal. Other data suggest that these assumptions are reasonable. Note that the molecular weight of acetohexamide is 324, that of hydroxyhexamide, 326.

Table 10-2

Time (hours)	0	0.5	1	1.5	2	3	4	6	8	10
Acetohexamide (mg/liter)	0	25	32	30	32	16	7	4	—	—
Hydroxyhexamide (mg/liter)	0	12	22	27	44	42	32	25	16	11

4. The scheme below depicts the disposition of a drug

$$\text{Drug} \longrightarrow \text{Metabolite} \longrightarrow \text{Excreted metabolite}$$

The drug is converted to a single metabolite; the metabolite is excreted entirely into the urine unchanged. Figure 10-10 is a semilogarithmic plot of the plasma concentration of metabolite (Cm) with time following an intravenous bolus dose of drug. Complete the boxes in Table 10-3, by denoting ↑ for increase, ↓ for decrease, and ↔ for no change, when the total clearance of metabolite is decreased. Also draw a curve on the figure that shows the changes you have indicated in the boxes. Assume that the administered dose and all other clearance and volume terms remain unchanged.

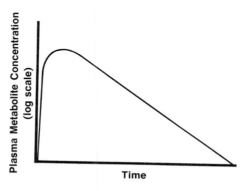

Figure 10-10.

Table 10-3

Plasma Metabolite Concentration	Rate-Limiting Step	
	A. Drug Elimination	B. Metabolite Elimination
Time to peak Peak height Area Terminal $t_{1/2}$		

11

integration of concepts and kinetics

Objectives

The reader will be able to:

1. **List examples of physiologic factors that may alter the primary pharmacokinetic parameters: absorption rate constant, hepatic clearance, renal clearance, and volume of distribution.**

2. **Given plasma (or blood) concentration versus time data in normal and altered states, determine the changes in the primary and secondary pharmacokinetic parameters that have occurred and list the physiologic mechanism(s) by which the changes may have occurred.**

3. **Predict and graphically demonstrate the effects of alterations in either plasma-protein or tissue binding, blood flow, or metabolic activity on the time course of drug in blood, when the appropriate primary pharmacokinetic parameters are known.**

4. **Predict the therapeutic consequences of the alterations given in objective 3.**

IN previous chapters the pharmacokinetic parameters of a drug have been assumed to be constant. For example, one frequently refers to *the* value of the half-life of a drug or to *the* value of its clearance. The pharmacokinetic parameters of a drug may, however, change—with disease, with concomitant drug therapy, and even within the same individual. Indeed, such changes permit an insight to be gained into the interrelationships between the drug and the body. In this context, drugs may be viewed as molecular probes. They help to define physiologic and pathophysiologic processes, in much the same way as they are used in

pharmacodynamics to characterize receptor sites.

The goal of this chapter is to integrate physiologic principles and pharmacokinetic concepts and so to serve as a basis for dealing in subsequent chapters with variability in drug response and with individualization of drug therapy. To achieve this goal each pharmacokinetic parameter is now treated as a variable instead of as a constant. It is assumed, however, that, within each period of measurement, the value of a parameter is constant; it only varies between circumstances, e.g., disease, presence of another drug, or between individuals. For this purpose, the parameter either has a control (or normal) value or an altered value.

Interrelationships Among Pharmacokinetic Parameters and Physiologic Variables

The physiology of the body dictates that several pharmacokinetic parameters are related to each other, e.g., half-life depends upon volume of distribution, and availability depends upon hepatic clearance. Furthermore, the values of many of these parameters are dependent on physiologic variables, for example, blood flow, which, in turn, is influenced by a number of other factors such as diseases and other drugs. A summary of the interrelationships between pharmacokinetic parameters and physiologic variables is in order.

Dependence of Primary Parameters on Physiologic Variables

As discussed in Chapters 3 through 6, drug absorption and disposition depend upon many physiologic variables. Absorption may be affected by blood flow at the absorption site, gastric emptying, and gastrointestinal motility. Distribution is influenced by binding to plasma proteins and to tissue components; and elimination may depend upon hepatic and renal blood flow, plasma-protein binding, hepatocellular enzyme activity, renal secretion (active transport), urine pH, and urine flow. Each of these physiologic variables is affected by numerous factors, including those listed in Table 11-1. Thus, rubbing increases subcutaneous and muscle blood flow, food slows stomach emptying, while diseases and drugs produce many effects.

The pharmacokinetics of a drug often can be described by relatively few parameters. One should recall that absorption can be characterized by availability and by an absorption rate constant, if absorption is first order; distribution can be characterized by the volume of distribution; and elimination can be characterized by hepatic and renal clearance. Each of these parameters may be directly affected by changes in one or more of the physiologic variables listed in Table

Table 11-1. Some Factors Affecting Physiologic Variables

Physiologic Variable	Factors Affecting Variable
Blood flow at absorption site	Stress, rubbing, drugs, posture (intestine), food (intestine), disease
Gastric emptying; motility	Food, drugs, electrolytes, disease
Hepatic blood flow	Cardiac output, posture, drugs, disease
Renal blood flow	Cardiac output, disease
Fractions unbound in blood and tissue	Binding component concentration (plasma : albumin and globulins), drug concentration, other drugs, disease
Hepatocellular enzyme activity	Drugs (inhibition of enzyme synthesis and induction, enzyme inhibition), environmental factors, disease
Renal transport system	Drugs, disease
Urine pH	Diet, time of day, drugs, disease
Urine flow	Fluid intake, drugs, temperature, disease

11-1. Because of this direct relationship, these parameters may be referred to as *primary pharmacokinetic parameters,* with the exception of availability which also depends upon the value of hepatic clearance. The dependence of the primary pharmacokinetic parameters on selected physiologic variables is summarized in Table 11-2.

The relationships between the primary pharmacokinetic parameters and the physiologic variables were developed in Chapters 3 to 6. One of the principal considerations was the effect of some of these variables on renal and hepatic clearance, when the extraction in these organs is perfusion rate-limited (high extraction ratio). Here the concentration of drug in blood is of interest, whereas, when assessing the therapeutic consequences of altered pharmacokinetics, interest lies in the unbound drug concentration. Consequently, the parameters determined from these two sites of measurement are emphasized in this chapter.

Secondary Pharmacokinetic Parameters and Derived Values

The half-life, the elimination rate constant, and the fraction renally excreted unchanged are examples of *secondary pharmacokinetic parameters,* in that their values

depend upon those of the primary pharmacokinetic parameters. Furthermore, there are several derived values that depend not only upon the primary pharmacokinetic parameters, but also upon either the dose, the rate of constant infusion, or the hepatic blood flow. These dependencies are summarized briefly in Table 11-3.

To integrate pharmacokinetic principles with physiologic concepts, consider the three hypothetic drugs listed in Table 11-4. Hypothetic drugs were chosen because, to date, there are no drugs with sufficient data to illustrate all facets of the interrelationships. Drug H (hepatic), which has a high extraction ratio, is eliminated almost entirely in the liver. Drug K (kidney) also has a high extraction ratio, but is eliminated exclusively by the kidney. Drug L (low) is eliminated by the liver and kidney, but it has a low extraction ratio in both of these organs. Propranolol, phenylpropanolamine, and nitrofurantoin have characteristics similar to those of drugs H, K, and L, respectively.

The consequences of an alteration in plasma protein binding, in tissue binding, in blood flow to the eliminating organs, and in metabolic activity are now examined in turn. Rather than cover all combinations of alterations, effects, and observations, three

Table 11-2. Dependence of Primary Pharmacokinetic Parameters on Physiologic Variables

Primary Pharmacokinetic Parameter	Independent Physiologic Variables
Absorption rate constant	Blood flow at absorption site, gastric emptying, motility of gastrointestinal tract
Hepatic clearance	Hepatic blood flow, binding in blood, intrinsic hepatocellular activity (Vm,Km)
Renal clearance	Renal blood flow, binding in blood, active secretion, active reabsorption, urine pH, urine flow
Volume of distribution	Binding in blood, binding in tissues, body composition, body size

Table 11-3. Dependence of Secondary Pharmacokinetic Parameters and Derived Values on Primary Pharmacokinetic Parameters

	Equation
Secondary Pharmacokinetic Parameters	
Elimination half-life	$0.7 \times \dfrac{\text{Volume of distribution}}{\text{Clearance}}$
Fraction excreted unchanged	Renal clearance/Total clearance
Derived Values	
Area under curve (i.v.)	Dose/Clearance
Oral availability[a]	$1 - \dfrac{\text{Hepatic blood clearance}}{\text{Hepatic blood flow}}$
Area under curve (oral)	$\dfrac{\text{Dose} \times \text{Availability}}{\text{Clearance}}$

[a]Hepatic elimination is assumed to be the only cause of a decrease in the oral availability.

situations have been chosen to serve as examples. The first is displacement, whereby another drug reduces binding of a drug to either plasma or tissue constituents, that is, *fu* or *fu_T* is increased. The second is increased hepatic and renal blood flow produced, for example, by increased cardiac output. The last situation is induction, an increase in the synthesis rate and hence in the amount of enzymes responsible for drug metabolism. Many of these facets are discussed in greater depth in subsequent chapters, particularly in Chapter 17, Drug Interactions.

Influence of Displacement

Changes in Pharmacokinetic Parameters

Recall from Chapters 4 to 6 that displacement of drug from plasma proteins alone always produces an increase in the volume of distribution, but that clearance only changes (increases) when the extraction ratio of the drug is low. Consequently, the half-life increases with displacement, only if a drug is highly extracted. With a drug of low extraction, the half-life should show no change, or decrease only slightly,

an observation perhaps best understood by considering the unbound drug. Thus, unbound clearance is unaffected, and the unbound volume of distribution tends to decrease, but only marginally, with changes in binding within blood (see Eq. 25, Chap. 4, and Eq. 6, Chap. 6), unless displacement in tissues also occurs.

Displacement in plasma should decrease oral availability, particularly when a drug has a high hepatic extraction ratio, in which case there is a substantial first-pass effect. This last statement may, at first, appear to contradict the statement made above, that for a highly cleared drug the extraction ratio is unaffected by displacement. These apparently conflicting statements can be reconciled by realizing that, in fact, displacement does increase the extraction ratio of a highly cleared drug, but marginally. However, since availability is 1 minus the hepatic extraction ratio ($1 - E_H$, Table 11-3), these small changes in the extraction ratio produce substantial changes in availability. For example, had displacement of drug within plasma increased the extraction ratio of Drug H from 0.95 to 0.98, clearance would increase by only 3 percent, but availability would be reduced from 5 to 2 percent, that is, a 60 percent decrease.

Table 11-4. Pharmacokinetic Parameters of Three Hypothetical Drugs

	Primary				Secondary			Other Parameters		
Drug	Availability[a] (oral)	Absorption Half-life (hours)	Volume[b] of Distribution (liters)	Total Clearance (liters/hours)	Elimination Half-life (hours)	Fraction Excreted Unchanged	Fraction Unbound in Blood	Extraction Ratio[c]		
								Hepatic	Renal	
H	0.05	1.38	430	100	3	0.05	0.10	0.95	0.06	
K	1.00	1.38	330	76	3	1.0	0.10	0	0.95	
L	0.97	1.38	26	6	3	0.6	0.01	0.03	0.05	

[a] Availability is accounted for by hepatic first-pass metabolism only; it is a secondary parameter in this respect.
[b] Based on measurement of drug in blood.
[c] Hepatic and renal blood flows are 100 and 80 liters/hour, respectively.

Displacement of drug from tissue binding sites always diminishes the volume of distribution. Since no change is anticipated in clearance, half-life decreases regardless of the value of the extraction ratio. Availability is unaffected.

Kinetic Consequences

Figure 11-1 summarizes the kinetic consequences of displacement of Drug L and Drug K following administration of single intravenous or oral doses.

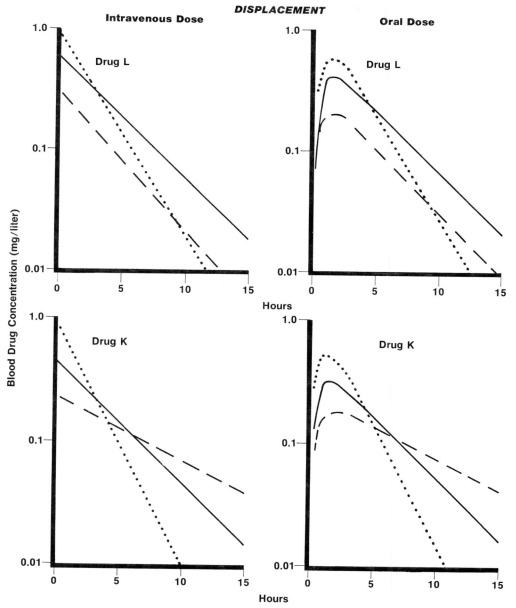

DISPLACEMENT

Figure 11-1. *Displacement of drug from binding sites in blood (---) or in the tissues (···) affects the concentration-time curve expected after single intravenous and oral doses of Drug L (15 mg), a poorly extracted drug, and of Drug K (150 mg), a drug highly cleared by the kidneys; normal condition (—). Note the changes in the initial concentration, the peak concentration, the half-life, and the corresponding (linear plot) area under the curve.*

Consider first the poorly cleared Drug L, given intravenously. With displacement within blood, both the initial concentration and the area under the curve are reduced, because both the volume of distribution and clearance are increased, but as discussed, half-life remains essentially unchanged. The picture is the converse when displacement occurs within tissues. Now, the initial concentration is higher because the volume of distribution is smaller, but, clearance and consequently the area under the curve are unaltered.

Consider next the two highly cleared drugs, Drug K and Drug H, given intravenously. The picture is essentially the same as seen with Drug L, when displacement occurs within the tissues. The observations differ only when displacement occurs within blood. Then, although the initial concentration is reduced, area remains unchanged because clearance is unaffected by displacement.

The kinetic picture seen following a single oral dose is much the same as that observed following an intravenous dose of Drug L and Drug K, respectively. However, for Drug H, which is highly extracted in the liver, the picture is different. As shown in Figure 11-2, displacement in blood lowers the peak concentration, partly because the volume of distribution is increased and partly because availability is decreased. Decreased availability primarily accounts for the smaller area; clearance, the other determinant of area, is essentially unchanged.

Figure 11-3 depicts the time course of both blood and unbound concentration of Drug L and Drug K following a constant rate intravenous infusion. Both being highly cleared, the events seen with Drug H would be qualitatively identical to those seen with Drug K. With all three drugs, displacement within tissues, by reducing the half-life, shortens the time to approach the plateau, but does not alter either the unbound or total plateau concentration, since the clearance values are unaltered. Differ-

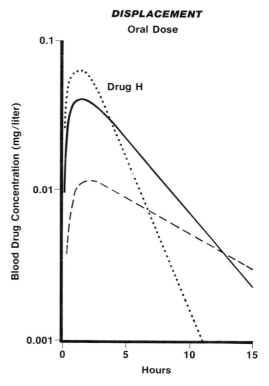

Figure 11-2. *Displacement of drug from binding sites in blood (---) or in the tissues (· · ·) affects the concentration-time profile after a single oral dose of Drug H (500 mg), a drug highly extracted by the liver; normal condition (—). Note the effect of displacement in blood on the corresponding (linear plot) area under the curve; the decreased area is a consequence of decreased availability. (The change in availability was calculated using Model I of Pang, S., and Rowland, M.: Hepatic clearance of Drugs I. J. Pharmacokin. Biopharm., 5: 625–653, 1977.)*

ences between the drugs are only seen when displacement occurs within blood. Let us consider first Drug L and then Drugs K and H.

Since the half-life is unchanged, so is the time for Drug L to approach the plateau. Likewise, as unbound clearance is unaltered, so too is the unbound concentration at steady state. Thus, in general, displacement should produce little or no change in the response at plateau of a low extraction ratio drug. In contrast, for the highly cleared drugs, K and H, since clearance and

DISPLACEMENT

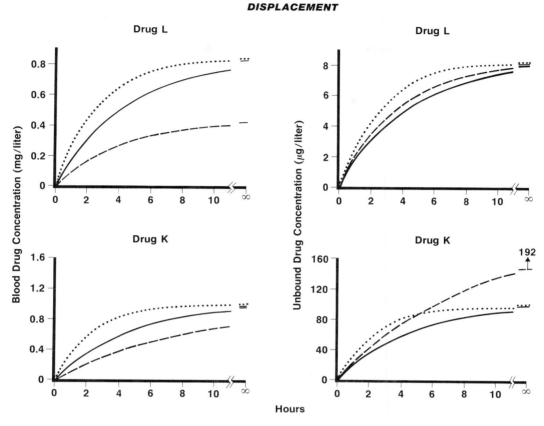

Figure 11-3. *The blood and unbound concentrations are altered by displacement of drug from binding sites in blood (---) or in tissue (· · ·) during the intravenous infusion of Drug L (5 mg/hour) and Drug K (75 mg/hour); normal condition (—). Note the effect of displacement on the blood concentration of Drug L and on the unbound concentration of Drug K at steady state.*

hence the total concentration in blood are unaffected by displacement, the steady-state unbound concentration, and therefore response, must be elevated when displacement occurs in blood. The time to approach the plateau is also increased, a consequence of an increased half-life.

Influence of Blood Flow

Changes in Pharmacokinetic Parameters

As presented in Chapter 5, changes in organ blood flow only affect clearance when the extraction ratio of a drug is high. This conclusion is based on the concept of a perfusion limitation. This concept is used in the following discussion of the consequence of an increase in blood flow. It should be borne in mind, however, that there are secondary effects of altered blood flow, particularly when decreased, that may supersede perfusion considerations alone. For example, a decreased blood flow may produce anoxia, which in turn may affect drug metabolism. Furthermore, because every blood vessel in the organ may not provide the same exposure of the drug to parenchymal cells, the extraction ratio may be altered. A change in the pattern of distribution of blood flow within the elimination organ may be associated with a change in blood flow. This alteration in the degree of shunting or bypassing of the parenchymal cells may occur in certain hepatic diseases and under a variety of conditions.

Oral availability of a drug with high hepatic extraction is expected to increase with elevated hepatic blood flow, because the blood remains in the liver for a shorter period of time. However, how much the availability changes depends upon the mechanism(s) of hepatic extraction. Unfortunately, at present, there is insufficient information to make quantitative conclusions.

Kinetic Consequences

Figure 11-4 shows the effect of a doubling of the blood flow to the organ(s) of elimination for a poorly cleared drug, Drug L, and for one highly cleared by the kidneys, Drug K. Because Drug L has a low extraction ratio in both the kidneys and the liver, the altered blood flow has little to no direct effect on the pharmacokinetics of the drug following administration by the routes shown. For Drug K, however, the increased renal clearance decreases the half-life, the

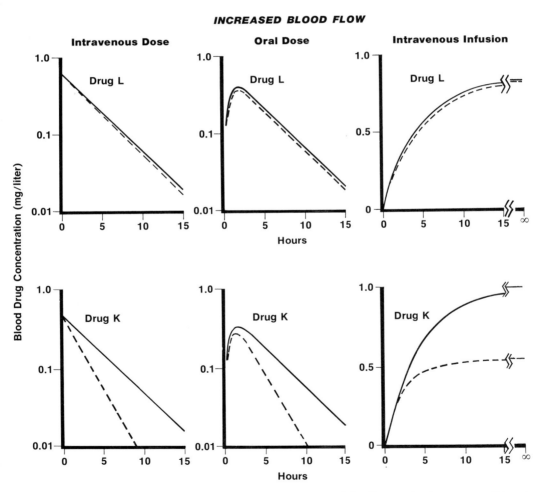

Figure 11-4. *Increased blood flow to the eliminating organ has very little effect on the time course of Drug L, but a pronounced effect on Drug K, following single intravenous and oral doses and following intravenous infusion: altered condition (---); normal condition (—). Administration is identical to that indicated in Figures 11-1 and 11-3.*

plateau concentration of both total and unbound concentration, and, presumably, the response following an intravenous infusion.

The events following intravenous administration of Drug H, when hepatic blood flow is altered, are readily apparent. Being well extracted, as clearance is increased, the infusion rate will need to be raised to maintain the same steady-state concentration when liver blood flow is elevated; and, as half-life is correspondingly shortened, the plateau is reached sooner. Not so apparent are the likely events that follow when Drug H is given as a single oral dose. Although half-life is decreased, clearance and availability are simultaneously increased. The result may be little or no change in the area under the curve (Fig. 11-5). The outcome depends primarily upon whether or not, with an elevated hepatic blood flow, the factor by which availability is increased exactly matches that for clearance (see Eq. 11, Chap. 9).

Influence of Induction

Changes in Pharmacokinetic Parameters

For a drug with a low hepatic extraction ratio, clearance increases and half-life decreases with induction, but the availability is essentially unaltered. For a drug with high hepatic extraction, the clearance and hence the half-life remain essentially unchanged. The oral availability, however, is reduced when induction occurs. These changes are evident from the relationships between extraction ratio and both clearance and availability. To demonstrate the point, assume that the hepatic extraction ratio (E_H) of a drug is increased from 0.98 to 0.99 with a twofold increase in enzyme activity. Then, clearance is increased by about only 1 percent while the fraction escaping metabolism on the first pass through the liver ($F_H = 1 - E_H$) is decreased by one-half.

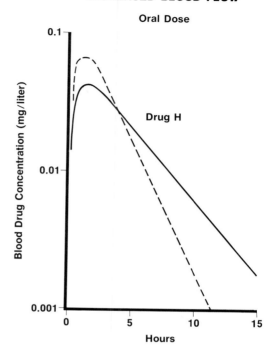

INCREASED BLOOD FLOW

Oral Dose

Figure 11-5. *Increased hepatic blood flow alters the blood drug concentration-time profile after an oral dose of Drug H (500 mg); altered condition (···); normal condition (—). Note that the corresponding (linear plot) area under the curve is not altered. This is a consequence of clearance and availability being equally affected. [Model I of Pang and Rowland (see Fig. 11-2) was used for this simulation.]*

Kinetic Consequences

Figure 11-6 demonstrates the anticipated pharmacokinetics of Drug L and Drug H before and after inducing drug-metabolizing enzymes. For Drug L, being poorly extracted, clearance is increased, and half-life is shortened as expected, although the changes are not as great as they would be were the drug eliminated solely by the liver. The decreased steady-state concentration is particularly noteworthy.

The disposition kinetics of Drug H are essentially unaltered when the drug is given intravenously; since, for this highly extracted drug, perfusion rather than enzy-

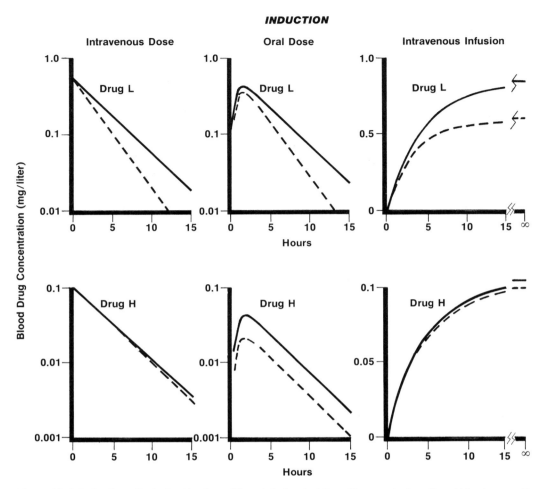

Figure 11-6. *Induction affects the kinetics of Drug L but not of Drug H, except when Drug H is given orally: altered condition (---); normal condition (—). The single intravenous dose, single oral dose, and infusion rate of Drug L and Drug H are: 15 mg, 15 mg, 5 mg/hour and 50 mg, 500 mg, and 10 mg/hour, respectively.*

matic activity is rate-limiting elimination, neither clearance nor half-life is appreciably affected by induction. On oral administration, however, the availability is reduced, which results in a lower area. Larger oral doses would, therefore, be needed to attain the same maximum effect. It should be noted that the consequences of induction are the reverse of those for an increased hepatic blood flow, with respect to both clearance and availability, following intravenous and oral administration.

The effect of induction on the kinetics of a drug with a high hepatic extraction ratio

is exemplified by alprenolol (Fig. 11-7). Pretreatment with pentobarbital appears to have little effect on the pharmacokinetics of alprenolol when given intravenously. Following oral administration, however, the peak concentration and the area under the curve are dramatically reduced, although there is little apparent change in the half-life. These observations on first glance would appear to be inconsistent. Knowing, however, that this drug is metabolized in the liver, and on calculating the clearance, 1.2 liters/min in this subject, an explanation can be offered. Pentobarbital induces the

Table 11-5. Anticipated Effects of *Increased* Values of Physiologic Variables on Various Parameters and Observations for a Drug Eliminated Exclusively by the Liver

Administration / Parameter or Observation	Low Extraction Ratio Drug				High Extraction Ratio Drug			
	Increased Unbound Fraction in Blood	Increased Unbound Fraction in Tissue	Increased Hepatic Blood Flow	Increased Enzyme Activity[a]	Increased Unbound Fraction in Blood	Increased Unbound Fraction in Tissue	Increased Hepatic Blood Flow	Increased Enzyme Activity[a]
Single Dose								
Intravenous								
Half-life	↔[b]	↓	↔	↓	↑	↓	↓	↔
Area under Curve	↓	↔	↔	↓	↔	↔	↓	↔
Oral								
Availability	↔	↔	↔	↔	↓	↔	↑	↓
Area under Curve	↓	↔	↔	↓	↓	↔	↔[c]	↓
Intravenous Infusion								
Plateau								
Total Concentration	↓	↔	↔	↓	↔	↔	↓	↔
Unbound Concentration	↔	↔	↔	↓	↑	↔	↓	↔

[a] Enzyme activity is increased by one of several mechanisms, such as enzyme activation, enzyme induction, or increased availability of cofactors, if rate-limiting.

[b] ↑ Increase, ↓ decrease, ↔ no significant change.

[c] The increase in availability is assumed to be countered by an equal increase in clearance.

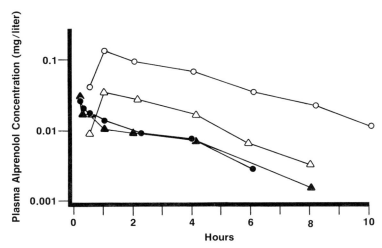

Figure 11-7. *Induction of alprenolol metabolism by pentobarbital treatment produces observed differences in the plasma concentration when the drug is given orally (200 mg), but not when given intravenously (5 mg). Alprenolol was administered before (●, i.v.; ○, oral) and 10 days into (▲, i.v.; △, oral) a pentobarbital regimen of 100 mg at bedtime. (From Alvan, G., Piafsky, K., Lind, M., and von Bahr, C: Effect of pentobarbital on the disposition of alprenolol. Clin. Pharmacol. Ther., 22: 316–321, 1977.)*

metabolism of alprenolol and thereby decreases its availability. In this subject the hepatic extraction ratio increased from 0.78 to 0.94, giving a fourfold decrease in availability with only a minor increase in hepatic clearance.

Table 11-5 summarizes the effects expected from displacement of drug from either blood or tissue binding sites, from increased blood flow or from induction of metabolism for a drug eliminated exclusively by the liver. Both low and high extraction ratio drugs are considered, in turn. The expectations are similar for a drug eliminated only by the kidneys; however, increased enzyme activity does not apply, and the oral availability of a highly extracted drug is unaffected by changes in these variables.

Study Problems

(*Answers to Study Problems can be found in Appendix G.*)

1. The total clearance of the β-blocker, propranolol, is high (approximately 1.1 liters/min) and relatively constant in man. However, the elimination half-life varies, being proportionately longer in individuals in whom the fraction of drug in plasma unbound is higher (see Table 11-6).

   Present a brief explanation that is consistent with the aforementioned observations.

Table 11-6. Half-life and Percent Unbound in a Group of Subjects

Percent Unbound	5	6	7	7.5	8	8	8.5	9	11
Half-life (hours)	2.4	2.2	2.9	2.6	3.1	3.6	3.2	3.3	4.0

2. On the same graph, draw curves (control and alteration) that demonstrate each of the situations below. Assume that all other physiologic parameters remain unchanged.

Situation	Drug Administration	Physiologic Alteration
A	Intravenous infusion of Drug H	Decreased hepatic blood flow
B	Single intravenous bolus of Drug K	Decreased renal blood flow
C	Single oral dose of Drug L	Increased tissue binding

3. Complete Table 11-7 below by marking: ↑ for increase, ↓ for decrease, and ↔ for little or no change in the empty spaces. Assume that the drug is only eliminated in the liver and that the volume of distribution is greater than 100 liters.

Table 11-7

Hepatic Extraction Ratio	Hepatic Blood Flow	Fraction in Blood Unbound	Fraction in Tissue Unbound	Total Clearance[a]	Volume of Distribution[a]	Half-life	Oral Availability
High	↑	↔	↔				
High	↔	↓	↔				
High	↔	↔	↑				
Low	↑	↔	↔				
Low	↔	↔	↑				
Low	↔			↑	↔ *		

[a]Based on drug concentration in blood.

4. The values for the clearance and for the fraction excreted unchanged in the urine in normal patients are given for three different drugs in Table 11-8. The subsequent columns contain data observed for patients with a particular condition in comparison with normal patients. Fill in the empty space with a ↑ = increased value, ↓ = decreased value, or ↔ = little or no change. Assume no change in blood flow and that no enzyme inhibition or enzyme induction occurs. Also assume that each drug has a large volume of distribution (greater than 50 liters) and that the observation may be a consequence of a change in more than one physiologic variable.

Table 11-8

Drug	Total Clearance[a] (ml/min)	Fraction Excreted Unchanged	Total Clearance[a]	Renal Clearance[a]	Half-life	Fraction in Blood Unbound	Fraction in Tissue Unbound	Urine Flow
Drug A	240	0.5	↓		↔	↔		↓
Drug B	100	0.01				↑[b]	↑[b]	↔
Drug C	1400	0.005	↔		↑		↔	↔

[a] Based on drug concentration in blood.
[b] By the same factor.

Unifying Problem

(Answer to Unifying Problem can be found in Appendix G.)

A highly bound drug ($fu = 0.01$) has a volume of distribution of 240 liters. The liver is the only organ of elimination. The hepatic extraction ratio is 0.95, despite the fact that the fraction in blood that is unbound, fu_b, is only 0.005. Assume an hepatic blood flow of 90 liters/hour.

(a) Estimate the following parameters for this drug: total clearance (Cl), total blood clearance (Cl_b), volume of distribution based on blood (V_b), and half-life.

(b) In uremic patients the volume of distribution and the fraction unbound in plasma, fu, average 140 liters and 0.03, respectively. Is there any evidence that the uremic state affects the tissue binding? If so, in what direction and by what factor is the tissue binding altered?

(c) When this drug is infused intravenously at the same constant rate to a patient who is and has been receiving another drug, the value of fu_b is now found to be 0.03. Assuming steady-state conditions for both drugs, calculate the ratio of the unbound concentration of the drug in the presence of, to that in the absence of, the other drug.

therapeutic regimens

12

therapeutic response and toxicity

Objectives

The reader will be able to:

1. **Explain why the effect (desired or toxic) of a drug is often better correlated with plasma concentration than with dose.**

2. **Define the terms: "minimum therapeutic dose," "therapeutic concentration range," and "utility curve."**

3. **List the range of plasma concentrations associated with therapy for any of the drugs given in Table 12-1.**

4. **Describe why both intensity and duration of effect are often proportional to the logarithm of the amount of drug in the body.**

5. **Calculate the minimum effective dose and the elimination rate constant of a drug, given data on the duration of action following various intravenous doses.**

6. **Calculate the intravenous dose necessary to achieve a given duration of action, and the converse, given the half-life and the minimum effective dose.**

7. **Show graphically how duration and intensity of effect are increased on the second dose but no further on subsequent doses, when each dose is given just as the response falls to a predetermined level.**

8. **With equations, show why, for reversibly acting drugs, the response varies linearly with time when the effect is proportional to the logarithm of the amount of drug in the body.**

9. **Devise a dosage regimen given appropriate dose-response-time information.**

THE concepts and basic principles of pharmacokinetics have been dealt with in the first two sections. The application of such information to the rational design of safe and efficacious dosage regimens is now examined. In this section, fundamental as-

pects of dosage regimens are covered from the point of view of treating a patient population with a given disease. It is realized, of course, that individuals vary in their response to drugs, and subsequently, in Section IV, attention is turned toward the

155

establishment of dosage regimens in individual patients.

The objective of most drug therapy is to produce and maintain a therapeutic response. The response may be as vague as a general feeling of improvement or as precise as a prothrombin time of 24 seconds in anticoagulant therapy. Attempts are made to minimize undesirable and toxic effects and to prevent ineffective therapy by an appropriate adjustment in the dosage regimen. At present, optimization of drug therapy is most commonly achieved, sometimes at considerable expense, time, and occasional toxicity, by relating response to the dose administered. In recent years, a considerable body of evidence has been accumulated from animal experiments and to a much lesser extent from studies in man, indicating that response is better correlated with the plasma concentration or with the amount of drug in the body than with the dose administered. In this chapter, some of this evidence as well as various elements of the level-response-time interrelationships is explored. Principles for attaining and maintaining a therapeutic level of drug in the body are discussed in Chapter 13.

Response and Concentration

Information relating concentration to response has been obtained at three levels: *in vitro* experiments, animal studies, and investigations in both human volunteers and patients. The last level is the most relevant to human drug therapy but, unfortunately, only limited information is obtainable here about the nature of the drug-receptor interaction. *In vitro* experiments, which include studies of the action of drugs on enzymes, on other proteins, on microorganisms, and on isolated tissues and organs, serve this purpose best. However, in isolating the variables, many of the complex interrelationships that exist *in vivo* are destroyed. Animal studies bridge the gap between *in vitro* experimentation and human investigation. Studies in animals introduce both the variable, time, with all that it connotes, and the elements of absorption and disposition as well as the feedback control systems that operate to maintain homeostasis. Animal studies are most useful for evaluating the pharmacologic spectrum of activity of a (potential) therapeutic agent and for determining its toxicity profile. Irrespective of the level of information, however, the conclusion is the same: A positive correlation, although sometimes complex, exists between the concentration of drug at the site of measurement and the response. Let us look at some of the information gathered.

Graded Response

The relaxant effect of terbutaline in an isolated human bronchial muscle strip (contracted with carbachol) is shown in Figure 12-1A as a function of the concentration of terbutaline in the fluid bathing the strip. The plot is characteristic of most response-concentration curves. Notice the nearly linear relationship between the intensity of response and the concentration at low concentrations, and the tendency to reach a maximal response at high concentrations. A more common form of representation of the data in Figure 12-1A is a plot of the intensity of response against the logarithm of the concentration (Fig. 12-1B). This transformation expands the early part of the curve, where response is changing rapidly with a small change in concentration, and contracts the latter part where a large change in concentration produces only a slight change in response. It also shows that, between 20 and 80 percent of the maximum, the response appears to be proportional to the logarithm of the concentration.

The reduction of exercise tachycardia by propranolol is proportional to the logarithm of its plasma concentration (Fig. 12-2). This straight-line relationship, instead of the expected S-shaped or sigmoidal curve seen in Figure 12-1B, arises in part because the

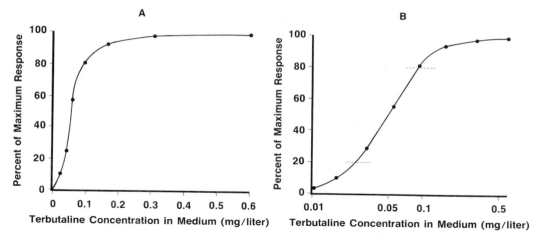

Figure 12-1. *Arithmetic,* A, *and semilogarithmic,* B, *concentration-response curves for the relaxant effect of terbutaline on an* in vitro *preparation of a human bronchial muscle previously contracted with carbachol. At low terbutaline concentrations, the relaxant effect is proportional to the concentration of terbutaline. Between 20 and 80 percent of maximal response, the response is proportional to the logarithm of the concentration. (Redrawn from Svedmyr, N., and Thiringer, F.S.: The effects of salbutamol and isoprenaline on beta-receptors in patients with chronic obstructive lung disease. Postgrad. Med. J., 47; (March Supplement): 44–46, 1971.)*

results were obtained in man, not in an isolated preparation. To illustrate this point, consider a drug that increases heart rate through sympathetic stimulation. In an isolated heart preparation, the baseline heart rate can be controlled precisely so that the response to small concentrations of drug can readily be measured. *In vivo,* in response to internal and external stimuli, the baseline heart rate is much more variable, making it more difficult to detect the minor changes in heart rate observed *in vitro.* Perhaps the response can only be measured accurately when it is at least 10 to 20 percent different from the baseline rate, that is, in the linear part of the response-log concentration curve. At the other extreme, the greatest response that may be produced *in vivo* is often less than 80 percent of the maximum pharmacologic response. The entire cardiovascular system may deteriorate and the animal (or the patient) may die long before the heart rate approaches the maximum rate capable of being produced. Other toxicities of the drug or metabolite(s) may further limit the maximally tolerated concentration *in vivo.*

Both the relaxant effect on the bronchial muscle produced by terbutaline and the reduction of exercise tachycardia by propranolol are examples of *graded responses,*

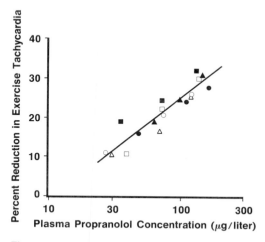

Figure 12-2. *The percent reduction in exercise tachycardia is proportional to the logarithm of the plasma concentration of propranolol. The solid line is the line of best fit. Each symbol denotes observations in a subject. (From McDevitt, D.G., and Shand, D.G.: Plasma concentrations and the time-course of beta blockade due to propranolol. Clin. Pharmacol. Ther., 18: 708–713, 1975.)*

so called because a continuously changing drug concentration, in the *same* preparation or person, produces a continuously changing response. Both drugs also act *reversibly* in that the effect is reversed upon reducing the concentration of drug at the site of action. The majority of drugs used clinically act reversibly and many elicit a graded response.

All-or-None Response

Many pharmacologic and toxic responses cannot be measured on a continuous basis. An obvious but extreme example is death. Another is the suppression of an arrhythmia. The arrhythmia either is or is not suppressed. Such effects are known as *quantal* or *all-or-none* responses. Unlike a graded response, the correlation between a quantal response and concentration is explored by examining the *frequency* of the event with the concentration. The frequency of the suppression of ventricular tachyarrhythmias as a function of the serum procainamide concentration is shown in Figure 12-3. It should be noted that in most patients the arrhythmia is suppressed at concentrations of 2 to 8 mg/liter.

Another form of representation of this information is a plot of the percent of responders against either the concentration or the logarithm of the concentration. Figure 12-4 shows this type of transformation. Note that of those patients who responded, 20 to 80 percent did so when the procainamide concentration was between 2 and 8 mg/liter. However, this belies the entire picture.

Therapeutic Plasma
Concentration Range

Figure 12-4 also shows the percent of those patients who did not respond to procainamide, those who responded, those who exhibited minor side effects, and those who exhibited serious toxicity. Side effects were considered minor when cessation of the

drug was unnecessary and serious when disturbances of cardiovascular function or other adverse effects necessitated discontinuation of the drug. Serious toxic effects included severe hypotension, atrioventricular and intraventricular conduction disturbances, appearance of major new ventricular arrhythmias or cardiac arrest. It should be noted in particular that serious toxicity begins to appear above 8 mg/liter and occurs with increasing frequency at higher concentrations. Above 16 mg/liter, the toxic effects may prove fatal. From these data, it can be concluded that the

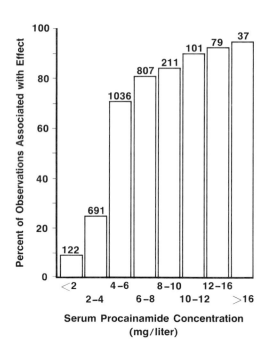

Figure 12-3. *The concentration of procainamide was determined in over 3000 serum samples obtained from 291 patients receiving this drug for the treatment of cardiac arrhythmias. The frequency, expressed as a percent of the number of serum samples with which a serum concentration correlates with effective therapy, increases with each interval of increasing concentration. The value above each bar refers to the number of samples within the respective concentration range. (From Koch-Weser, J.: In Pharmacology and the Future: Problems in Therapy. Edited by G.T. Okita, and G.H. Archeson. Karger, Basel, 1973, Vol. 3, pp. 69–85.)*

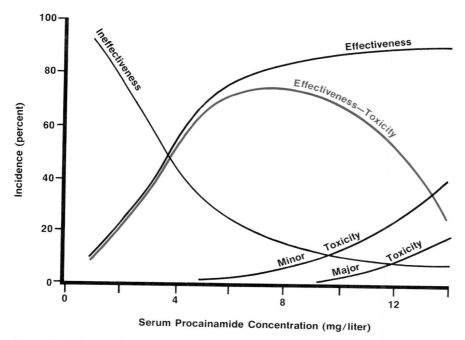

Figure 12-4. *Schematic representation of the frequency of ineffective therapy, effective therapy, minor side effects, serious toxicity, and "therapeutic effectiveness" with serum concentration of procainamide in patients receiving this drug for the treatment of arrhythmias. Therapeutic effectiveness is defined arbitrarily as the difference in the frequency between effective therapy and toxic effects; the therapeutic effectiveness of procainamide reaches a peak at 8 mg liter. (Adapted from the data of Koch-Weser, J.: In Pharmacology and the Future: Problems in Therapy. Edited by G.T. Okita, and G.H. Archeson. Karger, Basel, 1973, Vol. 3 pp. 69–85.)*

range of plasma concentrations of procainamide associated with effective therapy and without undue toxicity is 4 to 8 mg/liter. This range is commonly known as the *therapeutic concentration range* of the drug.

Clearly, not all patients receiving procainamide for the treatment of ventricular arrhythmias need plasma concentrations between 4 and 8 mg/liter. In a few, the arrhythmias are suppressed at concentrations below 4 mg/liter; in others, toxicity occurs before efficacy can be demonstrated. Thus, a therapeutic concentration is most appropriately defined in terms of an individual patient's requirements. Usually this information is unknown and, on initiating therapy, the therapeutic concentration must be estimated from consideration of the probability of therapeutic success within the patient population.

The frequency of various effects of pro-

cainamide in the patient population is shown schematically in Figure 12-4. A curve is also shown that represents the frequency of therapeutic effectiveness, that is, the frequency of effective therapy minus the frequency of toxic effects. This may be an inappropriate means of estimating the concentration at which therapeutic success is most probable. Perhaps the minor toxic effects should not be weighted equally against the desired response. Certainly, the major toxic effects should be given more weight. These are considerations of judgment.

Let us expand this concept philosophically using the information in Figure 12-4, adding hypersensitivity and assigning values to the responses according to our best judgment. Figure 12-5 shows the probabilities of each of the responses weighted by a judgmental factor versus the logarithm of

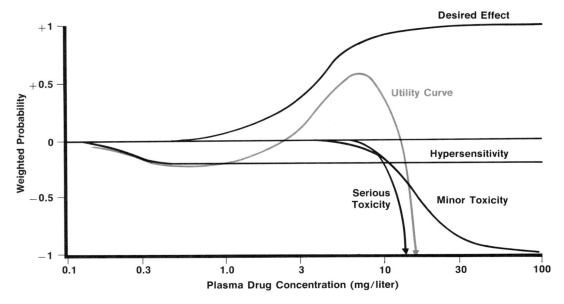

Figure 12-5. *Schematic diagram of the weighted probabilities of responses to procainamide versus the plasma concentration. The probabilities from Figure 12-4 (plus a hypothetical hypersensitivity reaction) are weighted by the following factors: desired effect, 1; hypersensitivity, −5; minor toxicity, −1; serious toxicity, −5. The algebraic sum of the weighted probabilities is the utility curve. According to this scheme, the highest probability of therapeutic success occurs at 7 mg/liter and concentrations below 2 mg/liter and above 12 mg/liter are potentially more harmful than beneficial.*

the plasma concentration. The factor is negative for undesirable effects and the converse. On algebraically adding the weighted probabilities a *utility curve* is obtained that simply shows the chance of therapeutic success as a function of the plasma concentration. Both the low and high concentrations have a negative utility, that is, at these concentrations the drug is potentially more harmful than helpful. There is an optimum concentration (7 mg/liter) at which therapeutic success is most likely, and there is a range of concentrations (about 4–10 mg/liter) in which the chances of successful therapy are high. This is the *therapeutic window* or *therapeutic concentration range*. Precise limits, of course, are not definable, particularly considering the subjective nature of the utility curve. Each drug has its own peculiar responses and the values assigned to these responses differ, but both the incidence of the drug effects and the relative importance

of each effect must be evaluated to determine the therapeutic concentration range.

There are problems associated with the acquisition of the incidence of the various responses. For example, the procainamide data were obtained in patients who were sometimes titrated with the drug. That is, the dosage was adjusted when the patient had not adequately responded or when toxicity was present. However, patients even on the usual dosage show a wide range of concentrations, leading one to question if selection of patients showing toxicity might have occurred. To avoid this bias, each of the patients should be titrated through all the responses. This is, of course, unacceptable. Our information on toxicity must come from the patient who, for one reason or another, exhibits toxicity because the drug concentration is excessive or who has an unusual response at a low concentration.

For the majority of patients, knowledge

of a drug's therapeutic plasma concentration and pharmacokinetics allows rapid establishment of a safe and efficacious dosage regimen. However, the narrower this range, the more difficult is the maintenance of the concentration of drug within it. The plasma concentration ranges associated with successful therapy of specific diseases are shown in Table 12-1 for a number of representative drugs. Relevant pharmacokinetic data for many of these drugs are also contained in Table 7-2.

Several points are worth noting about the data in Table 12-1. First, for most of these drugs, the therapeutic concentration range is very narrow; the upper and lower limits differ by a factor of only 2 or 3. Second, some drugs are used to treat several diseases, and the therapeutic plasma concentration range may differ with the disease. For example, a much higher plasma concentration of salicylic acid is needed to treat rheumatoid arthritis than is needed to relieve headache pain. Next, the upper limit of the plasma concentration may be either, like nortriptyline, a result of diminishing effectiveness at higher concentrations without noticeable signs of increasing toxicity, or, like digoxin, a result of the possibility of life-threatening toxicity. The upper limit may also be due to limiting effectiveness of the drug, as with the use of salicylic acid to relieve pain. Finally, toxicity may be either an extension of the pharmacologic property of the drug or totally dissociated from its therapeutic effect. The hemorrhagic tendency associated with an excessive plasma concentration of the oral anticoagulant, warfarin, is an example of the former; the ototoxicity caused by the antibiotic, gentamicin, is an example of the latter.

Therapeutic Correlates

So far, the plasma concentration has been assumed to be a better correlate of a

Table 12-1. Representative Drugs and the Ranges of Their Plasma Concentration Usually Associated with Successful Therapy

Drug	Disease	Concentration Range (mg/liter)
Acetazolamide	Glaucoma	10–30
Digitoxin	Congestive heart failure	0.01–0.02
Digoxin	Congestive heart failure	0.0006–0.002
Gentamicin	Gram-negative infection	1–10
Lidocaine	Ventricular arrhythmia	1.2–5.6
Lithium	Manic and recurrent depression	0.4–1.4mEq/liter[a]
Nortriptyline	Endogenous depression	0.05–0.14
Phenobarbital	Epilepsy	10–25
Phenytoin	Epilepsy	10–20
	Ventricular arrhythmias	10–20
Procainamide	Ventricular arrhythmias	4–8
Propranolol	Angina	0.01–0.1
Quinidine	Cardiac arrhythmias	3–6
Theophylline	Asthma and chronic obstructive airway disease	6–20
Warfarin	Thromboembolic diseases	1–4
Salicylic Acid	Aches and pains	20–100
	Rheumatoid arthritis	100–300
	Rheumatic fever	250–400

[a]Milliequivalents/liter.

drug's therapeutic response and toxicity in a population of patients needing a drug than any other parameter. The unbound plasma concentration should be an even better correlate, because it more accurately reflects the concentration at the site of action. However, since doses are administered, why not use dose as a therapeutic correlate? Certainly, in most cases, response, total and unbound plasma concentrations, and amount of drug in the body all increase with dose. Still, plasma concentration is expected to be a better correlate than dosage. This must be true following a single dose of drug, since with dose no account is taken of time. It is also true for continuous drug administration but for a different reason.

The objective of most drug therapy is to maintain a stable therapeutic response, usually by maintaining an effective plasma concentration. It should be recalled that a plateau concentration depends on the rate of entry of drug into the body and on total clearance (Chap. 8). In turn, the rate of entry is governed by the dosing rate and, if the drug is given extravascularly, by the availability. A smaller variability in the plasma concentration than in the dosing rate to achieve a given therapeutic effect gives credence to the use of plasma concentration as a therapeutic correlate. Studies with phenytoin illustrate this point.

Recall that Figure 1-5 showed the relationship between the steady-state serum concentration and the rate of administration of phenytoin, expressed as the daily dose, per kilogram of body weight. There are large deviations in the plasma concentration at any dosing rate; the serum concentration ranges from nearly 0 to 50 mg/liter, when the dosing rate is 6 mg/day/kg body weight. Had no correction been made for body weight, the deviations would have been even greater. In contrast, plasma concentration correlates reasonably well with effect. Thus seizures are usually effectively controlled at concentrations between 10 and 20 mg/liter; side

effects occur with increasing frequency and severity as the plasma concentration exceeds 20 mg/liter, as shown in Figure 12-6. The first sign of toxicity is usually nystagmus, which appears with a concentration of approximately 20 mg/liter; gait ataxia usually appears with a concentration approaching 30 mg/liter, and prolonged drowsiness and lethargy may be seen with concentrations in excess of 40 mg/liter.

An alternative way of looking at the level of drug is in terms of the amount in the body. Moreover, it may also be argued that the amount in the body is a better reflection of the pharmacologically active unbound plasma concentration than is the total plasma concentration (Chap. 4). Now, instead of a therapeutic plasma concentration range, one may refer to a range of the amount of drug in the body associated with efficacy and with minimal toxicity. While the idea of correlating response with the amount in the body is attractive, the problem is that in contrast to the plasma concentration the amount in the body is rarely known and cannot easily be measured.

Complicating Factors

Measurement of the plasma concentration of a drug, while useful, is not the universal panacea; often it correlates poorly with the measured response. Some examples of poor correlations and their explanations, where known, follow.

Active Metabolites. Unless these are also measured, poor correlations may exist. For example, based on its plasma concentration, propranolol is more active as a β-blocker when given as a single oral dose than when administered intravenously. This drug is highly cleared by the liver, and so in terms of the parent drug, the oral dose is poorly available. However, large amounts of metabolites, including an active species, 4-hydroxypropranolol, are formed during the absorption process, which explains the apparent discrepancy discussed previously.

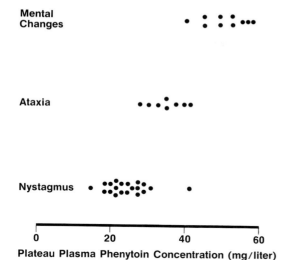

Figure 12-6. *The severity of the untoward effects of phenytoin increases in proportion to its concentration in plasma. (Modified from Kutt, H., Winters, W., Kokenge, R., and McDowell, F.: Diphenylhydantoin metabolism, blood levels, and toxicity, Arch. Neurol., 11: 642–648, 1964. Copyright 1964, American Medical Association.)*

Other examples of active metabolites are given in Table 10-1.

Tolerance and Acquired Resistance. The effectiveness of a drug can diminish with continual use. Acquired resistance denotes the diminished sensitivity of a population of cells (microorganisms, neoplasms) to a chemotherapeutic agent; tolerance denotes a diminished pharmacologic responsiveness to a drug. The degree of acquired resistance varies; it may be complete, thereby rendering the agent, e.g., an antibiotic, ineffective against a microorganism. The degree of tolerance also varies but is never complete. For example, within days or weeks of its repeated use, subjects develop a profound tolerance but not total unresponsiveness to the pharmacologic effects (euphoria, sedation, respiratory depression) of morphine. Tolerance can develop slowly; for example, tolerance to ethanol takes weeks. It can also occur acutely (tachyphylaxis). Thus, tolerance, expressed by a diminished cardiovascular responsiveness, develops within min-

utes following repetitive administration of many β-phenethylamine-type sympathomimetics. At any moment, a correlation might be found between the intensity of response and the plasma concentration of the drug, but the relationship varies with time.

Single-Dose Therapy. One dose of aspirin can often relieve a headache, which does not return even when all the drug has been eliminated. Other examples of effective single-dose therapy include the use of isoproterenol to relieve an acute asthmatic attack, colchicine to treat an acute gouty attack, nitroglycerin to relieve angina, and morphine to relieve acute pain. Although the specific mechanism of action is often poorly understood, the overall effect is known; the drug returns an out-of-balance physiologic system to within normal bounds. Thereafter, feedback control systems within the body maintain homeostasis. The need for the drug has now ended. In these instances of single-dose therapy, a correlation between the effect and the peak plasma concentration of the drug may exist, but beyond the peak, any such correlation is unlikely.

Time delays. It often takes some time for a measured response to reflect fully a given plasma concentration of drug. Until then, the continuously changing response makes any correlation between response and plasma concentration extremely difficult to establish. One source of the delay is the time required for equilibration to occur between drug in plasma and that at the site of action, usually in a tissue. This delay may be short if the site is well perfused and freely accessible; when effective, lidocaine suppresses ventricular arrhythmias within a few minutes of giving a bolus dose; thiopental induces anesthesia in about the same time. When the target organ resides in a poorly perfused tissue, or when the drug diffuses slowly into the site, the delay may be many hours. For example, the maximum cardiac effects of digoxin are not seen for an hour or more after administering an intravenous bolus of the drug.

Another source of delay can arise when the response monitored is an indirect measure of drug effect. A change in blood pressure is an indirect measure of either a change in peripheral resistance, cardiac output, or both. Plasma uric acid is another example; here, the direct effect is an alteration in uric acid synthesis or elimination. The delay between the attainment of a plasma concentration and the maximal indirect effect varies. Full response in blood pressure to a change in peripheral resistance or in cardiac output occurs within minutes, whereas full response of plasma uric acid to changes in its synthesis or elimination takes hours.

Yet another example of an indirect effect is the change in the one-step prothrombin time to coumarin oral anticoagulants. The more direct effect of these agents, of which warfarin is the most widely prescribed, is to inhibit synthesis of the four vitamin K-dependent clotting factors (Factors II, VII, IX, X). Anticoagulant therapy is followed with the one-stage prothrombin time, a test that measures three of these factors (II, VII, X). When the one-stage prothrombin complex activity is measured, the maximal effect is seen one to two days after a bolus dose of warfarin (Fig. 12-7).

In many of these examples of time delays, once the cause of the delay has been identified, it is possible, by analysis of the data, to establish the relationship between drug concentration and the direct effect. For example, appropriate treatment of the data in Figure 12-7 yields the classical relationship for the direct effect of warfarin; that is, the inhibition of synthesis of the prothrombin complex is directly related to the logarithm of the plasma concentration of warfarin (Fig. 12-8).

The responses to standard doses of warfarin change in disease states and following the coadministration of other drugs. By ascertaining the relationship between the plasma concentration and the direct effect,

distinctions can be made between changes in the pharmacokinetics of warfarin and changes in the responsiveness of the clotting system to this drug. For example, the diminished response to doses of warfarin, when coadministered with heptabarbital, was found to be caused by increased elimination of and not by a change in the direct response to the drug (Fig. 12-8).

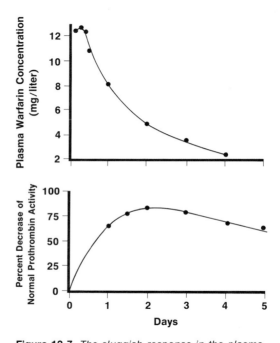

Figure 12-7. *The sluggish response in the plasma prothrombin complex activity to inhibition of its synthesis by warfarin reflects the slow elimination of this complex. For the first two days after giving warfarin, the complex activity steadily decreases. During the first day, the concentration of warfarin is sufficient to almost completely block complex synthesis. As warfarin levels fall, the synthesis rate of the complex increases and by 48 hours equals the rate of degradation of the complex. Thereafter, with the synthesis rate exceeding the rate of degradation, the complex activity rises and eventually, when all the warfarin has been eliminated, it will return to the normal pre-warfarin steady-state level. The data points are the average following the oral administration of 1.5 mg warfarin sodium/kg body weight in 5 male volunteers. (From Nagashima, R., O'Reilly, R.A., and Levy, G.: Kinetics of pharmacologic effects in man: The anticoagulant action of warfarin. Clin. Pharmacol. Ther., 10: 22–35, 1969.)*

Level-Duration-Intensity Relationships

An effect lasts as long as the minimum effective level at the site of action is exceeded. The duration of effect is, therefore, a function of dose and of rate of drug removal from the site of action. Removal can result either from redistribution of drug from the site to less well-perfused tissues, or from its elimination from the body. Here, the discussion is limited to the second situation (where elimination solely controls loss from the site of action).

Single Bolus Dose

Consider a drug that is eliminated by first-order kinetics, characterized by a rate constant k, and whose metabolites are inac-

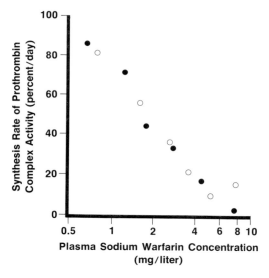

Figure 12-8. *Pretreatment with heptabarbital (400 mg daily for 15 days, starting 10 days before warfarin) decreased the response to a standard dose of warfarin, but failed to alter the linear relationship between the synthesis rate of prothrombin complex activity and the logarithm of the concentration of warfarin in a 21-year-old normal subject; control experiment (○); with heptabarbital (●). (From Levy, G., O'Reilly, R.A., Aggeler, P.M., and Keech, G.M.: Pharmacokinetic analysis of the effect of barbiturate on the anticoagulant action of warfarin in man. Clin. Pharmacol. Ther., 11: 372–377, 1970.)*

tive (Fig. 12-9). After a bolus dose, the amount of drug in the body falls exponentially, that is

$$Ab = \text{Dose} \cdot e^{-kt} \qquad 1$$

Eventually, a time is reached, the duration of action, t_D, when the amount of drug in the body falls to a value, Ab_{min}, below which the response is less than that minimally desired. The relationship between Ab_{min} and t_D is given by appropriately substituting into the preceding equation; thus,

$$Ab_{min} = \text{Dose} \cdot e^{-kt_D} \qquad 2$$

Upon rearrangement and taking logarithms an expression for t_D is thus obtained

$$t_D = \frac{2.3}{k} (\log \text{Dose} - \log Ab_{min}) \qquad 3$$

According to this relationship a plot of duration of effect against log dose should yield a straight line with a slope of $2.3/k$ and an intercept, at zero duration of effect, of log Ab_{min} (Fig. 12.9, inset). Evidence supporting these expectations is forthcoming. Thus, the duration of action of many local anesthetics is proportional to the logarithm of the injected dose. The muscle relaxant effect of succinylcholine also conforms to this last equation. Figure 12-10 shows the time to 10 (T_{10}), 50 (T_{50}), and 90 (T_{90}) percent recovery of muscle twitch (a measure of neuromuscular block) after the intravenous injection of 0.5, 1, 2, and 4 mg/kg bolus doses of succinylcholine in man. As expected, the slope, $2.3/k$, is independent of the end point chosen; the choice of end point only influences the value of Ab_{min}. The value of k, estimated from the slope, is 0.2 min^{-1}; the half-life is 3.5 min. Clinically, this short half-life is an asset in the use of succinylcholine. It is often given by constant infusion. Changes in the degree of muscle paralysis can be effected within 3 to 4 half-lives, that is, within approximately 10 min of changing the rate of infusion. This procedure allows for fine and continuous control of the effect. Also once the infusion is stopped, the patient promptly recovers.

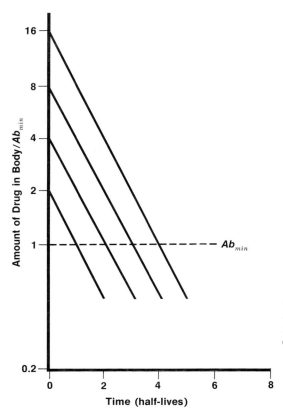

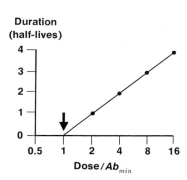

Figure 12-9. *The duration of action increases by one half-life with each doubling of the dose. Duration is proportional to the logarithm of the dose (inset).*

To further appreciate the last equation, consider the following statement: "The duration of action increases by one half-life with each doubling of dose." This must be true. To prove that this is so, let a dose, D, produce a duration of action, t_D. When twice the dose is given the level in the body falls by one-half in one half-life, that is, to D; the duration of action beyond one half-life must be t_D. The total duration of action produced by the larger dose is, therefore, $t_{1/2} + t_D$. The increase in the duration of action upon doubling the dose is, therefore, one half-life. For example, since a dose of 0.5 mg/kg of succinylcholine results in a T_{10} of approximately 4.5 min, the duration following 1 mg/kg is 8 min (Fig. 12-10). The increase in the time to recover, 3.5 min, is the half-life of succinylcholine at the site of action. Confirm that the same value is obtained with each doubling of dose on either the T_{10}, the T_{50}, or the T_{90} curve.

Multiple Bolus Doses

As noted previously, one way of extending the duration of action is to increase the dose. This approach, however, rapidly results in a condition of diminishing returns, especially for a drug with a short half-life and a low therapeutic index. For example, when the duration of action is extended by two half-lives, the quadrupled dose required may produce too great a response or substantially increase the chance of toxicity.

Instead of increasing the dose, a safer approach is to give the same dose each time the effect reaches a predetermined level, for example, just when the effect is wearing off (Fig. 12-11). With this alternative approach, an increase in duration of effect and, if the response is graded, an increase in intensity of effect with the second dose is expected. The reason is readily apparent. Immediately after giving the second dose, the

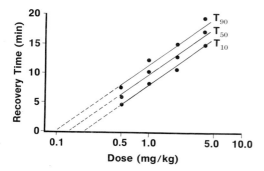

Figure 12-10. *The time to recover from succinyl-choline paralysis is proportional to the logarithm of the dose injected. T_{90}, T_{50}, and T_{10} indicate 90, 50, and 10 percent recovery of muscle twitch (a measure of the degree of return of muscle function). (Redrawn from the figure by Levy, G.: Kinetics of pharmacologic activity of succinylcholine in man. J. Pharm. Sci. 56: 1687–1688, 1967. The original data are from Walts, L.F., and Dillon, J.B.: Clinical studies of succinylcholine chloride. Anesthesiology, 28: 372–376, 1967.)*

the dose, very little remains from the first dose when the second dose is given, and little increase in effect, or duration of action, is expected. In contrast, large increases in effect and duration are expected when the effect from the first dose wears off before much drug is lost.

No further increase in the intensity of the effect or the duration of action is anticipated with subsequent doses, because the amount of drug in the body always returns to the same value, Ab_{min}, before the next dose. Stated differently, from the second dose onward, during each dosing interval, the amount lost equals the dose given. When the duration of action does increase with the third and subsequent doses, the effect is probably terminating during the distribution phase of the drug.

Level-Intensity-Time Relationships

An effect subsides when the concentration of drug at the site of action falls. How the intensity of effect varies with time therefore depends, as does the duration of

amount of drug in the body is not the dose, but Dose + Ab_{min}. How much the intensity or the duration of effect increases, therefore, depends upon the magnitude of the dose and Ab_{min}. If Ab_{min} is small relative to

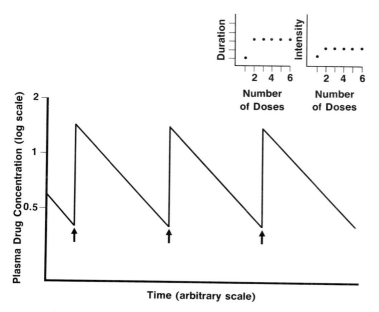

Figure 12-11. *The duration and the intensity of a graded response increase with the second, but not with subsequent bolus doses, when each dose is given, indicated by an arrow, at the time the effect (or concentration) reaches a predetermined value.*

effect, upon the dose and the rate of removal of drug from the active site. The intensity also depends upon the region of the response-concentration curve covered during the decline. Here, as before, the discussion is limited to the situation in which the response-concentration relationship is maintained at all times and in which the drug is distributed in a single compartment and is eliminated by first-order kinetics.

To appreciate the relationship between dose, effect, and time, consider the events, depicted in Figure 12-12, that follow the intravenous administration of a 10-mg bolus dose of a drug that has a half-life of 1 hour. A plot of the intensity of the response against the logarithm of the amount of drug in the body is shown in the inset; for convenience the plot is divided into three regions. In *region 1,* up to 20 percent maximal

response, the intensity of response is proportional to the amount of drug in the body; in *region 2,* covering 20 to 80 percent maximal response, it is proportional to the logarithm of the amount of drug in the body; and in *region 3,* the response slowly approaches the maximal value despite large changes in the amount of drug in the body. Since the size of dose given lies in region 3, although the amount of drug in the body falls rapidly within the first hour, the intensity of response remains almost constant and maximal. Only after 2 hours, when the amount of drug in the body falls below 3 mg and response falls below 80 percent of maximal response, does response begin to decline more rapidly. Then, for the next $2\frac{1}{2}$ hours, on passing through region 2, response declines at an almost constant rate of 22 percent/hour. The reason for this constant decline in response, as the drug

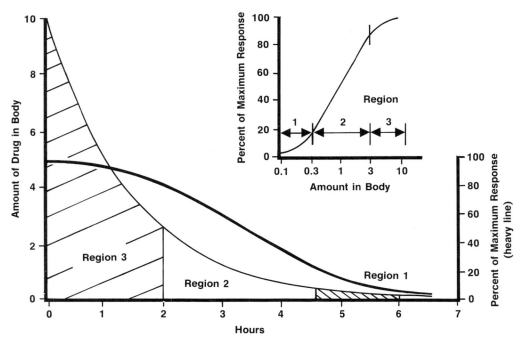

Figure 12-12. *The decline in the intensity of pharmacologic effect with time, following a single large dose, has three parts corresponding to the regions of the dose-response curve (inset). Initially, in* region 3, *the response remains almost maximal despite a 50 percent fall in the amount of drug in the body. Thereafter, as long as the amount of drug in the body is within* region 2, *the intensity of response declines linearly with time. Only when the amount of drug in the body falls into* region 1, *does the decline in response parallel that of drug in the body.*

levels decay exponentially, is apparent from the inset of Figure 12-12 in that during region 2

$$\text{Intensity} = m \cdot \log Ab + c \qquad 4$$

where m is the slope of the intensity-log (amount of drug in the body) curve. The value of the constant, c, is obtained by extrapolating the linear regression of the intensity versus logarithm of Ab to zero intensity. The constant is the intercept on the log Ab axis and may be defined as the minimum effective dose, assuming that the intensity of a response is always proportional to the logarithm of the amount of drug in the body.

Substituting $Ab_o \cdot e^{-kt}$ for Ab in Equation 4, where Ab_o is the amount of drug in the body upon entering region 2 from region 3, and collecting terms, therefore yields:

$$\text{Intensity} = (m \cdot \log Ab_o + c) - \frac{m \cdot k \cdot t}{2.3} \qquad 5$$

Letting I_o be the intensity of response when the amount, Ab_o, is in the body,

$$\text{Intensity} = I_o - \frac{m \cdot k \cdot t}{2.3} \qquad 6$$

Thus, *the intensity of effect falls linearly with time* in region 2. It should be noted that the rate of decline, $m \cdot k/2.3$, depends on both the slope of the intensity-log (amount of drug in the body) curve and the half-life of the drug. In this instance, for example, $m = 72$ (in region 2, the intensity of response changes by 72 percent of maximal response for a 1-log change in Ab), and since $k = 0.7$ hour^{-1}, a constant rate in the decline of activity of 22 percent/hour is anticipated.

Beyond 5 hours, when the amount of drug in the body has fallen below 0.3 mg and entered region 1, the fall in response parallels that of the drug. In theory, the drug's half-life can be determined from the intensity of response-time data in this region; it is the time for the intensity of a response to fall by one-half. In practice,

however, measurements in this region are too imprecise, being too close to a variable baseline to permit accurate assessment of the half-life. Let us now extend the foregoing considerations to two examples: the degree of muscle paralysis produced by succinylcholine and the lowering of blood pressure produced by minoxidil.

Changes in the degree of muscle paralysis with time, following a 0.5 mg/kg bolus dose of succinylcholine to a subject, are shown in Figure 12-13. The one-minute delay, before onset of action, is probably accounted for in part by the time taken for the drug to circulate from the injection site to the muscle and in part by the time taken for succinylcholine to diffuse into the neuromuscular junction. Once at the site, however, full response ensues promptly; the time between onset and total paralysis is less than one minute. Total paralysis is then maintained for a full two minutes despite the continual rapid hydrolysis of this agent. Subsequently, the effect subsides. As predicted, between 80 and 20 percent of maximal response, the effect declines at a constant rate: in this instance, 22% per min. At higher doses, the duration of action is longer (Fig. 12-14), but once 80 percent of maximal response is reached, the amount of drug in the body should be the same and independent of the dose administered, and the subsequent rate of decline in the intensity of effect should be constant. This is indeed so. Knowing the rate of decline ($m \cdot k/2.3$) and also the value of k (from the duration-log dose plot, Fig. 12-10), the value for m, the slope of the intensity of the response-log (amount of drug in the body) curve can be calculated; for succinylcholine, $m = 250$. By separating k from m in this manner, the distinction between elimination and receptor interactions, as the cause for a prolongation in the rate of decline in the intensity of response following a dose of succinylcholine, can be made.

Figure 12-15 shows the lowering of the mean arterial blood pressure (MAP) in a patient with a baseline MAP of 157 mm Hg

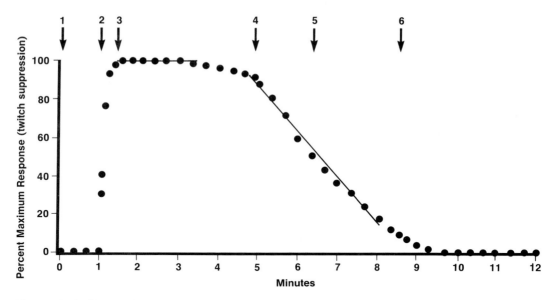

Figure 12-13. *Changes in the degree of muscle paralysis (assessed as the suppression of a twitch produced in response to ulnar nerve stimulation) following an intravenous bolus dose of 0.5 mg/kg succinylcholine to a patient. 1, Time of injection; 2, onset of twitch suppression; 3, complete twitch suppression; 4, 5, 6, recovery of twitch to 10 percent (T_{10}), 50 percent (T_{50}), and 90 percent (T_{90}) of the maximum twitch height. The straight lines cover the region of maximum response and that where the response declines essentially linearly with time. (Modified from Walts, L.F., and Dillon, J.B.: Clinical studies on succinylcholine chloride. Anesthesiology, 28: 372–376, 1967.)*

following 10- and 25-mg oral doses of minoxidil, a potent antihypertensive drug. A constant decay in the effect, given by the return of the MAP toward the baseline value of approximately 1 mm Hg/hour, is evident following each dose; the intensity of the response lies between 20 and 80 percent of the maximal value. The single dose information given in Figure 12-15 can be used to plan a dosage regimen for minoxidil.

Dosage Regimens and Response

Regimens are designed to maintain a therapeutic response for the duration of therapy. Several schemes for determining the appropriate regimen are discussed in the next and subsequent chapters. These schemes use pharmacokinetic information derived from single-dose studies. A similar approach may be taken using only phar-

macologic data. For example, assume that the objectives of minoxidil therapy are to give an initial dose to immediately reduce the MAP to 95 mm Hg and then to give supplementary doses at a frequency that maintains the MAP between 95 and 105 mm Hg. A dosage regimen to meet these objectives can be estimated using the limited information in Figure 12-15. The baseline MAP in the patient is 157 mm Hg. The initial dose must lower the MAP by approximately 60 mm Hg, which is achieved by giving 10 mg minoxidil orally. Since the effect wears off at the rate of approximately 1 mm Hg/hour, by 12 hours the MAP has risen to the upper limit of 105 mm Hg. A supplementary dose must then be given to reduce the MAP by 10 mm Hg back down to 95 mm Hg. The required supplementary dose may be estimated from the response-log dose plot, admittedly constructed with limited data, shown in the inset in Figure 12-15. By in-

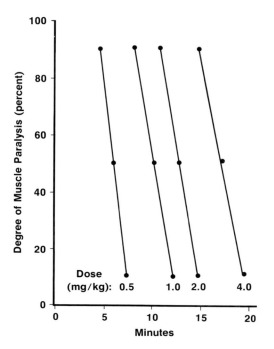

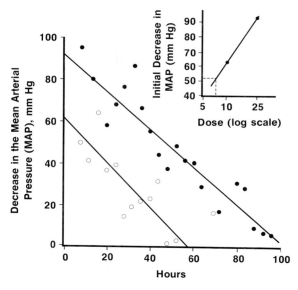

Figure 12-14. *Irrespective of the dose of succinyl-choline administered, once 90 percent of maximal paralysis is reached, the rate of decline in muscle paralysis is constant at 22 percent/min. (Redrawn from the figure by Levy, G.: Kinetics of pharmaco-logic activity of succinylcholine in man. J. Pharm. Sci., 56: 1687–1688, 1967. The original data are from Walts, F., and Dillon, J.B.: Clinical studies on succinylcholine chloride. Anesthesiology, 28: 372–376, 1967.)*

Figure 12-15. *The degree of lowering of the mean arterial blood pressure (MAP), in a patient with a baseline MAP of 157 mm Hg, falls at a constant rate following 10(○) and 25(●) mg single oral doses of minoxidil. In the inset, the extrapolated value for the initial lowering of the MAP is plotted against the logarithm of the dose. (From Shen, D., O'Malley, K., Gibaldi, M., and McNay, J.L.: Phar-macodynamics of minoxidil as a guide for individ-ualizing dosage regimens in hypertension. Clin. Pharmacol. Ther., 17: 593–598, 1975.)*

terpolation, it can be seen that the amount of drug in the body at 105 mm Hg, that is, when the MAP is depressed by 52 mm Hg, is 7.5 mg. Thus, the supplementary dose is 2.5mg, and it must be given every 12 hours if the MAP is to be maintained between 95 and 105 mm Hg.

Study Problems

*(**Answers to Study Problems can be found in Appendix G.**)*

1. An experimental anesthetic agent, CI-581, produces coma in human subjects. Table 12-2 shows the mean duration of coma as a function of the intravenous dose of CI-581 administered (Domino, E.F., Chodoff, P., and Corssen, G.: Clin. Pharmacol. Ther., 6: 279–291, 1965).

Table 12-2

Dose (mg/kg)	0.5	1.0	1.5	2.0
Duration of coma (min)	1.7	5.8	9.0	10.0

Several subjects, immediately after the initial coma had ended following the 1.0 mg/kg dose, received a second 1.0 mg/kg dose. The duration of coma associated with this second dose was 8.0 min.

(a) Determine the minimum dose of CI-581 required to produce coma.

(b) Is the increase in duration of coma seen with the second dose consistent with the information obtained following the single dose?

2. A compound is given as an intravenous bolus to a patient requiring a minimum plasma concentration of 40 mg/liter for a therapeutic effect. Given that: Dose = 1000 mg; $k = 0.10$ hour^{-1}; $V = 8$ liters,

(a) Calculate how long the clinical effect will last with this dose.

(b) Calculate how long the clinical effect will last following a 2000-mg dose.

(c) Determine the duration of effect following a 1000-mg dose, if $k = 0.05$ hour^{-1} and the change in the k is a result of (1) a twofold decrease in clearance; (2) a doubling of the volume of distribution by increased nonspecific tissue binding.

(d) Does doubling the dose of a drug yield the same change in duration of clinical effect as doubling the half-life?

3. The following average data (Table 12-3) for hexobarbital sleeping time were obtained in various animal species after intraperitoneal administration of 100 mg/kg:

Table 12-3

	Species		
	Mouse	Rabbit	Rat
Duration of action (min)	12	49	90
Hexobarbital plasma half-life (min)	19	60	140

(a) Assuming (1) that an intraperitoneal injection approximates an intravenous injection; (2) that the drug is eliminated by simple first-order kinetics; and (3) that the extrapolated initial plasma concentration is the same in all species, prepare a plot of the relative plasma concentrations with time in each species on one-cycle semilogarithmic graph paper.

(b) From the graph find the relative plasma concentration in each species when the animal awoke (sleeping time or duration of action). Comment on your findings with reference to the statement "species variations for many drugs can be decreased considerably if plasma concentration rather than doses are compared with the pharmacologic effect."

(c) What ratio of hexobarbital doses is needed to ensure that the sleeping time in both the mouse and the rat is (1) 12 min; (2) 90 min.?

4. Assuming that the data presented in Figure 12-15 are applicable, design a suitable dosage regimen of minoxidil to reduce immediately a patient's MAP of 180 mm Hg to 95 mm Hg and then to maintain the MAP between 95 and 105 mm Hg.

13

dosage regimens

Objectives

The reader will be able to:

1. **Develop a dosage regimen from knowledge of the pharmacokinetics of a drug.**

2. **Evaluate a dosage regimen of a drug from a pharmacokinetic point of view.**

3. **Predict the rate and extent of drug accumulation for a given regimen of fixed dose and fixed interval.**

4. **Evaluate a prolonged-release formulation from a kinetic point of view.**

5. **Derive pharmacokinetic parameters for a drug from plasma concentration (or urine) data following multiple-dosing therapy.**

IN the previous chapter, relationships between the amount of drug in the body or the plasma drug concentration and the pharmacologic or toxic responses were established. This chapter covers the pharmacokinetic principles upon which the appropriate dosage regimens for drugs are established. The overall aims and objectives of drug therapy are also considered.

Empirical and Kinetic Approaches to Drug Therapy

The questions of how much drug and how often to administer it for a given therapeutic purpose are not easily answered. Basically two approaches have been used to answer these questions: empirical and kinetic.

Empirical Approach

The empirical approach involves the evaluation of therapeutic response following the adjustment of both dose and dosing interval. The merit of each regimen is frequently compared first to no regimen at all, to determine if a drug is of value, and then to alternative regimens to determine which regimen is preferred. Appropriate consideration must be given to side effects and to toxicity. After experience with a sufficient number of subjects, fairly accurate predictions can be made. However, much information must be gathered and in the process some dosage regimens may have produced toxicity while others may have been ineffective. Such certainly has been the history of a number of drugs including the digitalis glycosides.

Kinetic Approach

The kinetic approach is based on the hypothesis that therapeutic and toxic responses are related to the amount of drug in the body or to the plasma drug concentration. Given pharmacokinetic data following a single dose, the levels of drug in the body following multiple doses can be estimated. The appropriateness of a particular dosage regimen can then be evaluated in terms of the resultant time course of drug in the body and the known relationships among drug levels, therapeutic response, and toxic effects. Ultimately, however, the value of a dosage regimen must be assessed by the therapeutic response produced. Pharmacokinetics simply facilitates the rapid achievement of an appropriate dosage regimen and serves as a useful means of evaluating existing dosage regimens.

What Constitutes a Therapeutic Dosage Regimen

A therapeutic dosage regimen is basically derived from the kinds of considerations shown in Table 13-1. One consideration includes those factors that relate to both efficacy and safety of the drug, that is, its pharmacodynamics and toxicology. Another consideration is how the body acts on the drug and its dosage form, the essence of biopharmaceutics-pharmacokinetics. A third consideration is that of the clinical state of the patient and his total therapeutic regimen. A fourth category includes all other factors such as genetic differences, tolerance, and drug interactions. All of these considerations are, of course, interrelated and interdependent.

The usual dosage regimen is either one in which the drug is administered continuously to maintain therapeutic levels or one in which therapeutic levels are achieved intermittently. Intermittent levels may be called for in maintenance therapy if only periodic therapeutic levels are required (this has been argued as a desirable condition for antibiotic treatment of some infectious diseases), if tolerance develops to the drug, or if the therapeutic effects of the drug persist and increase in intensity even though the drug rapidly disappears.

For the continuous maintenance of therapeutic amounts of drug in the body, the initial and maintenance doses must be given at dosing intervals that keep the amount above a minimum effective level and below a level producing excessive side effects and toxicity. To design a dosage regimen to maintain therapeutic amounts the following factors must be considered: the minimum therapeutic dose, the therapeutic index (ratio of toxic dose to therapeutic dose), availability and the half-life of the drug.

Drug Accumulation

Drugs are most commonly prescribed to be taken on a fixed-dose, fixed-time-interval basis: e.g., 100 mg daily or 25 mg three times a day. In association with this kind of intermittent administration, the levels in the body fluctuate and, similarly to an infusion, rise toward a plateau.

Consider the simplest situation of a dosage regimen composed of equal bolus doses administered intravenously at fixed and equal time intervals. Curve A of Figure 13-1 shows how the amount of drug in the body varies with time when each dose is given successively twice every half-life. Under these conditions the drug accumulates substantially. Accumulation occurs because drug from previous doses has not been completely removed. The rate and extent of accumulation can be ascertained from reasonably uncomplicated pharmacokinetic relationships.

Maxima and Minima on Accumulation to the Plateau

To appreciate the phenomenon of accumulation, let us examine what happens to a drug when given intravenously, in a 100-mg

Table 13-1. Factors That Determine a Dosage Regimen

Activity-Toxicity		Pharmacokinetics
Minimum therapeutic dose		Absorption
Toxic dose		Distribution
Therapeutic index		Metabolism
Side effects		Excretion
Dose-response relationships		

Dosage Regimen

Clinical Factors		Other Factors
Clinical state of patient	Management of therapy	Tolerance-dependence
Age, weight, urine pH	Multiple drug therapy	Pharmacogenetics-idiosyncrasy
Condition being treated	Convenience of regimen	Drug interactions
Existence of other disease states	Compliance of patient	

bolus dose, every elimination half-life. Table 13-2 lists the amounts of drug in the body just after each dose and just before the next dose is given; these values correspond to the maximum (Ab_{max}) and the minimum (Ab_{min}) amounts obtained within each dosing interval. The corresponding values during the first dosing interval are 100 mg and 50 mg, respectively. The maximum amount of drug in the second dosing interval ($Ab_{2,max}$), 150 mg, is the dose (100 mg) plus the amount of drug remaining from the previous dose (50 mg). The amount of drug remaining at the end of the second dosing interval ($Ab_{2,min}$), 75 mg, is the amount remaining from the first dose, 25 mg (100 mg × ½ × ½), because two half-lives have elapsed since administration), plus the amount remaining from the second dose, 50 mg. Alternatively, the value, 75 mg, may simply be calculated by recognizing that one-half of the amount just

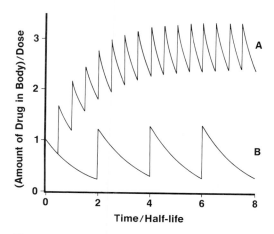

Figure 13-1. *Dosing frequency controls the degree of drug accumulation, but not the time to reach a plateau. Curve A, Intravenous bolus dose administered once twice every half-life; curve B, same bolus dose administered once every two half-lives. Note that time is expressed in half-life units.*

Table 13-2. Amount in Body When 100 mg of Drug Is Given Every Half-life

Dose	1	2	3	4	5	6	7	8
Maximum amount in body (Ab_{max}), mg	100	150	175	188	194	197	199	200
Minimum amount in body (Ab_{min}), mg	50	75	88	94	97	99	100	100

after the second dose, 150 mg, remains at the end of that dosing interval. Upon repeating this procedure, it is readily seen that drug accumulation, viewed in terms of either the maximum or the minimum amount in the body, continues until a limit is reached. At the limit, the amount lost in each interval equals the amount gained, the dose. For this reason drug in the body is said to be at *steady state* or at *plateau*. In this example, the maximum, denoted by $Ab_{ss,max}$, and the minimum, denoted by $Ab_{ss,min}$, amounts in the body at steady state are 200 mg and 100 mg, respectively. This must be so since at plateau, the difference between the maximum and minimum amounts is the dose, 100 mg, and since at the end of the interval, one half-life, the amount must be half that at the beginning.

The foregoing considerations can be expanded for the more general situation in which a drug is given at a dosing interval, τ, which may be different from the half-life. The corresponding general equations for the maximum and minimum amounts of drug in the body after the Nth dose ($Ab_{N,max}$; $Ab_{N,min}$) and at plateau ($Ab_{ss,max}$; $Ab_{ss,min}$) are

$$\text{Maximum amount in body after } N\text{th dose} = \text{Dose} \cdot \left[\frac{1 - (\frac{1}{2})^{N\epsilon}}{1 - (\frac{1}{2})^{\epsilon}} \right] \quad 1$$

$$\text{Minimum amount in body after } N\text{th dose} = \text{Dose} \cdot \left[\frac{1 - (\frac{1}{2})^{N\epsilon}}{1 - (\frac{1}{2})^{\epsilon}} \right] (\tfrac{1}{2})^{\epsilon} \quad 2$$

$$\text{Maximum amount in body at plateau} = \frac{\text{Dose}}{1 - (\frac{1}{2})^{\epsilon}} \quad 3$$

$$\text{Minimum amount in body at plateau} = \text{Dose} \cdot \left[\frac{1}{1 - (\frac{1}{2})^{\epsilon}} - 1 \right] \quad 4$$

where ϵ is the dosing interval expressed in elimination half-lives, that is, $\epsilon = \tau/t_{1/2}$. The derivation of these general equations is given in Appendix E.

For the simple situation in which drug is given every half-life, $\epsilon = 1$, it can readily be seen from Equations 3 and 4, that the maximum amount at plateau is twice the dose and that the minimum amount at plateau is the dose itself, a conclusion previously drawn.

To further appreciate the phenomenon of accumulation, consider the example of digitoxin, used in the treatment of congestive heart failure. For the purpose of the following calculation, consider an oral dosage regimen of 0.1 mg daily (the usual rate associated with the therapeutic use of this drug). Furthermore, assume that absorption is complete and virtually instantaneous, simulating intravenous bolus administration.

Let us now examine one aspect of digitoxin accumulation, the conditions at plateau. The solution of the mathematical operations of Equations 1 through 4 becomes simple with the use of the table of $(\frac{1}{2})^n$ functions in Appendix F-II. One first calculates a value of ϵ. The average half-life of digitoxin is 6 days, therefore, $\epsilon = (1 \text{ day})/(6 \text{ days})$ or 0.17. The value of the function $1/[1 - (\frac{1}{2})^{\epsilon}]$, that is, the maximum amount at plateau divided by the dose, $Ab_{ss,max}/\text{Dose}$, is 9.0. Thus the maximum amount of digitoxin at plateau is 0.9 mg and the minimum amount at plateau is 0.8 mg, since the dose (0.1 mg) is the amount lost during a dosing interval. Digitoxin clearly undergoes considerable accumulation when given daily. Accumulation is sufficiently extensive, so that distinction between the maximum and minimum amounts of drug in the body at the plateau is perhaps not meaningful.

These calculations of the maximum and minimum values at plateau are strictly only applicable to intravascular bolus administration. They are also applicable to extravascular administration when the absorption is complete and virtually instantaneous. The discussion that follows deals with a less restrictive view of accumulation, which applies to all routes of administration.

Average Amount in Body at Plateau and Accumulation Ratio

In many respects the accumulation of digitoxin or for that matter of any drug on administering multiple doses, is the same as that observed following a constant intravenous infusion. The average amount in the body at steady state, plateau, is readily calculated using the steady-state concept; the average *rate in* must equal the average *rate out*. That is, during each dosing interval the amount eliminated from the body is equal to the amount absorbed. The average rate in is $F \cdot (Dose/\tau)$. The average rate out is $k \cdot Ab_{av}$, where Ab_{av} is the average amount of drug in the body over the dosing interval at plateau. Therefore,

$$\frac{F \cdot \text{Dose}}{\tau} = k \cdot Ab_{av} \qquad 5$$

or

$$\frac{F \cdot \text{Dose}}{\tau} = Cl \cdot C_{av} \qquad 6$$

where C_{av} is the average plasma concentration at the plateau. Since $k = 0.7/t_{1/2}$, it also follows that

$$Ab_{av} = 1.44 \cdot F \cdot t_{1/2} \cdot (\text{Dose}/\tau) \qquad 7$$

and

$$C_{av} = \frac{F}{Cl} \cdot \frac{\text{Dose}}{\tau} \qquad 8$$

These are useful relationships; they show how the average amount of drug in the body at steady state depends upon rate of administration, $Dose/\tau$, availability, and half-life, and how the corresponding average concentration depends upon the first two factors and upon clearance.

Drug accumulation is not a phenomenon that depends upon the property of a drug, nor are there drugs that are cumulative and others that are not. Accumulation, in particular the extent of it, is a result of the frequency of administration (half-life of the drug relative to the dosing interval), as shown in Figure 13-2.

If the average amount of drug at plateau is related to the amount absorbed from each dose, an *accumulation index* or *accumulation ratio*, R_{AC} is obtained. This index is readily derived from Equation 7 by dividing by $F \cdot \text{Dose}$.

$$R_{AC} = \frac{Ab_{av}}{F \cdot \text{Dose}} = 1.44 \cdot t_{1/2}/\tau \qquad 9$$

As an example, again consider the accumulation of digitoxin. For this drug,

$$R_{AC} = \frac{1.44 \times 6 \text{ days}}{1 \text{ day}} = 8.6$$

Therefore, the average amount in the body at plateau, assuming $F = 1$, is $R_{AC} \cdot \text{Dose}$ or 0.86 mg.

From Equations 3 and 4 the maximum and minimum amounts of digitoxin at plateau are 0.91 mg and 0.81 mg, respectively. Notice that the average amount lies midway between these amounts. Since calculating the average value is the much simpler of the procedures, under these circumstances the maximum and minimum values can easily be calculated by adding and subtracting one-half the maintenance dose absorbed, respectively, to the average value. With digitoxin, for example, $Ab_{ss,max}$ is $0.86 + 0.05 = 0.91$ mg; $Ab_{ss,min}$ is $0.86 - 0.05 = 0.81$ mg. This simple

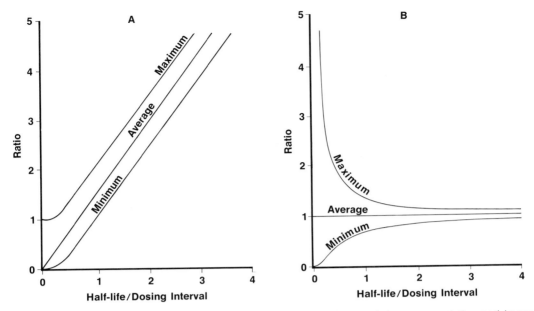

Figure 13-2. *More frequent administration results in a greater degree of drug accumulation and hence smaller relative differences among the maximum* ($Ab_{ss,max}$)*, average* (Ab_{av})*, and minimum* ($Ab_{ss,min}$) *amounts of drug in the body at plateau. Note that frequency is the reciprocal of the dosing interval expressed here in half-life units. A, Ratios of the maximum, average, and minimum amounts of drug at plateau to the maintenance dose following chronic intravenous bolus administration, as a function of the dosing frequency. B, Ratios of maximum to average, and minimum to average amounts of drug in the body as a function of the dosing frequency.*

method can be used as long as the dosing interval does not exceed the half-life.

According to the definition of R_{AC}, accumulation may be avoided by giving a dose of drug every 1.44 half-lives or less often. For example, to avoid accumulation, a drug with a half-life of 16 hours should be given once daily. Giving the drug less frequently results in an accumulation index of less than 1, but obviously, in terms of maximum and minimum levels, drug still accumulates on such regimens. Any index of accumulation, based upon peaks or troughs, is sensitive, however, to the rate of drug absorption and often is not as convenient as the definition of R_{AC} which, being based on the average value, is independent of route of administration and rate of absorption.

Comparison of Maximum, Average, and Minimum Amounts at Plateau

Fluctuation in the amount of drug in the body, like accumulation, depends upon both the frequency of drug administration and the half-life of the drug. Fluctuation also depends upon the rate of absorption; it is greatest for intravascular bolus administration. Figure 13-2A illustrates how the maximum, minimum, and average amounts of drug in the body at plateau depend upon the frequency of administration. Several observations are pertinent: (1) The average amount increases in direct proportion to the frequency of administration (the inverse of the dosing interval). (2) The maximum amount is not much greater than the dose if the drug is administered less frequently than once every three half-lives, $t_{1/2}/\tau = 0.33$ or less. Most of the drug from all previous doses has been eliminated before the next dose is administered. (3) Defining fluctuation as the ratio, $Ab_{ss,max}/Ab_{ss,min}$, the greater the frequency of administration the smaller is the fluctuation.

Figure 13-2B also demonstrates how the fluctuation at plateau depends upon the frequency of administration. The maximum and minimum amounts are each compared with the average amount of drug in the body. Note that the average is arithmetically closer to the minimum than to the maximum value. This is particularly evident for low frequencies of administration.

Rate of Accumulation to the Plateau

The amount in the body rises on multiple dosing just as it does following a constant rate intravenous infusion (Chap. 8); that is, the approach to the plateau depends solely on the drug's half-life. The data in Table 13-3, which shows the ratio of the maximum amount during various dosing intervals to the maximum amount at plateau, illustrate this point for digitoxin. Observe that it takes one half-life (6 days), or 6 doses, to be at 50 percent of the maximum at plateau, two half-lives (12 days), or 12 doses, to be at 75 percent of the maximum at plateau, and so on. The same holds true for accumulation with reference to the minimum and average amounts of drug in the body. The proof of these statements is given in Appendix E.

The accumulation of digitoxin takes a long time because of its long half-life. The degree of accumulation is extensive, because of frequent administration. The frequency of administration also determines the small fluctuation in the amount of drug in the body at plateau; 0.1 mg is lost in every dosing interval, but there are about 0.9 mg in the body.

Change in Regimen

Suppose that the decision is made to reduce the amount of digitoxin in the body by one-half by reducing the rate of administration twofold, for example, to 0.05 mg a day. This reduction follows from Equation 7.

As with intravenous infusion, it takes one half-life to go one-half the way from 0.90 to 0.45 mg, two half-lives to go three-quarters of the way, and so on. For digitoxin it would take about 12 days to go 75 percent of the way to the new plateau. (The same principle operates for an increase in the rate of digitoxin administration.) The fastest way of achieving the level of 0.45 mg would be to discontinue the drug for one week (approximately one half-life) before initiating the reduced rate of administration.

Relationship Between Initial and Maintenance Doses

It might be therapeutically desirable to establish the required amount of digitoxin in the body on the first day. When the first or initial dose is intended to be therapeutic it is referred to as the *priming* or *loading dose*. In this case, the patient would require 0.9 mg initially, followed by 0.1 mg daily. For digitoxin the initial dose is often administered in divided doses. Several procedures are followed, but the divided dose is commonly given every 6 hours until the desired therapeutic response is obtained. In this way each patient is titrated to the initial therapeutic dose required.

Instead of determining the loading dose when the maintenance dose is given, it is more common to determine the maintenance dose required to sustain a therapeutic amount of drug in the body. The initial dose rapidly achieves the therapeutic re-

Table 13-3. Approach to Plateau on Daily Administration of Digitoxin

Time (days)	0	1	2	3	6	12	18	24	30	∞
Number of doses (N)	0	1	2	3	6	12	18	24	30	∞
$\left[\dfrac{\text{Maximum amount}}{\begin{array}{c}\text{Maximum amount}\\ \text{at plateau}\end{array}} \right]^{a}$	0	0.11	0.21	0.29	0.5	0.75	0.875	0.94	0.97	1.00

$^{a}Ab_{N,max}/Ab_{ss,max} = 1 - (\tfrac{1}{2})^{0.17N}$

sponse; subsequent doses maintain the response by replacing drug lost during the dosing interval. The maintenance dose, D_M, therefore, is the difference between the initial dose, D_L, and the amount remaining at the end of the dosing interval, $D_L e^{-k\tau}$ or $D_L \cdot (\frac{1}{2})^\epsilon$, where ϵ is the dosing interval expressed in half-lives. That is,

$$\text{Maintenance} \atop \text{dose} = \left[\text{Loading} \atop \text{dose} \right] \cdot (1 - e^{-k\tau}) \quad 10$$

or

$$\text{Maintenance} \atop \text{dose} = \left[\text{Loading} \atop \text{dose} \right] \cdot (1 - (\tfrac{1}{2})^\epsilon) \quad 11$$

Likewise, if the maintenance dose is known, the initial dose can be estimated:

$$\text{Loading dose} = \frac{\text{Maintenance dose}}{(1 - e^{-k\tau})} \quad 12$$

or

$$\text{Loading dose} = \frac{\text{Maintenance dose}}{[1 - (\tfrac{1}{2})^\epsilon]} \quad 13$$

Using the table of $(\frac{1}{2})^n$ functions in Appendix F-II, for a value $\epsilon = 0.17$ ($\epsilon = 1 \text{ day}/6$ days) and a daily maintenance dose of 0.1 mg, the initial dosage requirement is 0.9 mg.

The similarity between Equations 3 and 11 should be noted. From the viewpoint of accumulation, Equation 3 relates the maximum amount of drug in the body at plateau with a given dose administered repetitively. Conversely, if the maximum amount were put into the body initially, then Equation 11 indicates the dose needed to maintain that amount. The relationships are the same, although they were derived using different logic. These equations form the heart of multiple dose drug administration and might well be called the "dosage regimen equations."

The difference between the loading and maintenance doses depends upon the dosing interval and the half-life. For example, tetracycline has approximately an 8-hour half-life in man, and a dose in the range of 250 to 500 mg is considered to provide ef-

fective antimicrobial drug concentrations. Therefore, a reasonable schedule is 500 mg (two 250-mg capsules) initially, followed by 250 mg every half-life, as shown in Figure 13-3. A dosage regimen consisting of a priming dose equal to twice the maintenance dose, and a dosing interval of one half-life, are convenient for drugs with half-lives between 6 and 24 hours. The frequency of administration for such drugs varies from 4 times a day to once daily, respectively. For drugs with very short to short half-lives, less than 3 hours, or with very long half-lives, greater than 24 hours, this regimen is often impractical.

Maintenance of Drug Levels in the Therapeutic Range

Dosage regimens that achieve therapeutic amounts of drug in the body are listed in Table 13-4 for drugs with both medium to high and low therapeutic indices and with various half-lives.

Great difficulty is encountered in trying to maintain therapeutic levels of a drug with a short to very short half-life (less than 3 hours). This is particularly true for a drug

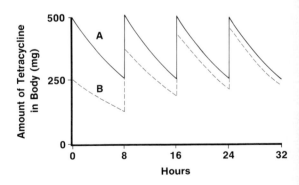

Figure 13-3. Sketch of the amount of tetracycline in the body with time; simulation of the intravenous administration of 500 mg initially and 250 mg every 8 hours thereafter, curve A. When the initial and maintenance doses are the same, curve B, it takes approximately 30 hours (3 to 4 half-lives) before the plateau is practically reached. Thereafter curves A and B are essentially the same.

Table 13-4. Dosage Regimens for Continuous Maintenance of Therapeutic Levels

Therapeutic Index:[a]	Half-life[b]	Ratio of Initial Dose to Maintenance Dose	Ratio of Dosing Interval to Half-life (ε)	Comments	Drug Examples
Medium to High					
	Very short (<20 min)	—	—	Candidate for infusion and/or short-term therapy.	Nitroglycerin
	Short (20 min to 3 hours)	1	3–6	To be given any less often than every 3 half-lives, drug must have very high therapeutic index.	Penicillin
	Intermediate (3 to 8 hours)	1–2	1–3	Very common and desirable regimen.	Tetracycline Sulfamethoxazole
	Long (8 to 24 hours)	2	1		
	Very long (>24 hours)	>2	<1	Once daily is practical. Occasionally given once weekly. Initial dose may need to be much greater than maintenance dose.	Chloroquine (suppression of malaria)
Low					
	Very short (<20 min)	—	—	Not a candidate except under very closely controlled infusion.	Succinylcholine
	Short (20 min to 3 hours)	—	—	Only by infusion.	Lidocaine Procainamide
	Intermediate (3 to 8 hours)	1–2	~1	Requires 3–6 doses per day, but less frequently with prolonged release formulation.	
	Long (8 to 24 hours)	2–4	0.5–1	Requires careful control, since once toxicity is produced, drug level and toxicity decline very slowly.	Lithium Digitoxin
	Very long (>24 hours)	>2	<1		

[a] Usually toxic maintenance dose/usual therapeutic maintenance dose.
[b] Descriptions of half-life are arbitrary.

that also has a low therapeutic index, e.g., heparin. Such a drug must either be infused or must be discarded unless intermittent levels are permissible. Drugs with a high therapeutic index may be given less frequently, but the greater the dosing interval the greater is the dose required to ensure that the level of drug in the body stays above a minimum effective value. Penicillin is a notable example of a drug for which the dosing interval (4–6 hours) is many times longer than its half-life (approximately 0.7 hour). The dose given greatly exceeds that required to yield plasma concentrations of antibiotic equivalent to the minimum inhibitory concentration for most microorganisms.

For a drug of short to intermediate half-life (20 min–8 hours) the major considerations are therapeutic index and convenience of dosing. A drug with a high therapeutic index need only be administered once every 1 to 3 half-lives. A drug with a low therapeutic index must be given approximately every half-life, or more frequently, or be given by infusion. Lidocaine, for example, has a half-life of only 90 min, and the range of plasma drug concentrations associated with the treatment of cardiac arrhythmias is only about threefold (Table 12-1): This drug must be given by infusion to ensure prolonged suppression of arrhythmias and minimal toxicity.

For a drug with a long half-life (8–24 hours) the most convenient, common, and desirable regimen is one in which a dose is given every half-life ($\epsilon = 1$). It is often also desirable to achieve the maintenance levels at once instead of waiting for accumulation to occur. Then, as previously mentioned, the initial dose must be twice the maintenance dose, and the minimum and maximum amounts in the body are equivalent to one and two maintenance doses, respectively.

For drugs with very long half-lives (greater than 1 day), administration once daily is convenient and promotes patient compliance. If an immediate therapeutic effect is desired the therapeutic dose is given initially. Otherwise the initial and maintenance doses are the same, in which case several doses may be necessary before the drug accumulates to therapeutic levels. The decision whether or not to give larger initial doses is often a practical matter. Side effects to large oral doses (gastrointestinal side effects) or to acutely high concentrations of drug in the body may necessitate a slow accumulation.

To summarize the foregoing discussion, consider tetracycline, phenylpropanolamine, and phenobarbital and their common dosage regimens, given in Table 13-5. The fraction of the initial amount remaining at the end of a dosing interval, the average amount of drug in the body at steady state, and the maximum and minimum levels can be calculated knowing the half-life and the regimen. These quantities, listed in Table 13-6, are readily estimated using the table of $(\frac{1}{2})^n$ functions. Some values were obtained by interpolation. Instantaneous and complete absorption is assumed.

Table 13-5. Dosage Regimens and Half-lives of Three Drugs

Drug	Loading Dose (mg)	Maintenance Dose (mg)	Dosing Interval (hours)	Half-life (hours)
Tetracycline	500	250	8	8
Phenyl- propanolamine	30	30	8	4
Phenobarbital	30	30	8	120

Table 13-6. Estimates of Amount of Drug in Body on Regimens Given in Table 13-5

Drug	Fraction Remaining at τ[a]	Average at Steady State Ab_{av} (mg)[b]	Maximum at Steady State $Ab_{ss,max}$ (mg)[c]	Minimum at Steady State $Ab_{ss,min}$ (mg)[d]
Tetracycline	0.5	360	500	250
Phenyl-propanolamine	0.25	22	40	10
Phenobarbital	0.95	650	665	635

[a]Calculated by $(\frac{1}{2})^{\epsilon}$.
[b]$1.44 \cdot F \cdot t_{1/2} \cdot D_M / \tau$.
[c]$D_M / [1 - (\frac{1}{2})^{\epsilon}]$.
[d]$Ab_{ss,max} - D_M$.

The dosing intervals for all three drugs are identical. The doses of phenylpropanolamine and phenobarbital are also the same, but the amounts of them in the body with time are certainly not identical. The explanation is readily visualized with a sketch.

As with any graph, consideration should first be given to scaling the axes. The amount of drug in the body should be scaled to the maximum amount at steady state. The time axis should be scaled to 4 to 5 half-lives, by which time the levels are virtually at plateau.

For tetracycline the amount in the body immediately after the first dose is 500 mg. At the end of the dosing interval the fraction remaining is 0.5, and the amount therefore is 250 mg. A maintenance dose of 250 mg returns the level to 500 mg and so on. Figure 13-3, curve A, is thus readily drawn. Now consider the sketch, had no loading dose been given. The initial amount, 250 mg, would then decline to 125 mg at the end of the first interval. The amount in the body immediately after the next dose would be 375 mg. At the end of the second interval 187 mg would remain and so on (curve B of Fig. 13-3).

For phenylpropanolamine the maximum and minimum amounts in the body at plateau are 40 mg and 10 mg, respectively, and 4 half-lives is 16 hours. The fraction remaining at the end of each dosing interval is 0.25; therefore,

Dose	Time (hours)	Ab (mg)
1	0	30
	8	7.5
2	8+	37.5
	16	9.4
3	16+	39.4

By the third dose (24 hours) the levels are virtually at plateau. Being given every two half-lives the accumulation of phenylpropanolamine is minimal. Figure 13-4 is the sketch of phenylpropanolamine levels in the body with time.

The same dosage regimen for phenobar-

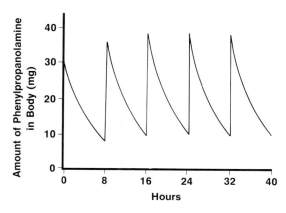

Figure 13-4. *Sketch of the amount of phenyl-propanolamine in the body with time; simulation of 30 mg given intravenously every 8 hours. Because the half-life, 4 hours, is short relative to the dosing interval, the degree of accumulation is small and the fluctuation is large.*

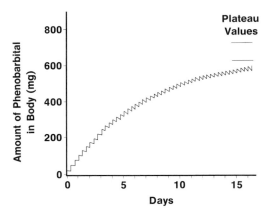

Figure 13-5. *Sketch of the amount of phenobarbital in the body with time; simulation of 30 mg given intravenously every 8 hours. Because the half-life, 5 days, is extremely long relative to the dosing interval, the degree of accumulation is large and the fluctuation is low.*

bital produces dramatically different results. At the end of each dosage interval the fraction remaining is approximately 0.95. Accumulation then occurs until the 5 percent lost in each interval is equal to the dose, and the amount in the body at steady state is therefore about 20 times the dose. From the calculated value of the maximum amount at plateau (650 mg) and the half-life, it is apparent that a sketch must be scaled to 700 to 1000 mg and to 15 to 20 days (Fig. 13-5). The curve is similar to that obtained with constant infusion. The amount of drug in the body at 5 days (120 hours) is one-half of the steady-state amount, and at 10 days (240 hours) the level is 75 percent of the plateau amount and so on. Practically, there is little need to consider the minor fluctuations.

The clinical implications of these regimens are manifold. The tetracycline regimen is designed to attain and maintain therapeutic levels. The phenylpropanolamine regimen gives rise to large fluctuations that may be desirable. Tolerance to the drug develops readily. The maintenance of high, effective, decongesting levels is questionable. With phenobarbital several questions come to mind, depending on whether this regimen is used for sedation or for

anticonvulsant therapy. For sedation the lack of a loading dose has logic in that tolerance to the sedative effect develops with time and a large priming dose, 600 mg, causes too great a central depressive effect. As an anticonvulsant, however, a loading dose may be appropriate. For both purposes chronic administration of the drug three times daily is illogical, except perhaps for its psychologic value.

Practical Aspects of Multiple Dose Administration

So far, consideration has been given primarily to the amount of drug in the body following multiple intravenous bolus injections, or their equivalent, at equally spaced time intervals. In practice, chronic administration is usually by the oral route. Furthermore, only drug concentration in plasma or in blood can be measured and not the amount of drug in the body. In addition, the dosage regimen is often one in which the dosing interval and the maintenance dose are not constant. Let us look at each of these practical considerations in turn.

Extravascular Administration

The oral (also intramuscular, buccal, subcutaneous, and rectal) administration of drugs requires the added step, absorption. The previous equations, Equations 1 to 4, are applicable to extravascular administration, provided that absorption is essentially completed within a small fraction of a dosing interval, a condition similar to intravenous bolus administration. Even so, a correction must be made in the dose if the availability is less than 1. When absorption continues throughout a dosing interval, or longer, then the relationships of Equations 7 to 9 are still applicable. These relationships allow estimation of the average plateau concentration, the average plateau amount in the body, and the accumulation ratio, respectively. The rapidity of drug absorption affects the degree of fluctuation around, but not the value of, the average level. However, if absorption is too slow, e.g., because of poor dissolution from an oral solid dosage form or slow diffusion through the gastrointestinal membranes, some drug will appear unchanged in the feces.

Fluctuations in the level of drug in the body within a dosing interval may be very small following oral or other extravascular routes of administration because of continuous absorption. Furthermore, the maximum level at plateau is always close to the average plateau value when the dosing interval is less than one-half of a half-life, irrespective of the route of administration or the rate of absorption. In both instances, the relationship between initial and maintenance doses becomes a simple one, namely,

$$\frac{\text{Maintenance}}{\text{dose}} = 0.7 \times \epsilon \times \frac{\text{Loading}}{\text{dose}} \quad 14$$

where $\epsilon = \tau/t_{1/2}$. This simple relationship is derived from Equation 11. As ϵ approaches zero (less than 0.5), the function $[1 - (\frac{1}{2})^{\epsilon}]$ approaches the value of 0.7ϵ.

Thus, if a drug is administered more frequently than twice every half-life the error in using Equation 14 is less than 20 percent. This error may appear large, but in practice it is acceptable when viewed against the normal variability in human drug response.

Plasma Concentration Versus Amount in Body

After multiple dosing, the maximum and minimum concentrations can be calculated by dividing the corresponding equations defining amount by the volume of distribution of the drug. It should be recalled, however, from Chapter 4 that distribution equilibrium between drug in the tissues and that in the plasma takes time. Thus, for some drugs, observed and calculated maximum concentrations may be disparate.

The average plateau concentration may be calculated using Equation 8. This equation is applicable to any route, method of administration, or dosage form, as long as availability and clearance remain constant with both time and dose. Often clearance can be approximated from the half-life and the volume of distribution, $Cl = 0.7 \, V/t_{1/2}$, in which case

$$C_{av} = 1.44 \cdot F \cdot \frac{t_{1/2}}{V} \cdot \frac{Dose}{\tau} \quad 15$$

Although this last relationship is an alternative, often convenient, way of estimating the average concentration, it should be used with caution. The half-life is commonly measured; the volume of distribution is not. A change in half-life is usually associated with a change in clearance, in which case adjustment of the dosing rate to the change in half-life maintains the same average plateau concentration. Sometimes, however, altered distribution is the cause of a change in half-life (see Chap. 11), and no adjustment in the rate of administration is necessary. Nor is it usually necessary to adjust dosage when changes in plasma protein binding are responsible for the change in clearance. That drug effects are best related to the unbound concentration should always be kept in mind.

Active Metabolites

Thus far, the inherent assumption has been made that only the drug is pharmacologically active. However, often a metabolite is active (Table 10-1), and it should also be considered. As discussed in Chapter 10, the accumulation of metabolite may depend as much upon its half-life as upon that of the parent drug. For example (Fig. 13-6), the accumulation of desmethyldiazepam, the primary metabolite of diazepam, lags behind the parent drug because this metabolite has the longer half-life. In addition the plateau desmethyldiazepam concentration is higher than that of diazepam, because of the lower clearance of the metabolite. The metabolite also appears to inhibit its own

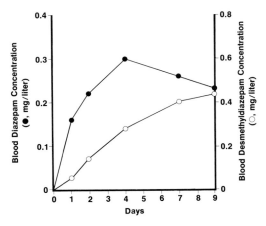

Figure 13-6. *Diazepam and its primary metabolite, desmethyldiazepam, accumulate on a dosage regimen of 5 mg at 6 A.M., 11 A.M. and 4 P.M. daily. Drug concentrations in blood just before the 6 A.M. doses are shown for one subject in the study. Note the slow accumulation of the metabolite. (Adapted from Eatman, F.B., Colburn, W.A., Boxenbaum, H.G., Posmanter, H.N., Weinfeld, R.E., Ronfeld, R., Neissman, L., Moore, J.D., Gibaldi, M., and Kaplan, A.: Pharmacokinetics of diazepam following multiple-dose oral administration to healthy human subjects. J. Pharmacokin. Biopharm., 5: 481–494, 1977.)*

formation and thereby decreases the clearance of diazepam.

Dosage Regimens of Unequal Doses and Unequal Dosing Intervals

Although there is no simple mathematical method of doing so, the plasma concentration with time, following dosage regimens of different maintenance doses and of varying dosing intervals, can be predicted or evaluated, if the plasma concentration-time curve is known for one dose. The underlying concept here is that each successive dose does not influence the time course of drug from a previous dose. Consequently, the amount or the concentration of drug in the body following multiple doses is simply the sum of what remains from each of the previous doses. The summation is readily accomplished for multiple intravascular

doses, or their equivalent, by using semi-logarithmic graph paper. As an example, consider the following regimen of unequal dose and unequal dosing interval for a drug (Table 13-7).

To determine graphically the amount of drug in the body with time only one more piece of information is needed—the half-life; assume it to be 5 hours. A sketch is prepared by placing a point on the graph corresponding to the value of each dose at the respective time when administered. A straight line is then drawn for drug remaining in the body with time from each of the respective doses using the half-life. The amount in the body at any time is then simply obtained by adding the amount that remains from all the preceding doses. Figure 13-7 is such a sketch of drug in the body on the regimen above.

Alternatively, the amount in the body at a specific time can be numerically determined. For example, the amount in the body at 8:00 A.M. on day 2, 23 hours after the first dose, is the sum of what remains from each of the three previous doses. The fraction remaining is e^{-kt} or $e^{-(0.7/5) \cdot t}$, therefore, amount remaining is

$$200e^{-0.14 \times 23} + 100e^{-0.14 \times 19} + 100e^{-0.14 \times 13}$$

| 8.0 mg | 7.0 mg | 16.2 mg |

Thus, 31 mg remains in the body, assuming that the availability is 1. The expected plasma concentration at this time is estimated by dividing by the volume of distribution.

No dose at night clearly produces a dramatic drop in the level of drug. If this were a drug with a low therapeutic index the therapeutic effect may well vanish by morning. The larger dose on day 2, presumably to compensate for inadequate therapy overnight, may produce toxicity. This regimen demonstrates the importance of the dosing schedule in maintaining an adequate therapeutic response.

Oral dosage regimens may be simulated

Table 13-7. An Example of an Uneven Dosage Regimen

	Dose	Time	
No.	Amount (mg)	O'clock	From First Dose (hours)
1	200	Day 1 9:00 A.M.	0
2	100	1:00 P.M.	4
3	100	7:00 P.M.	10
4	100	Day 2 9:00 A.M.	24
5	200	3:00 P.M.	30
6	300	6:00 P.M.	33
7	100	Day 3 11:00 A.M.	50

in a manner analogous to that just discussed if the plasma level-time curve is known for a single dose. In this case, however, it is usually easier to draw a rough sketch on regular Cartesian graph paper. The curve for each dose is placed on the graph at the appropriate time, and the total level of drug is obtained again by adding what remains from previous doses.

Use of Plasma Concentration to Design Dosage Regimens

A dosage regimen may be developed to keep the plasma concentration of drug within limits, e.g., between a minimum effective concentration, lower limit (C_{min}), and a potentially toxic concentration, upper limit (C_{max}). The relationship between these limits is expressed by

$$C_{min} = C_{max} \cdot e^{-k \cdot \tau_{max}} = C_{max} \cdot (\tfrac{1}{2})^\epsilon \quad 16$$

where τ_{max} is the maximum dosing interval that ensures that the plasma concentration at steady state is kept within these limits. By rearrangement of Equation 16 the value of τ_{max} is given by

$$\tau_{max} = \frac{\ln(C_{max}/C_{min})}{k} \quad 17$$

or from the relationship, $k = 0.7/t_{1/2}$,

$$\tau_{max} = 1.44 \cdot t_{1/2} \cdot \ln(C_{max}/C_{min}) \quad 18$$

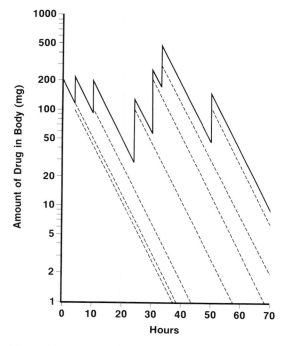

Figure 13-7. *The amount of drug in the body with time following the uneven dosage regimen in Table 13-7 may be determined graphically. First, knowing the half-life, draw lines (dashed) on semilogarithmic paper representing the amount of each dose remaining in the body with time. The total amount in the body (solid line) is then simply constructed by adding the amount remaining at each time from the preceding doses. Note that the amount remaining from doses administered more than four half-lives (20 hours) prior to the last dose contributes very little and can therefore be ignored.*

The corresponding maximum maintenance dose, D_{max}, that can be given every τ_{max} is therefore

$$D_{M,max} = \frac{V}{F}(C_{max} - C_{min}) \qquad 19$$

and the required rate of dosing (Equation 19 divided by Equation 17) is

$$\frac{D_{M,max}}{\tau_{max}} = \frac{Cl}{F} \cdot \left[\frac{(C_{max} - C_{min})}{\ln(C_{max}/C_{min})}\right] \qquad 20$$

By substituting Equation 20 into Equation 8 it is apparent that the corresponding value of C_{av} is

$$C_{av} = \frac{C_{max} - C_{min}}{\ln(C_{max}/C_{min})} \qquad 21$$

The calculated maintenance dose and dosing interval may not be practical. Both values may need to be adjusted to make the frequency of administration convenient for patient compliance and to accommodate the doses of the drug products available. The guiding principle is to maintain the same rate of administration and therefore the same average steady-state concentration. In addition, a loading dose of a size approximating $V \cdot C_{ss,max}/F$ may be appropriate to attain the steady-state concentration initially. One major consideration is how quickly distribution takes place; the preceding relationships were developed assuming instantaneous equilibration of drug in the tissues with that in plasma.

Following extravascular administration, fluctuations in the plasma concentration of drug are less than those after intravascular administration. Depending upon the slowness of the absorption process, it may be possible to administer the drug less frequently than every τ_{max}. Again, the guiding principle should be to maintain the same dosing rate and the same average plateau concentration.

Oral dosage regimens can also be designed, without determining the availability. This is accomplished using the area under the plasma concentration-time curve following a single dose. From the relationship $F \cdot \text{Dose} = Cl \cdot \text{Area}$ after a single dose (Equation 7, Chap. 9) and the relationship $F \cdot \text{Dose}/\tau = Cl \cdot C_{av}$ during steady state after multiple doses (Equation 6), it follows that

$$C_{av} = \text{Area (single dose)}/\tau \qquad 22$$

Consequently, either the dosing interval necessary to achieve a desired average steady-state concentration or the concentration resulting from administering the dose every dosing interval can be calculated.

By definition of C_{av}, the value of $\tau \cdot C_{av}$ is the area under the curve within a dosing interval at steady state. Thus, this area is equal to that following a single dose. This principle is illustrated in Figure 13-8.

Useful relationships have been derived for designing and evaluating a dosage regimen in which the dose and the dosing interval are fixed. Table 13-8 contains some of the more important relationships and their limitations. Table 13-9 summarizes the relationships for developing such a dosage regimen to keep the concentration of drug in plasma within defined limits.

Prolonged Release

The maintenance of a constant plasma concentration of drug is achieved by constant intravenous infusion (Chap. 8). This method of administration is not practical in an outpatient setting and is of limited value in an inpatient setting. For many drugs given in multiple doses, it would seem desirable to design a dosage form that mimics the infusion situation by releasing drug at a controlled rate so that absorption is maintained (see drug delivery systems, Chap. 3). This design applies to oral as well as to other extravascular routes of administration. In principle the idea is simple; in practice the problems associated with the preparation of such prolonged release formulations are many and beyond the scope of this book.

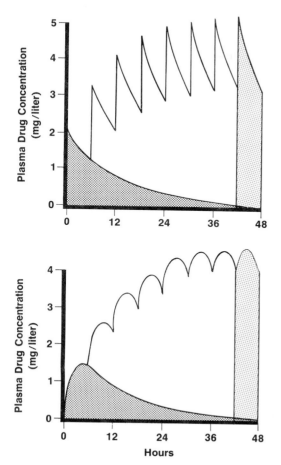

Figure 13-8. *Plasma concentration of a drug given intravenously (top) and orally (bottom) on a fixed dose of 50 mg and fixed dosing interval of 8 hours. The half-life is 12 hours. Note that the area under the plasma concentration-time curve during a dosing interval at steady state is equal to the total area under the curve for a single dose. The fluctuation of the concentration is diminished when given orally (half-life of absorption is 1.4 hours) but the average steady-state concentration is the same as that after intravenous administration, since F = 1.*

Prolonged-release preparations are potentially useful in situations in which maintenance of therapeutic levels with a usual multiple dosage regimen is difficult or inconvenient. They can be used to reduce local irritation caused by high concentrations at the absorption site, to reduce the chances of side effects associated with ex-

cessively high peak plasma concentrations, and to reduce the frequency of drug administration. The principal criterion of the last is the half-life. For oral administration, once or twice daily is an optimal schedule. For drugs with half-lives beyond 12 hours, oral prolonged-release dosage forms may be of little value, not only because the usual regimen is convenient but because prolongation of the release puts the drug in the lower intestines or perhaps out of the body before the release is complete. Availability thus becomes a major concern.

For a drug that is usually given intramuscularly or subcutaneously, multiple injections are inconvenient and a prolonged-release injectable dosage form may be advantageous. Depending on the total dose required and on the local effects of the injection mixture, it may be possible to administer the injection weekly, monthly, or perhaps as a single dose.

To maintain a constant steady-state level of drug in the body, Ab_{ss}, the rate of release from a prolonged-release formulation must match the rate of drug elimination; therefore,

$$\text{Rate of drug release} = k \cdot Ab_{ss} \qquad 23$$

and so, the amount required to maintain a level for h hours is,

$$\text{Amount in formulation} = k \cdot Ab_{ss} \cdot h \qquad 24$$

The longer the period over which the level is to be maintained, the greater is the amount required.

When the amount to be maintained is small the resulting size of the formulation is reasonable. If the amount is large, however, a problem exists. Consider a drug with a half-life of 3 hours for which 250 mg is required in the body. If the prolonged-release dosage form is designed to be administered twice daily, each formulation must contain 700 mg:

Amount in formulation

$$= \frac{0.7}{3 \text{ hours}} \times 250 \text{ mg} \times 12 \text{ hours} = 700 \text{ mg}$$

Table 13-8. Relationships for Evaluating a Dosage Regimen and Their Usefulness[a]

	Relationship	I.V. Bolus	Rapid Absorption $(k_a \gg k)$	Slow Absorption $(k_a > k)$	$(k > k_a)$
Maintenance dose	$D_M = D_L \cdot (1 - e^{-k\tau})$	***[b]	***	**	N
Accumulation ratio	$R_{AC} = \dfrac{1.44 \cdot t_{1/2}}{\tau}$	***	***	***	***
PLATEAU					
Average amount	$Ab_{av} = 1.44 \cdot F \cdot D \cdot \left(\dfrac{t_{1/2}}{\tau}\right)$	***	***	***	***
Average concentration	$C_{av} = \dfrac{F \cdot D_M}{Cl \cdot \tau}$	***	***	***	***
	$C_{av} = \dfrac{\text{Area (single dose)}}{\tau}$	***	***	***	***
Maximum concentration	$C_{ss,max} = \dfrac{F \cdot D_M}{V(1 - e^{-k\tau})}$	**[c]	**	*	N
Minimum concentration	$C_{ss,min} = \dfrac{F \cdot D_M \cdot e^{-k\tau}}{V(1 - e^{-k\tau})}$	***	***	*	N

[a]If doses or dosing intervals are unequal none of the above holds.
[b]*** Generally useful.
** A reasonable approximation.
* Limited usefulness.
[c]Valid if distribution is very rapid.
N Not Valid.

Since the formulation must also contain nondrug materials (excipients) to provide the release desired, the total size of the product would probably exceed 1 gram, a horse capsule. A loading dose, D_L, to be released immediately may also be considered desirable, in which case, as a reasonable approximation,

$$\text{Total amount in formulation} = D_L \cdot (1 + k \cdot h) \quad 25$$

Needless to say, however, a constant level of drug in the body would not be maintained were such a formulation containing a loading dose administered repetitively.

A major limitation to prolonged release of some drugs is variability in kinetics and in response. Even if the release is perfectly controlled, the dosage requirement may vary from one individual to another. A standard formulation allows no easy adjustment in dosing rate, and changing the dosing interval does not give adequate therapy.

Assessment of Pharmacokinetic Parameters

Data obtained on multiple dosing may be used to calculate the pharmacokinetic parameters of a drug. In most instances, however, the estimates are crude.

Perhaps the most useful information derived from a multiple oral dosing study is the ratio of clearance to availability. It is obtained from

$$\frac{Cl}{F} = \frac{(\text{Dose}/\tau)}{C_{av}} \quad 26$$

where C_{av} is determined from the ratio of the area under the plasma concentration

Table 13-9. Dosage Regimen Design[a]

Step	Description	Relationship
1	Establish maximum (C_{max}) and minimum (C_{min}) plasma concentrations desired.	
2	Obtain population estimates of ka, F, V, Cl, and $t_{1/2}$.	
3	Calculate the maximum dosing interval to keep within the limits. Assume I.V. administration.	$\tau_{max} = 1.44 \cdot t_{1/2} \cdot \ln(C_{max}/C_{min})$
4	Calculate the maximum maintenance dose that can be given.	$D_{M,max} = \dfrac{V}{F}(C_{max} - C_{min})$
5	Calculate dosing rate.	$\text{Dosing rate} = \dfrac{D_{M,max}}{\tau_{max}}$
6	Adjust D_M and τ to doses available and to a convenient frequency of administration, keeping approximately the same dosing rate.	$\dfrac{D_M}{\tau} = \dfrac{D_{M,max}}{\tau_{max}}$
7	If τ chosen$/t_{1/2}$ is much less than one and rapid initiation of therapy is desired, calculate a loading dose.	$D_L = \dfrac{V}{F} \cdot C_{ss,max}$
8	Appropriately adjust for other factors, such as slow absorption after extravascular administration, slow distribution to tissues, side effects on administering the calculated loading dose, and so on.	

[a]To keep the plasma concentration of drug within prescribed limits.

curve within a dosing interval at plateau to the dosing interval. On multiple intravenous administration the ratio $(\text{Dose}/\tau)/C_{av}$ is simply clearance, since $F = 1$. The accuracy of the clearance estimate depends upon the number of plasma concentrations measured in the dosing interval, that is, on how close the concentration is to the true steady-state value, and on the ratio of $\tau/t_{1/2}$. The estimate, of course, can be improved by using several dosing intervals. Equation 26 is also useful for determining the availability of a drug administered extravascularly (orally). Assuming that clearance remains unchanged, the

$$\text{Availability} = \frac{(C_{av})_{\text{oral}}}{(C_{av})_{\text{i.v.}}} \times \frac{(\text{Dose}/\tau)_{\text{i.v.}}}{(\text{Dose}/\tau)_{\text{oral}}} \quad 27$$

The renal clearance and the fraction excreted unchanged, fe, can be estimated from the amount of drug excreted unchanged in a dosing interval at steady state, $Ae_{\tau,ss}$, the dose, and the value of C_{av}

$$\text{Renal clearance} = \frac{Ae_{\tau,ss}}{C_{av\tau}} \quad 28$$

$$\text{Fraction excreted unchanged} = \frac{Ae_{\tau,ss}}{\text{Dose}_{\text{i.v.}}} \quad 29$$

Again, the availability of an extravascular

dose may be determined from urine data if data from an intravenous (or intramuscular) regimen are also available.

$$F = \frac{(Ae_{\tau,ss})_{oral}}{(Ae_{\tau,ss})_{i.v.}} \times \frac{\left(\dfrac{Dose}{\tau}\right)_{i.v.}}{\left(\dfrac{Dose}{\tau}\right)_{oral}} \qquad 30$$

Otherwise, by comparing two routes or dosage forms, an estimate of the relative availability is made. The half-life and the volume of distribution of a drug are more difficult to assess from multiple dosing data. In general, the half-life may be determined only if the accumulation is extensive and the plasma concentration is followed to steady state or if the drug is discontinued and the decline in the concentration is observed. The former is based on the accumulation principle, i.e., it takes one half-life to reach 50 percent of the plateau, two half-lives to reach 75 percent, and so on (Chap. 8). The volume of distribution can then be estimated from the clearance and the half-life values.

Study Problems

(Answers to Study Problems can be found in Appendix G.)

1. On administering 1 gram sodium bromide (molecular weight 103) every 8 hours (a common regimen when formerly employed as an antiepileptic agent), accumulation occurs until an average plateau plasma concentration of 30 milliequivalents/liter is reached. Knowing that bromide distributes extracellularly, does not bind, and is rapidly and completely absorbed, calculate the following:
   (a) The accumulation ratio
   (b) The half-life of the drug
   (c) The maximum and mimimum amount of drug in the body at plateau
   (d) The minimum plasma concentration after one week (just before the 22nd dose)

2. The pharmacokinetics of acetozolamide has been determined in nine patients with glaucoma by following the plasma concentrations with time after an oral dose of 500 mg. Some of the results are presented below as average values:

   $$Age = 48 \text{ years}$$
   $$ka = 2.2 \text{ hours}^{-1}$$
   $$k = 0.18 \text{ hours}^{-1}$$
   $$V = 14 \text{ liters}$$
   $$F = 1$$

   If 600 mg is the maximum amount of drug desired in the body and 10 mg/liter is the minimum plasma concentration found to have a therapeutic effect in lowering intraocular pressure, suggest a rational therapeutic oral dosage regimen for this drug. Tablets are available in 125- and 250-mg strengths.

3. Chlorpropamide and tolbutamide are oral hypoglycemic agents. Given the following information and assuming instantaneous and complete absorption:

> Chlorpropamide: tablet size   = 250 mg
> half-life   = 36 hours
> dosage regimen = 250 mg once daily
> Tolbutamide: tablet size   = 500 mg
> half-life   = 6 hours
> dosage regimen   = 500 mg every 12 hours (before meals)

(a) Complete the table below:

Amount of Drug in Body

	Dose:	1	2	3	4	5	6	7	8
Chlorpropamide									
	$Ab_{N,max}$	250							
	$Ab_{N,min}$								
Tolbutamide									
	$Ab_{N,max}$	500							
	$Ab_{N,min}$								

(b) Determine for which drug the average amount in the body at plateau is greater.

4. The therapeutic dose of a rapidly (compared to elimination) and completely absorbed drug is 50 mg. A prolonged-release dosage form to be given every 8 hours is designed to release its contents *evenly* and *completely* (no loading dose) over this dosing interval. Given that the half life of the drug is 4 hours:
    (a) How much drug should the prolonged-release dosage form contain?
    (b) To achieve a prompt effect a rapidly absorbed dosage form is administered initially. When should the first prolonged-release dosage form be given?
    (c) Following the dosage regimen in (b) what is the total dose (i) for day one? (ii) for day two?
    (d) In tabular form or on the same graph roughly sketch the relative amounts of drug in the body versus time curves expected when the prolonged-release preparation only is given (i) every 4 hours; (ii) every 8 hours; (iii) every 12 hours.

Unifying Problem

(Answer to Unifying Problem can be found in Appendix G.)

Jenne et al. (Clin. Pharmacol. Therap. *13*: 349, 1972) studied the pharmacokinetics of theophylline, a mainstay in the treatment of acute and chronic obstructive airway disease. In this study the following average pharmacokinetic parameters were obtained:

> Half-life = 312 min
> Clearance = 72 ml/min
> Volume of distribution = 34 liters

"Trough" plasma concentrations, i.e., concentrations just before the next dose, following multiple oral doses given every 6 hours, were commonly found to be associated with nausea, vomiting, and anorexia when above 20 mg/liter. Theophylline plasma concentrations required for adequate bronchodilator effect ranged from 8 to 20 mg/liter. The drug is rapidly and completely absorbed.

(a) Calculate an oral dose to be given every 6 hours to achieve an average steady-state plasma concentration of 13 mg/liter.

(b) What is the "trough" concentration at steady state on the regimen in (a)?

(c) Does your suggested oral dosage regimen seem reasonable? Comment briefly.

(d) Mr. J., a 70-kg asthmatic, was placed on the regimen that you suggested in (a) above. However, he failed to respond adequately. He was then given an intravenous infusion of the drug at the same rate as he was given orally, but after 24 hours of infusion he still did not respond adequately to the drug. At 24 hours a plasma sample was obtained; the theophylline concentration was 5.8 mg/liter. If the desired plasma concentration was 13 mg/liter, at what rate should the drug have been infused in this patient?

(e) Evidently Mr. J. eliminates theophylline more rapidly than normal. If the volume of distribution is normal in this patient, what is the value of the half-life of the drug in him?

(f) Mr. J. responded dramatically to the new intravenous regimen you suggested. It is decided to return Mr. J. to oral maintenance therapy for subsequent discharge from the hospital. What oral dosage regimen would you give him?

SECTION FOUR

individualization

14

variability in drug response

Objectives

The reader will be able to:

1. **List major sources of variability in drug response.**

2. **Evaluate whether the variability in drug response is due to a variability in pharmacokinetics, in pharmacodynamics, or in both, given pharmacokinetic data.**

3. **Identify which pharmacokinetic parameters change in the presence of a given source of variability.**

4. **Suggest an approach to the establishment of a dosage regimen in an individual patient, given patient population pharmacokinetic data.**

THUS far, the assumption has been made that all people are alike. True, as a species, man is reasonably homogeneous but differences between people do exist including their responsiveness to drugs. Differences in size of body frame, color of hair, color of eyes, are but a few of the countless genetic expressions of our individuality. Add to the genetic component the variability introduced by disease, by other drugs, by pollutants, by location, as well as by differences in age and in sex, and the frequent need to tailor drug administration to the individual patient becomes apparent. A failure to do so can lead to ineffective therapy in some patients and toxicity in others.

The remainder of this book is devoted to individual drug therapy. A broad overview of the subject is presented in this chapter. Evidence for and causes of variation in drug response and approaches to individualized drug therapy are examined. Subsequent chapters deal in much greater detail with age and dosage requirements (Chap. 15), the tailoring of a dosage regimen in a patient with chronic renal function impairment (Chap. 16), and the problems introduced by the interactions between drugs within the body (Chap. 17). Chapter 18 is a discussion of the use of monitoring of the plasma concentration of a drug as an approach to individualizing drug therapy.

Before proceeding, a distinction must be made between the individual and the population. One should consider, for example, the results of a study designed to examine the contribution of an acute disease to variability in drug response. Suppose, of thirty patients studied during and after recovery, only two showed a substantial difference in response; in the remainder the difference was insignificant. Viewed as a whole, the disease would not be considered as a significant source of variability, but in the two affected patients it would. Moreover, to avoid toxicity, the dosage regimen of the drug may need to be reduced in these two patients during the disease. The lesson is clear: Average data are useful as a guide, but ultimately, information pertaining to the individual patient is all-important.

Expressions of Individual Differences

Evidence for interindividual differences in drug response comes from several sources. Variability in the dosage required to produce a given response was illustrated in Figure 1-4 (Chap. 1), which showed the wide range in the daily dose of warfarin needed to produce a similar degree of anticoagulant control. Variability in the intensity of response to a set dose is illustrated in

Figure 14-1, which shows a frequency distribution histogram of the blood glucose-lowering effects of intravenous tolbutamide. As illustrated in Figures 14-2 and 14-3, which show frequency distribution histograms of the plateau plasma concentration of nortriptyline to a defined daily dose of the drug and the plateau plasma concentration of warfarin required to produce the same degree of anticoagulant control, variability exists in both the pharmacokinetics and the pharmacodynamics of a drug. Variability in the pharmacokinetics of a drug was also illustrated by the wide scatter in the plateau plasma concentration of phenytoin seen following various daily doses of this drug (see Fig. 1-5).

Why People Differ

Genetics

Inheritance accounts for a large part of the differences between individuals, including much of the variation in the response to an administered drug. *Pharmacogenetics* is the study of hereditary variations in drug response.

Where distinguishable differences in a

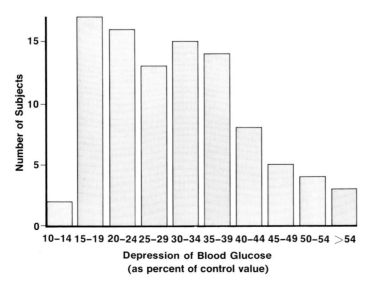

Figure 14-1. *The depression of blood glucose at 30 min, after a test dose of 1 gram tolbutamide I.V. in 97 subjects, varies widely. (Adapted from the data of Swerdloff, R.S., Pozefsky, T., Tobin, J.D., and Andres, R.: Influence of age on the intravenous tolbutamide response test. Diabetes, 16: 161–170, 1967; reproduced with permission from the American Diabetes Association, Inc.)*

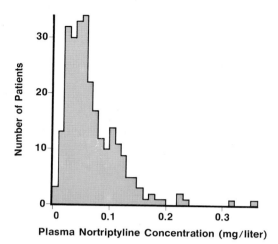

Figure 14-2. *The plateau plasma concentration of nortriptyline varies widely in 263 patients receiving a regimen of 25 mg nortriptyline orally three times daily. (Redrawn from Sjoqvist, F., Borga, O., and Orme, M.L'E.: Fundamentals of clinical pharmacology. In Drug Treatment. Edited by S.G. Avery. Churchill Livingstone, Edinburgh, 1976, pp. 1–42.*

given characteristic exist, it is called polymorphism. The mode of inheritance is either monogenic or polygenic depending upon whether it is transmitted by a gene at a single locus or by genes at multiple loci. Table 14-1 lists some genetic conditions that affect the pharmacokinetics and the pharmacodynamics of some drugs. Most of these are probably transmitted monogenically. Many, but not all, are rare events. Indeed, monogenically controlled conditions are usually detected as an abnormal drug response, that is, a *drug idiosyncrasy.* Occasionally they are detected from population studies. Polygenically controlled variations are usually detected from studies in twins.

Inherited Variation in Pharmacokinetics. Typically, muscle paralysis wears off within minutes of discontinuing succinylcholine (see Figs. 12-13 and 12-14) because it is rapidly hydrolyzed to inactive products, choline and monosuccinylcholine by plasma and liver pseudocholinesterases. In the occasional patient, however, neuromuscular blockade lasts up to several hours after stopping the infusion, because hydro-

lysis is much slower than usual. The reason is the existence of an atypical enzyme rather than a lower concentration of the typical cholinesterase; the atypical cholinesterase has only $\frac{1}{100}$ the usual affinity for succinylcholine, and it behaves differently from the typical cholinesterase to various enzyme inhibitors. These succinylcholine-sensitive patients are conveniently detected by adding the inhibitor, dibucaine, to a sample of plasma containing the cholinesterase substrate, benzoylcholine. Dibucaine inhibits the hydrolysis of benzoylcholine by the atypical cholinesterase to a lesser degree than it does with normal cholinesterase. Several aberrant forms of the enzyme are now known to exist, each determined by a different gene.

Individuals vary widely in their elimination kinetics of the antitubercular drug, isoniazid. The bimodality of the frequency distribution histogram of the 6-hour plasma isoniazid concentration following a single oral dose (Fig. 14-4) was taken as evidence of polymorphism. While subsequent evidence confirmed that polymorphic isoniazid elimination exists, the use of a single time-point measurement could have been misleading. One does not know, a priori, whether a low concentration reflects poor

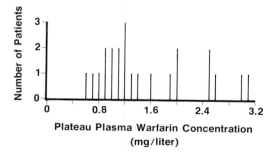

Figure 14-3. *The plateau plasma concentration of warfarin (expressed to the nearest 0.1 mg/liter), required to produce the same degree of anticoagulant control in 23 patients, varies widely. (Redrawn from Breckenridge, A., and Orme, M.L.E.: Measurement of plasma warfarin concentrations in clinical practice. In Biological Effect of Drugs in Relation to Their Plasma Concentrations. Edited by D.S. Davies, and B.N.C. Prichard. Macmillan, London and Basingstoke, 1973, pp. 145–154.)*

Table 14-1. Some Genetically Determined Drug Responses[a]

Inherited Variation in Pharmacokinetics

Condition	Response	Abnormal Enzyme and Location	Frequency	Drugs That Produce the Response
Slow and fast acetylation	Slow acetylators may show toxicity	N-Acetyltransferase in liver	50% of USA population are fast acetylators; higher percentage among Japanese and Eskimos	Isoniazid, procainamide, hydralazine, sulfasalazine, phenelzine dapsone, and many sulfonamides
Slow succinylcholine hydrohysis	Prolonged apnea	Cholinesterase in plasma	Several abnormal genes; most common disorder occurs 1 in 2500	Succinylcholine

Inherited Variation in Pharmacodynamics

Condition	Response	Abnormal Enzyme and Location	Frequency	Drugs That Produce the Response
Warfarin resistance	Resistance to anticoagulation	Altered receptor or enzyme in liver with increased affinity for vitamin K	2 large pedigrees	Warfarin
Favism or drug-induced hemolytic anemia	Hemolysis in response to certain drugs	Glucose-6-phosphate dehydrogenase (G6PD) deficiency	Approximately 100 million affected in world; occurs in high frequency where malaria is endemic; 80 biochemically distinct mutations	Variety of drugs, e.g., acetanilide primaquine, nitrofurantoin, chloramphenicol

Phenylthiourea taste insensitivity	Inability to taste certain drugs	Unknown	Approximately 30% of Caucasians	Drugs containing N-C-S group, e.g., phenylthiourea, methyl and propylthiouracil
Glaucoma	Abnormal response of intraocular pressure to steroid eye drops	Unknown	Approximately 5% of USA population	Corticosteroids
Malignant hyperthermia	Uncontrolled rise in body temperature with muscular rigidity	Unknown	Approximately 1 in 20,000 anesthetized patients	Various anesthetics, especially halothane
Methemoglobin reductase deficiency	Methemoglobinemia	Methemoglobin reductase deficiency	Approximately 1 in 100 are heterozygous carriers	Same drugs as listed above for G6PD deficiency

[a] Adapted from E.S. Vesell, TRIANGLE, Sandoz Journal of Medical Science, *14*: 125, 1975.

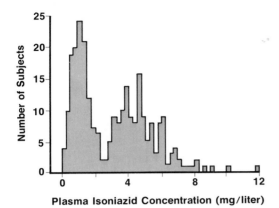

Figure 14-4. *The bimodal distribution of the 6-hour plasma isoniazid concentration in 483 subjects after 9.8 mg/kg isoniazid orally results from acetylation polymorphism. (Redrawn from Evans, D.A.P., Manley, K.A., and McKusick, V.A.: Genetic control of isoniazid metabolism in man. Br. Med. J., 2: 485–491, 1960.)*

availability, slow absorption, with perhaps the concentration still rising, or rapid elimination, with the concentration falling. Moreover, if the measurements had been taken at 2 hours, when the concentration primarily reflects absorption rather than elimination, one might have obtained a unimodal frequency distribution and excluded polymorphism. Isoniazid is primarily acetylated to N-acetylisoniazid, a precursor of an hepatotoxic compound; the differences in the elimination kinetics of isoniazid reflect polymorphism of the N-acetyltransferase involved. Whether these differences lie in the synthesis, in the catabolism, or in the activity of this enzyme is unknown. Interest in acetylation polymorphism is not just academic. Peripheral neuropathy, associated with elevated concentrations of isoniazid, occurs more prevalently in slow acetylators unless adjustment is made in the dosage of isoniazid or vitamin B_6 is concomitantly administered. Acetylation polymorphism also occurs and is important for several other drugs including procainamide and hydralazine (Table 14-1). For both drugs the N-acetyl derivative is the major metabolite. A

systemic lupus erythematous syndrome, a generalized inflammatory response, often limits procainamide use; it occurs on long-term therapy more frequently in slow than in rapid acetylators. The mechanism remains obscure but does appear to be associated with an elevated plasma procainamide concentration. Rapid acetylators require higher doses of hydralazine to control hypertension.

The elimination kinetics of many drugs that primarily undergo hepatic metabolism, particularly by oxidation and by reduction, varies widely within the population. Studies in twins indicate that the variability is often primarily under genetic control. Figure 14-5 illustrates such an investigation with antipyrine. Variability in the elimination half-life among identical twins is much less than among fraternal twins or, indeed, among any randomly selected age-matched group. Similar data exist for phenylbutazone, bishydroxycoumarin, and nortriptyline. Although the evidence presented in

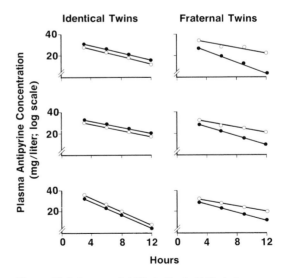

Figure 14-5. *Less variability in the half-life between identical twins than between fraternal twins proves that antipyrine elimination is predominantly genetically controlled. (Redrawn from Vessel, E.S., and Page, J.G.: Genetic control of drug levels in man: Antipyrine. Science, 161: 72–74, 1968. Copyright 1968 by the American Association for the Advancement of Science.)*

Figure 14-5 is striking, analysis based solely on the unchanged drug in plasma may be misleading. Consider, for example, a drug that is eliminated by several metabolic pathways of which only a minor one is under genetic control. Looking solely at the elimination half-life or at the total clearance of the drug may fail to detect this genetically controlled source of variability. Yet, if the affected metabolite is very potent or toxic, identifying this source of a variability may be therapeutically important. The need to measure both drug and metabolites under these circumstances and to calculate the clearance associated with the formation of each metabolite is self-evident.

In contrast to many metabolic pathways, the renal handling of drugs does not appear to be under genetic control. Thus, the renal clearance value for any drug is essentially the same in age and weight-matched healthy subjects. This last observation suggests that much of the interindividual variability in pharmacokinetics could be avoided if drugs were entirely excreted unchanged. A notable exception to the absence of genetic control is the excretion of drugs in renal tubular acidosis, a genetic disorder characterized by a constant alkaline urine. The renal clearance of pH-sensitive drugs should be different in patients with this disorder than in the normal population. Whether any of the variations in drug absorption and distribution are also under genetic control is poorly defined. Slow and fast gastrointestinal absorption of several drugs has been traced to differences in stomach emptying rate, but extensive twin studies and family studies to define this aspect further are lacking.

One drug can hasten the elimination of another drug by inducing the synthesis of metabolizing enzymes. Conversely, one drug can retard the elimination of another by competing for the metabolizing enzymes. Large interindividual variations exist in the degree of induction or inhibition produced by concurrent drug therapy; part of the variability is genetically controlled.

Evidence supporting this statement is illustrated by the data in Figure 14-6, which show the percentage lowering of the half-life of antipyrine in identical and fraternal twins following administration of phenobarbital. Several points are worth noting. First, antipyrine is both poorly cleared by hepatic enzymes and negligibly bound to plasma, or indeed to tissue proteins. Accordingly, as discussed in Chapter 11, the shortening in the elimination half-life directly reflects an increase in drug clearance caused, in this case, by induction with phenobarbital. Second, the longer the initial half-life, the greater the degree of induction, despite a comparable plasma concentration of phenobarbital in each subject. Perhaps those subjects with the shortest half-lives already have the maximum amount of enzyme and hence cannot be induced further. Third, identical twins not only have the same initial half-life but also the same degree of shortening of the half-life. The corresponding values are different in fraternal twins, strengthening the argu-

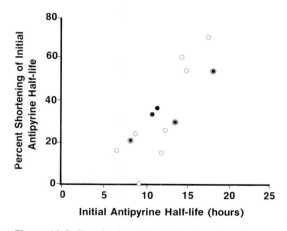

Figure 14-6. *The degree of induction by phenobarbital of antipyrine metabolism varies widely and is influenced genetically. Both the initial antipyrine half-life and the degree of shortening of the half-life are either the same (◉) or very similar (●) in identical twins, but they are different in fraternal twins (○). (Redrawn from Vessel, E.S., and Page, J.G.: Genetic control of the phenobarbital-induced shortening of plasma antipyrine half-lives in man. J. Clin. Invest., 48: 2202–2209, 1969.)*

ment that genetics is a major source of variability in enzyme induction.

Inherited Variability in Pharmacodynamics. As previously noted, patients vary in their dosage requirements of warfarin to produce adequate anticoagulant control. At most, the variation in dosage requirements is fivefold. In several members of two families, however, massive doses of warfarin were needed to achieve a therapeutic response. Figure 14-7 illustrates the findings in the two families. In common with other genetic traits, warfarin resistance is not found in all kindred. Analysis of the frequency of the resistance in several generations indicates that the resistance is a dominant characteristic transmitted as a single gene effect. A normal pharmacokinetic profile of warfarin in the resistant subjects points to a pharmacodynamic-based resistance. A probable mechanism is either a reduced affinity of warfarin at the site of

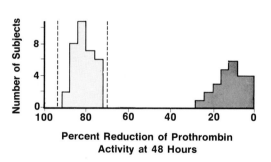

Figure 14-7. *Reduction of the one-stage prothrombin activity (an index of anticoagulability) from 0 to 48 hours, after an oral dose of 1.5 mg/kg sodium warfarin, for 59 members of two warfarin-resistant kindreds. The dotted lines represent the 99 percent confidence limits for the response in 50 normal subjects given the same dose. The 34 members of both kindreds with a normal response are indicated by the lightly shaded bars, and 25 of the 26 members with a resistant response are indicated by the darkly shaded bars. (Redrawn from O'Reilly, R.A.: Symposium on pharmacogenetics. Genetic factors in the response to the oral anticoagulant drugs in human genetics. Proceedings of the Fourth International Congress of Human Genetics, International Congress Series 250. Excerpta Medica, Amsterdam, 1972, pp. 428–438.)*

action, or an increased affinity of the receptor for vitamin K, with which warfarin competes to produce its anticoagulant effect.

Disease States

Despite a paucity of data, as the limited information in Table 14-2 shows, disease can be an added source of variation in drug response. Usual dosage regimens may need to be substantially modified in patients with renal function impairment, liver disorders, congestive heart failure, thyroid disorders, gastrointestinal disorders, and other diseases. The modification in the dosage may apply to the drug used to treat the specific disease, but may apply equally well to other drugs the patient receives. For example, to prevent excessive accumulation and so reduce the risk of toxicity, the dosage of the antibiotic, gentamicin, used to treat a pleural infection of a patient, must be reduced if the patient also has compromised renal function. Similarly, hyperthyroidic patients require higher doses of digoxin, a drug used to improve cardiac efficiency. Moreover, a modification in dosage may not only arise from the direct impairment of a diseased organ, but also from secondary events that accompany the disease. Drug metabolism, for example, may be modified in patients with renal disease; plasma and tissue binding of drugs may be altered in patients with uremia and with liver disorders.

In many diseases a change in response is due primarily to a change in the pharmacokinetics of a drug, and it is in this area that attention is principally focused. Discussion is also restricted primarily to the influence of renal function impairment, liver disorders, and cardiovascular disorders on pharmacokinetics, because more is known about the influence of these diseases on drug handling than any other group of diseases.

Renal Diseases. Consider the data in Figure 14-8, which show the frequency distribution of the half-life of kanamycin in pa-

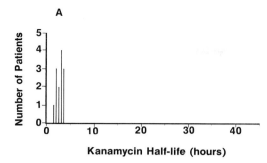

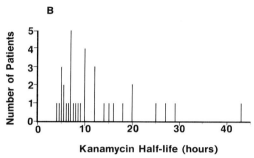

Figure 14-8. *The elimination half-life of kanamycin in a hospital population is much shorter and less variable in patients with normal renal function, A, than in patients with compromised renal function, B. It has been arbitrarily assumed that a patient has compromised renal function if his serum creatinine exceeds 1.2 mg/liter. (Adapted from data of Sørensen, A.W.S., Szaba, L., Pedersen, A., and Scharff, A.: Correlation between renal function and serum half-life of kanamycin and its application to dosage adjustment. Postgrad. Med. J. Suppl.: 37–43(May), 1967 and from data of Cutler, R.E., and Orme, B.M.: Correlation of serum creatinine concentration and kanamycin half-life. J.A.M.A., 209: 539–542, 1969. Copyright 1969, American Medical Association.)*

tients with normal kidney function and in patients with compromised kidney function. Contrast the narrow range in the half-life, 1.7 to 4 hours, when kidney function is normal, to the tremendously wide range in the half-life, 4 to 43 hours, when kidney function is impaired. Clearly, to avoid excessive accumulation, the dosage regimen of kanamycin must be reduced in patients with impaired kidney function, but by how much? A reasonable answer to this question is to reduce the dosage most in those patients with the longest half-life, but is there any way of knowing, prior to giving the

drug, how rapidly kanamycin will be eliminated in an individual patient? Fortunately, there is a means of estimating this value. The half-life of kanamycin is prolonged because the excretion of this drug is diminished in patients with impaired renal function. However, renal function impairment is not an all-or-none response: It is a graded one. Several convenient measures of renal function exist, the most popular being the renal clearance of creatinine. The corresponding measure of the renal handling of a drug is its renal clearance. When, as illustrated with kanamycin in Figure 14-9, the renal clearance of a drug is plotted against the renal clearance of creatinine in a population of patients with varying degrees of renal function impairment, a direct proportionality between the two variables is obtained. That is, the creatinine clearance is a satisfactory quantitative index of renal drug excretory function. How this and other measures of renal function are used to individualize dosage regimens in patients with renal function impairment is discussed in greater detail in Chapter 16.

Hepatic Disorders. Because the liver is the major site for drug metabolism, an impression prevails that special care should be taken in administering drugs to patients

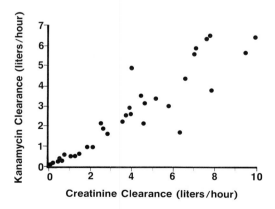

Figure 14-9. *Kanamycin clearance is directly correlated with creatinine clearance, an index of renal function. (From Orme, B.M., and Cutler, R.E.: The relationship between kanamycin pharmacokinetics: its distribution and renal function. Clin. Pharmacol. Ther., 10: 543–550, 1969.)*

Table 14-2. Examples of Increased Variability in Drug Response Associated with Concurrent Disease States

Condition	Drug	Class	Observation	Variation in Pharmaco-kinetics	Variation in Pharmaco-dynamics	Comments
Renal Disease						
Uremia	Gentamicin	Gram-negative antibiotic	Increased toxicity with usual dosage	+	–	Renal clearance diminished; reduce dosage to lessen risk of toxicity
Uremia	Thiopental	Anesthetic	Prolonged anesthesia	NS	NS	Reduce dose to avoid excessive sleeping time
Hepatic Diseases						
Cirrhosis	Theophylline	Bronchodilator	Slower fall in plasma concentration	+	–	Clearance reduced; reduce dosage to avoid toxicity
Acute viral hepatitis	Warfarin	Anticoagulant	Excessive anticoagulant response	–	+	Reduce dosage to lessen risk of hemorrhage
Cardiovascular Disease						
Congestive heart failure	Lidocaine	Antiarrhythmic agent	Elevated plasma concentration after usual dosage	+	–	Clearance and volume of distribution diminished; reduce dosage to lessen risk of toxicity
Gastrointestinal Diseases						
Celiac Disease	Fusidic acid	Antibacterial agent	Elevated plasma concentration after usual oral dose	+	–	Availability increased and/or clearance diminished
Crohn's Disease	Propranolol	β-blocker	Elevated plasma concentration after an oral dose	+	NS	Increased plasma binding, elevated α_1 acid glycoprotein suspected cause; observed only in active phase

Respiratory Diseases						
Asthma	Tolbutamide	Hypoglycemic agent	More rapid fall in plasma concentration	+	−	Therapeutic consequences uncertain
Emphysema	Morphine	Analgesic	Increased sensitivity to respiratory depressant effect	NS	NS	Reduce dose to diminish risk of respiratory complications
Cystic Fibrosis	Dicloxacillin	Antibiotic	Reduced area under plasma drug concentration-time curve	+	−	Renal clearance increased
Pneumonia	Theophylline	Bronchodilator	Elevated plasma concentration	+	−	Metabolic clearance decreased: reduce dose to lessen risk of toxicity
Endocrine Diseases						
Thyroid Disease	Digoxin	Cardioactive agent	Diminished response in hyperthyroidism; increased response in myxedema	+	+	Adjust dosage according to thyroid activity
Mongolism	Atropine	Spasmolytic	Heart rate increase to standard dose is greater than usual	NS	NS	
Fever	Quinine	Antimalarial agent	Plasma concentration of drug elevated, of metabolite depressed, after usual dosage	+	NS	Impaired metabolism suspected. May need to reduce doses in severe febrile states

+, established source of variability.
−, no evidence that variability is increased due to disease.
NS, not studied.

with disease states modifying hepatic function. Objective data, obtained primarily in patients with hepatic disorders, while generally supporting this impression, are surprisingly limited and occasionally in conflict. Let us examine some of the available data and explore some of the reasons for this apparent conflict.

One reason for the conflict arises from an attempt to classify liver disorders as a single entity. However, disorders of the liver, local or diffuse, are caused by many diseases; each disease affects the various levels of hepatic organization to a different extent. This is illustrated by the data in Table 14-3, which shows the changes in half-life or, where measured, in clearance of a number of drugs in patients with liver disease. Grouped together there appears to be no consistent relationship between disease and

drug handling. Many drugs show a decreased clearance, some drugs show no change. The clearance is even increased with tolbutamide. When, however, liver disease is divided into chronic (especially cirrhosis) and acute and reversible situations, e.g., acute viral hepatitis, a much clearer picture emerges. With the exception of tolbutamide, chloramphenicol, and oxazepam, there is a decreased clearance of drugs in cirrhosis. In contrast, in acute viral hepatitis, there appears to be a fairly even division between those drugs for which clearance is decreased, or half-life prolonged, and those for which no change is detected. With tolbutamide, an increased clearance was noted. The meager existing data suggest that drug elimination is diminished in chronic active hepatitis and obstructive jaundice.

Table 14-3. Changes in Total Clearance and Elimination Half-Life of Some Drugs in Liver Disease[a]

Disease	Decreased Clearance, Increased Half-Life	Unchanged	Increased Clearance, Decreased Half-Life
Cirrhosis	Ampicillin Amobarbital Antipyrine Chloramphenicol[b] Diazepam Isoniazid[b] Lidocaine Meperidine Phenobarbital[b] Phenylbutazone[b]	Tolbutamide[b] Chloramphenicol Oxazepam	
Acute viral hepatitis	Antipyrine Diazepam Hexobarbital Meperidine	Lidocaine Phenobarbital[b] Phenylbutazone[b] Phenytoin Warfarin Oxazepam	Tolbutamide[b]
Chronic active hepatitis	Antipyrine Diazepam		
Obstructive jaundice	Antipyrine		

[a]Adapted from Rowland, M., Blaschke, T.F., Meffin P.J., and Williams A.L.: Pharmacokinetics in Disease States Modifying Hepatic and Metabolic Function. *In* Symposium on the Influence of Disease States on Drug Pharmacokinetics. Edited by L.Z. Benet, Washington, D.C., American Pharmaceutical Association, 1976, pp. 53–75.
[b]Only half-life measured.

Another reason for the apparent conflict is the failure of many earlier workers to appreciate the influence of concurrent drug therapy. Consider, for example, the data displayed in Figure 14-10, which shows the half-life of phenylbutazone in normal subjects and in patients with liver disease (primarily cirrhosis). Initially, no difference was revealed between the two groups, except for a greater variability in the half-life among the patients with liver disease (Fig. 14-10A). When, however, both groups are further subdivided on the basis of whether they received other drugs, the picture is clearer (Fig. 14-10B). Of those receiving no other drugs, patients with liver disease handled phenylbutazone more slowly than did normal subjects. Evidently some of the drugs received can induce the enzymes responsible for phenylbutazone elimination.

Genetic factors can also obscure the picture. As seen previously, many metabolic pathways are under genetic control and when, as with phenylbutazone, metabolism is a major route of elimination, intersubject variability in the pharmacokinetics of a drug in the normal population can be wide. With such wide intersubject variability, a change in the pharmacokinetics of a drug associated with a disease is difficult to detect. This is particularly so when studying the effect of chronic disease on pharmacokinetics; assessment is usually made by comparing average drug handling in the

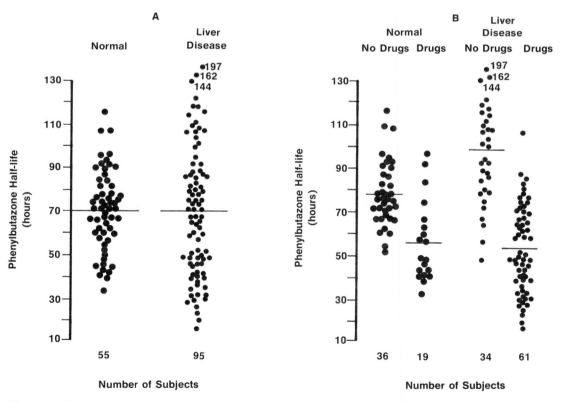

Figure 14-10. A, *No difference is seen between the average half-life of phenylbutazone (horizontal line) in normal subjects (●) and that in patients with liver disease (●). B, After separating drug takers from nondrug takers, the prolonged elimination of phenylbutazone in patients with liver disease becomes evident. (Redrawn from Levi, A.J., Sherlock, S., and Walker, D.: Phenylbutazone and isoniazid metabolism in patients with liver disease in relation to previous drug therapy. Lancet, 1: 1275–1279, 1968.)*

patient population with its average handling in an otherwise comparable population without the disease. Had, for example, the sample size in the phenylbutazone study been smaller and the effect of the disease less consistent, a difference between normal subjects and cirrhotic patients may not have been detected.

Often forgotten is that pharmacokinetics of a drug may also change with age (Chap. 15), and care should always be taken in population studies to age match the control group. In reversible diseases, such as acute viral hepatitis, genetic and other factors may be eliminated with a longitudinal study in which the kinetics of a drug is studied in the individual during and after recovery from the disease. Since each person now acts as his own control, the influence of disease can be assessed on an individual basis. It is also important to divide total clearance into hepatic and renal clearance before making any assessment of the influence of hepatic disease on drug handling. For example, if a drug is primarily renally excreted, a depressed formation of an important metabolite in liver disease may go undetected by measuring only the total clearance of the drug. Similarly, a lack of change in total clearance does not exclude the possibility of compensating changes in renal and hepatic clearance.

Another potential pitfall is to equate a prolonged half-life with a diminished hepatic drug-metabolizing activity. Half-life is controlled by both total clearance and volume of distribution, two independent parameters (Chap. 6). To assess clearance and volume of distribution, the drug should be given intravenously to ensure complete absorption. Unfortunately, in most studies the drug is given orally, thereby complicating the interpretation of plasma drug concentration data. In some of the few studies in which drug is given parenterally, the volume of distribution of some drugs remains unaltered in liver disease (Table 14-4). A change in half-life can then be ascribed to a change in clearance, a better index of the ability of an eliminating organ to remove drug. Nonetheless, a potential for misinterpreting the mechanism for a change in half-life does exist.

How complex the situation may become can be appreciated from an examination of the data in Table 14-5, which shows the disposition kinetics of amobarbital in healthy subjects and in patients with

Table 14-4. Influence of Liver Disease on the Volume of Distribution of Some Drugs[a]

Volume of Distribution	Drug	Disease
Unchanged	Chlorpromazine	Cirrhosis
	Hexobarbital	Acute viral hepatitis
	Lidocaine	Acute viral hepatitis
	Meperidine	Cirrhosis
	Meperidine	Acute viral hepatitis
	Phenytoin	Acute viral hepatitis
	Tolbutamide	Acute viral hepatitis
	Warfarin	Acute viral hepatitis
Increased	Ampicillin	Cirrhosis
	Amobarbital	Cirrhosis
	Diazepam	Cirrhosis
	Lidocaine	Cirrhosis
	Propranolol	Cirrhosis
	Propranolol	Chronic active hepatitis

[a]Adapted from the reference cited in Table 14-3.

Table 14-5. Disposition Kinetics of Amobarbital and Tolbutamide

Condition	Half-life (hour)	Fraction of Drug in Plasma Unbound (*fu*)	Volume of Distribution (liter/kg)		Clearance (ml/hour/kg)	
			Based on plasma	Based on unbound drug	Based on plasma	Based on unbound drug
Amobarbital[a]						
Healthy	20	0.39	0.97	2.5	34	88
Cirrhosis	36	0.69	1.46	2.1	28	38
Tolbutamide[b]						
Healthy	5.8	0.060	0.15	2.5	18	300
Acute viral hepatitis	4.0	0.10	0.15	1.5	26	260

[a]Adapted from Mawer, G.E., Miller, N.E., and Turnberg, L.A.: Metabolism of amylobarbitone in patients with chronic liver disease. Br. J. Pharmacol., *44*: 549–560, 1972.
[b]From Williams, R.L., Blaschke, T.F., Meffin, P.J., Melmon, K.L., and Rowland, M.: The influence of acute viral hepatitis on the disposition and plasma binding of tolbutamide. Clin. Pharmacol. Therap., *21*: 301–309, 1977.

chronic liver disease. Cirrhotic patients have an enlarged volume of distribution, while clearance, low and primarily hepatic, remains approximately constant at 30 ml/hour/kg. In addition, the fraction of drug unbound in plasma (*fu*) increases with disease. Amobarbital, in common with most acids, binds to albumin, and patients with chronic liver disease frequently have a low serum albumin concentration, reflecting a sustained depression of protein synthesis. As discussed in Chapters 4 and 6, altered plasma binding can mask changes in drug tissue distribution and drug-metabolizing activity. For instance, when corrections are made for the change in plasma binding, the volume of distribution of amobarbital, based on unbound drug, is unchanged. Evidently, no net change in tissue binding of this barbiturate occurs in cirrhosis. In contrast, although the clearance of amobarbital is essentially unaltered, its clearance based on unbound drug, reflecting hepatic metabolic activity, is decreased twofold, from the control value of 88 ml/hour/kg to 38 ml/hour/kg in cirrhotic patients. It appears then that prolonged half-life reflects a depressed drug-metabolizing activity. Recall from Chapter 6 (Eq. 21), however, that half-life only mirrors the unbound drug

clearance when the volume of distribution based on unbound drug remains constant. The half-life may also reflect changes in the volume of distribution based on unbound drug, as the study of the pharmacokinetics of the oral hypoglycemic agent, tolbutamide, in acute viral hepatitis (Table 14-5) shows.

The half-life of tolbutamide, a drug predominantly but poorly cleared by hepatic metabolism, is shortened during acute viral hepatitis. Because the volume of distribution (0.15 liter/kg) remains unchanged, the half-life reflects a corresponding elevation in the plasma clearance of this drug. However, contrary to initial appearances, hepatic metabolic activity is unchanged. The plasma binding of tolbutamide is also decreased and when a correction is made for the difference in binding, the clearance based on unbound drug remains unchanged. Also, because the diminished plasma binding of tolbutamide is not accompanied by a change in its volume of distribution, a diminished tissue binding (fu_T) is automatically implied. The cause of the diminished plasma and tissue binding is uncertain. Tolbutamide, an acidic drug, is primarily bound to albumin in plasma, but in acute viral hepatitis plasma albumin concentration is unchanged. Bilirubin, an end product of hemoglobin degradation, is an acidic compound that binds avidly to albumin and displaces some drugs from it. Bilirubin elimination is impaired in hepatitis and so it accumulates. When added to control plasma of healthy subjects at the same concentration as found in patients, bilirubin decreases the plasma binding of tolbutamide but not to the same extent as seen during viral hepatitis. Perhaps bilirubin also causes part of the diminished tissue binding of tolbutamide.

The influence of liver disease on drug absorption is poorly understood. The problem is complicated by the need to separate disposition from absorption when analyzing plasma drug concentration-time data. It is likely, though, that the oral availability of drugs highly extracted by the liver, and therefore exhibiting a high first-pass effect, is increased in cirrhosis. Many cirrhotic patients develop portal bypass, a condition where a significant fraction of the portal blood bypasses the liver and enters directly into the superior vena cava via esophagial varices.

From the foregoing discussion, it is apparent that drug dosage may need to be reduced in patients with hepatic function impairment. An adjustment in dosage is particularly warranted when the usual regimen results in the unbound drug concentration at the plateau approaching or exceeding the upper limit of the therapeutic concentration window. This condition arises when the clearance based on unbound drug is substantially depressed, since it is this clearance that controls the unbound drug concentration at the plateau (see Chap. 11). Like renal function impairment, hepatic dysfunction is a graded phenomenon, and theoretically a correlation should exist between changes in the pharmacokinetics of drugs, especially hepatic clearance, and an appropriate measure of hepatic function. Attempts to establish such relationships, while occasionally encouraging, have been generally unsuccessful. This failure probably arises because, unlike drug excretion, there are numerous pathways of drug metabolism, each with a different set of cofactor requirements, which appear to be affected to varying degrees by liver disorders. The contribution of each pathway to total drug elimination also varies with the drug.

Circulatory Disorders. Circulatory disorders, which include shock, malignant hypertension, and congestive heart failure, are generally characterized by diminished vascular perfusion to one or more parts of the body. Since blood flow may influence drug absorption, distribution, and elimination, it is not surprising that the pharmacokinetics of drugs may be altered in circulatory disorders.

A diminished perfusion of absorption sites, e.g., gastrointestinal tract and muscle, with an associated protracted and erratic drug absorption, tends to be seen in patients with depressed cardiovascular states; it may be necessary to give the drug intravenously if a prompt response is desired. However, in these conditions the distribution dynamics of the drug is also affected, with perfusion to many organs diminished. Exceptions are the brain and the myocardium, which consequently receive an increased fraction of an intravenous bolus dose, particularly in the earlier moments of administration. For centrally acting and cardioactive agents, the rate of administration of a bolus dose to patients with circulatory depression must be tempered if the risks of toxicity are to be reduced. In these depressed circulatory states, cardiac output and therefore liver blood flow and to a much lesser extent, renal blood flow, are also reduced. Therefore, the same response should be evident in the clearance of highly extracted drugs. Evidence supporting this concept is illustrated in Figure 14-11, which shows the relationship between the clearance of the highly hepatically cleared drug, lidocaine (see Table 7-2), and the cardiac output, normalized for weight, in patients of varying degrees of congestive heart fail-

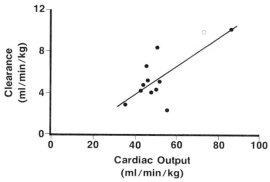

Figure 14-11. *Much of the variability in lidocaine clearance among patients with congestive heart failure can be accounted for by differences in cardiac output. The open circle represents the mean value for healthy volunteers (From Thomson, P.D., Melmon, K.L., Richardson, J.A., Cohn, K., Steinbrum, W., Cudihee, R., and Rowland, M.: Lidocaine pharmacokinetics in advanced heart failure, liver disease and renal failure in humans. Ann. Intern. Med., 78: 499–508, 1973.)*

ure. Potentially, liver blood flow is a more accurate correlate of lidocaine clearance, but cardiac output that determines liver blood flow is, to a large extent, both easier and safer to measure. Notice in Figure 14-11 that much, but not all, of the variability in lidocaine clearance can be accounted for by differences in cardiac output between patients. The hepatocellular enzymatic activity is perhaps also depressed, to a variable degree, by diminished hepatic perfusion. Notice also that the cardiac output varies between patients as much as threefold, and so therefore does lidocaine clearance. Since lidocaine has a narrow therapeutic window (see Table 12-1), dosage must be individualized if the risks of toxicity are to be reduced. These data suggest an approach to individualization, namely, adjust the dosage rate of lidocaine according to the patient's cardiac output, or indeed, any suitable index of liver blood flow.

Other Sources of Variability

Table 14-6 lists examples of other factors known to contribute to variability in drug response. Of these, age and concurrently administered drugs are more important sources of variability; these topics are covered in Chapters 15 and 17, respectively. Sex-linked differences in hormonal balance, body composition, and activity of certain enzymes manifest themselves in differences in both pharmacokinetics and responsiveness, but the effect of sex tends to be minimal.

Food, particularly fat, slows gastric emptying and so decreases the rate of drug absorption. Oral drug availability is not usually affected by food, but there are many exceptions to this statement. Food is a complex mixture of chemicals, each potentially capable of interacting with drugs. Recall, from Chapter 3, for example, that the availability of tetracycline is reduced when taken with milk, because of the formation of an insoluble complex with calcium. Recall also that a slowing of stomach emptying may increase the oral availability of a sparingly soluble drug, such as griseofulvin, and of some of the actively transported water-soluble vitamins. Diet may also affect drug metabolism. Enzyme synthesis is ultimately dependent on protein intake. When protein intake is severely reduced for prolonged periods, particularly because of an imbalanced diet, drug metabolism may be impaired. Conversely, a high protein intake may cause enzyme induction.

Chronopharmacology is the study of the influence of time on drug response. Many endogenous substances, for example hormones, are known to undergo cyclic changes in concentration in plasma and tissue with time. The amplitude of the change in concentration varies between the substances. The period of the cycle is often diurnal, approximately 24 hours, although there may be both shorter and longer cycles upon which the daily one is superimposed. The menstrual cycle and seasonal variations in the concentrations of some endogenous substances are examples of cycles with a long period. Drug responses may therefore

Table 14-6. Examples of Other Factors Known to Contribute to Variability in Drug Response

Factor	Observations and Remarks
Age	Pharmacokinetics and pharmacodynamics of many drugs vary with age.
Drugs	Pharmacokinetics and Pharmacodynamics of many drugs vary with concurrent drug therapy.
Food	Rate, and occasionally, extent of absorption are affected by eating. Effects depend on composition of food. Severe protein restriction may reduce the rate of drug metabolism.
Pollutants	Drug effects appear to be lessened in smokers and workers occupationally exposed to pesticides; enhanced drug metabolism is hypothesized.
Time of day and season	Diurnal variations are seen in pharmacokinetics and in drug response. Sufficiently important to lead to the development of a new subject, chronopharmacology.
Location	Dose requirements of some drugs differ between patients living in town and in the country.
Sex	Intramuscular absorption of some drugs is slower in females than in males; explained by differences in blood flow.

change with the time of day, with the day of the month, or with the season of the year.

Cigarette smoking tends to reduce the clinical and toxic effects of some drugs, including diazepam, theophylline, chlordiazepoxide, propoxyphene and chlorpromazine. The drugs affected are extensively metabolized by hepatic oxidation, and induction of the drug-metabolizing enzymes appears likely. The pesticide DDT and related compounds also induce microsomal enzymes, and induction may help to explain the more rapid elimination of certain drugs in workers occupationally exposed to these pesticides. Patients living in rural areas tend to be more sensitive to the analgesic effects of pentazocine than those living in towns. Enzyme induction may also explain this effect of location. Many compounds that are environmental pollutants and that exist in higher concentrations in

the city than in the country, can stimulate the synthesis of hepatic metabolic enzymes.

Accounting for Variability

Expressions and causes of variability in drug response have been examined. It remains to be seen how this information might profitably be used to devise an optimal dosage regimen of a drug for the treatment of a disease in an individual patient. Obviously, the desired objective would be most efficiently achieved if the individual's dosage requirements could be calculated, *prior to administering the drug.* While this ideal cannot be totally met in practice, some success may be achieved by adopting the following type of approach.

Assume that the patient population pharmacokinetics of a drug, partly metabolized in the liver and partly excreted unchanged, are: availability, 0.82; volume of distribution, 10.3 liters; renal clearance, 6.7 liters/hour; and metabolic clearance, 16.2 liters/hour. These data help to define the optimal population oral dosage regimen, but not necessarily that for an individual patient; the patient's pharmacokinetics may differ from those of the population. The objective then is to move from the population estimates to the individual patient's values. An approach to this problem is first to assess the variability within the patient population of each parameter and then to determine how much of the variability can be accounted for in terms of parameters, such as weight, age, renal function, and so forth, that are known or can be readily measured. The greater the variability that can be accounted for, the greater the likelihood of achieving the objective.

Figure 14-12 illustrates the approach. Depicted are four tablets, representing availability, volume of distribution, renal, and metabolic clearances. The size of each tablet is a measure of the variability of that parameter within the patient population. For this drug, availability is the least variable and hepatic clearance is the most variable parameter. Stated differently, the greatest confidence exists in assuming that the availability of the drug in the patient is the population value; the least confidence exists in assuming that the hepatic clearance in the patient is the corresponding population value. Moreover, since the population value for hepatic clearance is much greater than that for renal clearance, the variability in the value of the total clearance within the population is also high.

It should also be noted that, not unexpectedly, weight accounts for most of the variability in volume of distribution and for some of the variability in renal and hepatic clearance. Age, separated from its influence on body weight, accounts for some of the variability in renal and hepatic clearance and, to a much lesser extent, for some of the variability in the volume of distribution. A measure of kidney function, such as creatinine clearance, also, as expected, accounts for much of the variability in renal clearance. Indeed, together with age and weight, kidney function helps explain almost all the variability in this parameter. Surprisingly perhaps, kidney function helps to explain some of the variability in metabolic clearance and volume of distribution, but it should be recalled that drug distribution and metabolism can be altered in patients with renal function impairment. None of the variability in availability is accounted for but, as mentioned, this variability is small and is acceptable.

Finally, the inability to account for most of the variability in metabolic clearance should be noted. None of the characteristics included, or indeed any other known characteristic, can adequately account for the

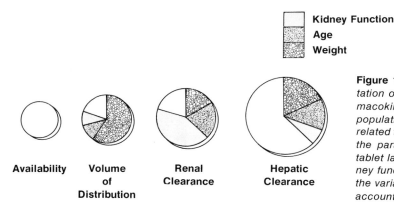

Kidney Function
Age
Weight

Availability   Volume of Distribution   Renal Clearance   Hepatic Clearance

Figure 14-12. *Schematic representation of variability in various pharmacokinetic parameters within a population. The size of each tablet is related to the degree of variability in the parameter. The portion of the tablet labeled weight, age, and kidney function reflects the fraction of the variability in a parameter that is accounted for by these factors.*

influence of genetics, disease, and other drugs on this parameter. A useful correlate may be found in the future.

Returning to the individual patient, correcting the population pharmacokinetics for the patient's weight, age, and renal function, should give reasonable individual estimates of F, V, and Cl_R, but poor estimates of Cl_H and hence total clearance. Since the ratio F/V strongly influences the peak plasma drug concentration after a single dose, assuming absorption is rapid relative to elimination, reasonable confidence can be expected in estimating the patient's loading dose, if required. However, since the ratio F/Cl controls the average plateau drug concentration, less confidence can be expected in estimating the patient's maintenance dose requirements. Nonetheless, the estimate of the maintenance dose should be better than using the population value. Clearly, if the drug had just been excreted unchanged, the probability of being able to estimate the correct dosage regimen for the patient would have been much higher.

Study Problems

(Answers to Study Problems can be found in Appendix G.)

1. Suggest which pharmacokinetic parameter is likely to be the most variable to explain the observations for nortriptyline in Figure 14-2. The drug is lipophilic, stable in the gastrointestinal tract, and little is excreted unchanged.

2. Explain the following observation: By coincidence, the weight, age, and renal function of the patient, discussed under the section, "Accounting for Variability," corresponded to the patient population values. Yet, when the pharmacokinetics of the drug was studied in the patient, the values of F, 0.42, and V, 22 liters, were considerably different (outside the 99 percent confidence intervals) from the population values: F, 0.82; V, 10.3 liters.

3. In a group of healthy subjects the average pharmacokinetic parameters of propranolol, a drug eliminated almost exclusively by hepatic metabolism, were found to be: volume of distribution, 180 liters; clearance, 0.82 liters/min; and half-life, 2.5 hours. After intravenous administration, values of these parameters differed little within this group; yet, when the drug was ingested orally, both the peak plasma concentration and the area were observed to vary over a fivefold range. Suggest why the variability in the observed plasma concentration–time curve is much greater after oral than after intravenous administration.

4. The following data (Table 14-7) were obtained in a study of the pharmacokinetic variability of a renally eliminated drug, $fu = 0.98$. The drug was intravenously infused at a constant rate of 20 mg/hour for 48 hours in five subjects. The value of the fraction unbound was found to be independent of drug concentration, but did vary among the subjects.

Table 14-7

Subject	1	2	3	4	5
Steady-state plasma concentration (mg/liter)	5.0	3.2	5.9	3.0	4.5
Postinfusion Half-life (hours)	14.4	5.9	4.7	9.9	8.2
Fraction unbound	0.1	0.15	0.09	0.16	0.11

(a) Analyze the data to identify the most and the least variable (use the *range/mean value* as your index of variability) of the following parameters:
Clearance based on unbound drug (Cl_u), fraction unbound in plasma (fu), fraction unbound in tissue (fu_T). Assume V_T to be 40 liters.
(b) Discuss briefly the therapeutic implications of these data with regard to the rate of attainment of and maintenance of a "therapeutic" concentration in the various subjects.

15

age and weight

Objectives

The reader will be able to:

1. **Determine those drugs for which the loading dose, normalized for body weight, is likely to be independent of age, given the values of the volume of distribution and the fraction of drug in plasma unbound.**

2. **Describe the likely changes with age in the pharmacokinetics of a drug that is predominantly excreted unchanged, from the neonate to the elderly.**

3. **Calculate the average dosage regimen of a drug for a child, given the child's weight and the usual adult dosage regimen.**

4. **Calculate the average dosage regimen of a drug that is predominantly excreted unchanged, for a geriatric patient, given the patient's weight and the usual adult dosage regimen.**

AGING, characterized by periods of growth, development, and senescence, is an additional source of variability in drug response, and the usual adult dosage regimen may need to be modified, particularly in both the young and the old, if optimal therapy is to be achieved. Unfortunately, the pharmacokinetic and therapeutic information required to make these necessary modifications in dosage is sparse. Controlled clinical trials in the elderly are rare; they are even rarer in children. The child is indeed a "therapeutic orphan." Yet it is the very young and the aged that often are in most critical need of drugs. It is against this background of limited data that this chapter, in which an attempt is made to develop a framework for making dosage adjustments for age, must be viewed.

The life of a human is commonly divided into various stages: that of the newborn, the infant, and so forth. For the purposes of this book the various stages are defined as follows: *newborn,* up to two months *post utero; infant,* between the ages of two months and one year; *child,* between one year and 12 years of age; *adolescent,* between the ages of 12 and 20 years; *adult,* between 20 and 70 years; and *geriatric,* older than 70 years of age. It is recognized, however, that this stratification of human life is arbitrary. Life is a continuous process with the distinction between one period and the next often ill-defined. It is also recognized that chronologic age does not necessarily define functional age, and, accordingly, statements made in this chapter pertain to the average person within the age bracket rather than to the individual.

Expediency and practicality dictate

against the use of longitudinal studies in individuals to examine the influence of age on pharmacokinetics. Rather, single observations are made in individuals of differing ages. The information obtained therefore pertains to the population and does not necessarily reflect how an individual may change with age.

A Point of Reference

Throughout this chapter reference is made to the "(usual) adult dosage regimen" of a drug. Before proceeding it is necessary to define this phrase more precisely. The word "adult" refers here to the average adult patient with the disease or condition. The "(usual) adult dosage regimen" is defined as that regimen which when given to this population, on the average, achieves therapeutic success. Clearly, the characteristics of the adult patient population vary with the disease. This is certainly true of age.

The data in Figure 15-1 show different age trends for the use of two drugs. Thus, patients taking digoxin, used to treat congestive heart failure, are generally older than those taking nitrofurantoin, used to treat urinary tract infections, a condition more evenly affecting people of all ages. Patients with incontinence are generally even older, 70 to 80 years, than those with congestive heart failure. However, there are few drugs for which pharmacokinetic data are obtained at the mean age of the adult patient population. Since most patients taking drugs tend to be middle-aged, for the purposes of subsequent calculations, an adult age of 55 years is assumed.

The data in Table 15-1 illustrate a point about age and disease. Listed are estimates of the population pharmacokinetics of digoxin in a group of young healthy adults and in a group of inpatients receiving digoxin for the treatment of severe congestive heart failure. Notice the differences in the values of the estimates, particularly for renal clearance, between the two groups. Clearly,

the estimates in the young healthy group are of less therapeutic value. Yet, most pharmacokinetic data on drugs are obtained in this selected group. Of greater clinical value are estimates of the pharmacokinetic parameters in the patient population requiring the drug.

Part of the difference in renal clearance of digoxin between the two groups is accounted for by the disease. Part, however, is accounted for by age. One objective of this chapter is to suggest means of correcting the values of pharmacokinetic parameters for age. The intent thereby is to permit a better estimate to be initially made of the dosage required to treat a disease in an individual patient or in a patient population whose age differs substantially from the mean age of the patient population in which the usual adult dosage regimen was established. It is assumed that the influence of all other factors on the pharmacokinetics of a drug, such as the disease being treated, concurrent diseases, and other drugs, is independ-

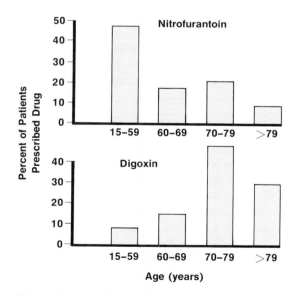

Figure 15-1. *Age distribution of drug consumption. Outpatients in the county of Jämtland, Sweden, taking digoxin are generally older than those taking nitrofurantoin. (Abstracted from Boethius, G., and Sjöqvist, F.: Doses and dosage intervals of drugs—clinical practice and pharmacokinetic principles. Clin. Pharmacol. Ther., 24: 255–263, 1978.)*

Table 15-1. Estimates of the Population Pharmacokinetics of Digoxin in Young Healthy Subjects and in Inpatients with Severe Congestive Heart Failure

	Age (years)	Weight (kg)	Availability (percent)	Volume of Distribution (liters)	Renal Clearance (liters/ hour)	Extrarenal Clearance (liters/hour)
Young healthy subjects[a]	28	71	40–70	760	8.52	3.48
Inpatients, severe congestive heart failure[b]	54	68	60	476	3.50	1.37

[a] Abstracted from the data of Koup, J.R., Greenblatt, D.J., Jusko, W.J., Smith, T.W., and Koch-Weser, J.: Pharmacokinetics of digoxin in normal subjects after intravenous bolus and infusion dose . J. Pharmacokinet. Biopharm. *3*: 181–192, 1975.
[b] Abstracted from the data of Sheiner, L.B., Rosenberg, B., and Marthe, V.V.: Estimation of population characteristics of pharmacokinetic parameters from routine clinical data. J. Pharmacokinet. Biopharm. *5*: 445–479, 1977.

ent of age or that the age-related effects are known and can be accounted for independently.

Pharmacodynamics

Throughout this chapter, the range of unbound plasma drug concentrations associated with successful therapy is assumed to be independent of the age of the patient. This assumption may well be substantiated for most drugs in the future, but, at present, data are very limited. At least for those antiepileptic drugs studied and for digoxin, effective plasma drug concentrations appear to be the same in both children and adults, although children appear to tolerate a higher concentration of these drugs before any toxic manifestations become apparent. It is likely, however, that differences in response with age do exist for certain drugs. For example, the observed increased sensitivity of elderly patients to the central nervous effects of the benzodiazepines cannot be explained on the basis of differences in the pharmacokinetics of this group of drugs.

Absorption

Although the subject has not been systematically studied, drug absorption does not appear to change dramatically with age. Nonetheless, all the factors discussed in Chapter 3 that affect drug absorption, including gastric pH, stomach emptying, intestinal motility, and blood flow, do change with age. Thus, in the newborn, a condition of relative achlorhydria persists for the first week of life, and it is not until after three years of age that gastric acid secretion approaches the adult value. Gastric emptying is also prolonged and peristalsis is irregular during the early months of life. Skeletal muscle mass is also much reduced, and muscle contractions, which tend to promote both blood flow and spreading of an intramuscularly administered drug, are relatively feeble. An elevated gastric pH, a delay in stomach emptying, and both diminished gastrointestinal motility and blood flow are also seen in old people. A difference in drug absorption between the adult and both the very young and the old is therefore expected. Generally, changes in rate (usually slower) rather than in extent of absorption are found. These changes tend to be less apparent in the elderly than in the very young. Children often appear to absorb drugs as completely and, if anything, more rapidly than adults. Accordingly, in subsequent calculations of dosage, absorption is assumed not to vary with age.

Body Weight

One aspect of aging is body weight. Weight, three kilograms at birth, increases rapidly in childhood and in adolescence and then declines slowly during later years. Because body water spaces, muscle mass, organ blood flow, and organ function are related to body weight, so too should be volume of distribution, clearance, and hence the dosage regimen of drugs. Owing to large variability in drug response, however, a weight adjustment is generally thought unnecessary unless the weight of an individual differs by more than 50 percent from the average adult weight (70 kg). Indeed, the dose strengths of most products usually do not differ by less than a factor of two or more. In practice, then, adjustments for weight are only made for the child and for the petite, emaciated, or obese adult patient.

Loading Dose

Clinically, correcting the adult loading dose proportionately for body weight appears reasonable. The volume of distribution based on unbound drug, V_u, is frequently both directly proportional to body weight and independent of age, but not always so. Much depends on the physicochemical properties of the drug and on the reason for the difference in weight.

Shown in Table 15-2 are values for the degree of plasma protein binding, the volume of distribution (V), the unbound volume of distribution (V_u), and the percent of drug in the body unbound, for a number of drugs in neonates and in adults. The last two parameters were calculated from the fraction unbound in plasma and the volume of distribution (see Chap. 4). As commonly found, plasma drug binding is lower in the neonate than in adults. Yet, for the first three drugs, phenobarbital and the two sulfonamides, the value of V_u, normalized for body weight, is the same because most of the drug is unbound in the body. Clearly, for these drugs a weight-normalized dose produces the same unbound drug concentration in both neonates and adults or in any other age group. In contrast, little of either diazepam, digoxin, or phenytoin is unbound in the body. Differences in tissue binding can now have a dramatic effect on the unbound drug concentration. Evidently for diazepam, the value of V_u, and hence tissue binding, is substantially higher in adults and, if this drug is needed, the neonate should require a much lower dose per kilogram of body weight. Muscle mass and

Table 15-2. Plasma Protein Binding and Distribution Data for Some Drugs in Neonates and Adults[a]

Drug	Fraction Unbound in Plasma (*fu*)		Volume of Distribution (*V*, liter/kg)		Unbound Volume of Distribution (V_u, liter/kg)		Percent of Drug in Body Unbound[b]	
	Neonate	Adult	Neonate	Adult	Neonate	Adult	Neonate	Adult
Phenobarbital	0.68	0.53	1.0	0.55	1.4	1.0	56	58
Sulfisoxazole	0.32	0.16	0.38	0.16	1.2	1.0	65	58
Sulfamethoxypyrazine	0.43	0.38	0.47	0.24	1.1	0.63	72	92
Diazepam	0.16	0.04	1.6	2.4	10	60	8	1
Digoxin	0.80	0.70	5–10	7.0	6–12	10	6–12	6
Phenytoin	0.2	0.1	1.3	0.63	6.5	6.3	12	9

[a] Adapted from the data collected by Morselli, P.L.: Clinical pharmacokinetics in neonates. Clin. Pharmacokinet., *1*: 81–98, 1976.

[b] Calculated from Equation 27, Chapter 4, assuming that the unbound drug distributes evenly throughout total body water.

fat are certainly higher in adults than in neonates, and diazepam partitions into both these tissues. Interestingly, for phenytoin, a difference in binding only occurs in plasma (V_u is the same), and so a weight-normalized loading dose, if required, should suffice.

Body composition should also be considered. A dose correction must be considered for emaciated and obese patients. However, the difference in the required loading dose may not be as great as initially anticipated. As with age-related changes in drug distribution, mucn depends upon the physicochemical properties of the drug. Digoxin, for example, and polar drugs do not partition well into fat. Accordingly, for these drugs the volume of distribution correlates better with lean body mass, which is similar between obese and average persons of the same height and frame, than with total body weight.

Disposition Kinetics

Figure 15-2 shows the changes with age in the half-life of creatinine and the clearance of creatinine expressed per kg body weight. Creatinine distributes into total body water spaces, is negligibly bound to tissue or plasma constituents, is eliminated almost entirely by renal excretion, and has a clearance equal to the glomerular filtration rate. The example of creatinine was chosen because changes in total body water and glomerular filtration rate with age are reasonably well understood. To the extent that creatinine mimics other drugs, the data displayed in Figure 15-2 further our understanding of age-related changes in the pharmacokinetics of drugs and suggest a means of individualizing dosage regimens for age. Let us consider the various parts of Figure 15-2 in some detail.

Clearance, if normalized for body weight, is depressed in the newborn and rapidly increases to reach a maximum value at 6 months, when it is almost twice that in the adult. Thereafter, weight-normalized clear-

ance falls but still remains, throughout childhood, considerably above the adult value. Also, an often forgotten point is that, throughout adulthood, creatinine clearance (glomerular filtration rate) diminishes at a rate of about 1 percent per year; therefore, as an approximation, beyond 20 years of age,

$$\text{Creatinine clearance (ml/min)} = [140 - \text{Age}] \times \frac{\text{Weight}}{70} \qquad 1$$

where age is expressed in years and weight in kilograms. Thus, in the average 95-year-old adult, who weighs 55 kg, the creatinine clearance is only one-third (35 ml/min) of that in the average young adult (120 ml/min). More exact relationships between creatinine clearance and age, for males and females, are given in Chapter 16.

Because total body water as a percent of body weight, and hence distribution, changes relatively little during life, the change in the half-life of creatinine inversely reflects the change in clearance. That is, the half-life is shortest at one year of age and longer in both the newborn and the elderly. Although extensive data are lacking, similar age-related changes in disposition of drugs seem to occur.

First, consider the data on diazepam, a drug metabolized primarily in the liver. As seen in Figure 15-3, the elimination half-life of diazepam is longest in the newborn, particularly in the premature neonate, and in adults of greater than 55 years of age. Infants eliminate the drug most rapidly. With creatinine, the long half-life in the newborn is due to depressed renal function, which takes several months to mature. With diazepam the long half-life in the newborn reflects an undeveloped drug-metabolizing activity. Metabolic activity may take months to mature; the time required for full maturation varies with the enzyme system. That the premature newborn has the longest half-life of diazepam is not surprising and stresses a point made earlier; chrono-

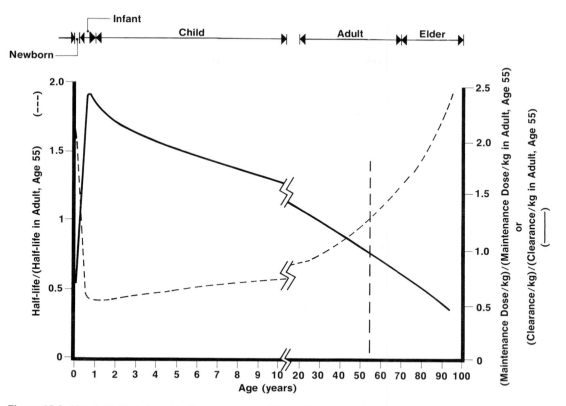

Figure 15-2. *How half-life (---) and both clearance and the maintenance dose rate (—) of a drug might vary with age. The values were calculated from data on creatinine. The drug, like creatinine, distributes into total body water, is eliminated entirely by renal excretion, and has a clearance equal to the glomerular filtration rate. The half-life is expressed as a fraction of the average value for a typical adult patient, 55 years old; the dosage regimen is calculated on the assumption that the desired average plateau concentration of drug remains constant throughout life. Notice that, because of poor kidney function, elimination is slow in the newborn, but function rapidly improves such that, by 1 year, the elimination half-life is only about one-half of the adult value. During childhood and adolescence the half-life becomes longer because, with growth, clearance, a function of surface area, increases more slowly than does volume of distribution, a function of body weight. Although body weight and therefore volume of distribution change only slightly beyond 30 years, because kidney function and therefore clearance progressively diminish, the half-life is longer in the aged. By 95 years the half-life is twice the adult value. These changes in clearance and weight with age explain why the maintenance dose per kg body weight is higher in the child and lower in both the newborn and the aged than in the adult.*

The data used in the calculations were obtained as follows: Half-life—Calculated from volume of distribution and clearance. The half-life in an average adult, 55 years, is 5.9 hours. Volume of distribution—Taken as 78 percent of body weight at birth, 67 percent of body weight at 6 months, and 60 percent of body weight thereafter (Friis-Hansen, B: Changes in body water compartments during growth. Acta Paediatr. (Supp.) 110: 1–68, 1956). Clearance—at birth, taken as the inulin clearance, 3 ml/min (Weil, W.B.: The evaluation of renal function in infancy and childhood. Am. J. Med. Sci., 229: 678–694, 1955); between 6 months and 20 years, calculated by multiplying the creatinine clearance 120 ml/min/1.8 m² in an average healthy adult, 21–29 years, by body surface area; between 30 and 99 years, taken from the data of Siersbaek-Nielsen (Siersbaek-Nielsen, K., Hansen, J.M., Kampmann, J., and Kristensen, M.: Rapid evaluation of creatinine clearance. Lancet, 1: 1133–1134, 1971). Surface Area—Calculated from body weight using the nomogram in Fig. 15-7.

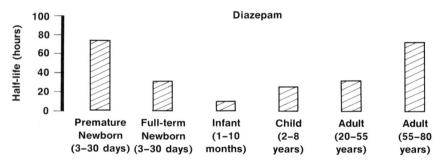

Figure 15-3. *The elimination half-life of diazepam is shortest in the infant and longest in the newborn and the elderly. (Adapted from the data of Morselli, P.L.: Drug Disposition During Development. Spectrum Publications, New York, 1977, pp. 311–360 and p. 456; and from the data of Klotz, U., Avant, G.R., Hoyumpa, A., Schenker, S., and Wilkinson, G.R.: The effect of age and liver disease on the disposition and elimination of diazepam in adult man. J. Clin. Invest., 55: 347–359, 1975.)*

logic and functional age must be distinguished, especially in newborns.

The shorter half-life of diazepam in the infant than in the adult, 20 to 55 years, reflects differences in clearance, because the volume of distribution of this drug is approximately the same (1.2 liters/kg) in both groups. One might be tempted to conclude that the further prolongation in half-life in the most elderly group is due to diminished drug metabolism. An excellent age-related increase in half-life is certainly found (Fig. 15-4A); however, clearance remains essentially constant from 20 to 80 years (Fig. 15-4B). Consequently, the change in half-life reflects a proportional decrease in the volume of distribution. Since no change in plasma drug binding with age was found, tissue binding must have increased. The mechanism responsible for this observation remains to be elucidated.

Next consider the observed smaller ratio of the plateau plasma drug concentration to dosing rate/kg determined after chronic oral dosing of several antiepileptic drugs in younger children (Fig. 15-5). All these drugs are completely available and since

$$\frac{C_{av}}{(\text{Dose}/\text{kg})/\tau} = \frac{1}{\text{Clearance}/\text{kg}} \qquad 2$$

it follows that the weight-normalized clearance must be higher in the younger, and

smaller, child. All these antiepileptic drugs are extensively metabolized, and in none studied does the protein binding appear to change substantially between the different age groups. Greater hepatic metabolic capacity per unit body weight is therefore implicated in the younger group.

Maintenance Dose Therapy

The Newborn. The lack of maturation of renal and hepatic function necessitates that the rate of administration of drugs to both the newborn and the young infant be reduced, even on a body weight basis, if toxicity is to be avoided. Unfortunately, events occur so rapidly in these stages of life that it is impossible to predict the clearance and hence the required dosage regimen. Caution must clearly be exercised in administering drugs to this patient population, and, besides carefully noting the effects, monitoring of the plasma concentration of drugs with narrow therapeutic indices should be helpful.

The Child. The evidence in Figures 15-2 and 15-5 suggests that a maintenance regimen, calculated by correcting the adult dosage for body weight, would prove inadequate for children, especially for the very young. *Body surface area* has been found to be a much better correlate than weight of dosage requirements, and indeed of cardiac output, of liver and renal blood flow, and of glomerular filtration rate in children and in adults of varying sizes. Because clearance relates dosing rate to the plateau plasma concentration of a drug, and because renal clearance is proportional to the glomerular filtration rate (see Fig. 14-9), the choice of surface area over weight as the method of calculating maintenance therapy has some

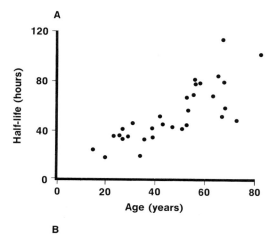

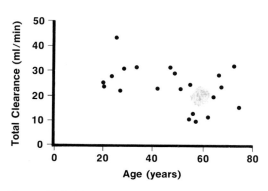

Figure 15-4. *Diazepam (0.1 mg/kg) was administered intravenously to 33 normal volunteers. Essentially all of the linear increase in half-life with age, A, can be accounted for by changes in the volume of distribution, since clearance varied little, B. (Redrawn from Klotz, U., Avant, G.R., Hoyumpa, A., Schenker, S., and Wilkinson, G.R.: The effects of age and liver disease on the disposition and elimination of diazepam in adult man. J. Clin. Invest., 55: 347–359, 1975.)*

justification. According to this concept a child's maintenance dosage is calculated from the formula:

Child's maintenance dosage

$$= \left[\frac{\text{Surface area of child (m}^2)}{1.8 \text{ m}^2} \right]$$
$$\times \text{Adult maintenance dosage} \quad 3$$

where 1.8 m² is the surface area of an average 70-kg adult. The surface area of a child may be obtained from the nomogram in Figure 15-6, which relates surface area to body weight. This nomogram has been constructed based upon the observation that surface area is proportional to body weight to the 0.7 power (weight$^{0.7}$). Alternatively, using this last relationship, Equation 3 may be rewritten as:

Child's maintenance dosage
$$= \left[\frac{\text{Weight of child (kg)}}{70} \right]^{0.7}$$
$$\times \text{Adult maintenance dosage} \quad 4$$

To illustrate the relationship expressed in Equation 3, consider the example of phenobarbital; the usual adult antiepileptic maintenance dose is 100 mg daily. Q. What is the phenobarbital dosage needed in a 15-kg child? A. 34 mg daily. This answer can be estimated from the ratio of surface areas (estimated from body weight using the nomogram) or from Equation 4.

Child's dosage of phenobarbital

$$= \frac{0.61 \text{ m}^2}{1.8 \text{ m}^2} \times 100 \text{ mg/day}$$

$$= \left(\frac{15}{70} \right)^{0.7} \times 100 \text{ mg/day}$$

$$= 34 \text{ mg/day}$$

Notice that the weight-normalized dosage of phenobarbital in the child, 2.3 mg/kg, is much higher than that in the adult, 1.43 mg/kg. The reason is that clearance is proportional to surface area, and surface area *increases* disproportionately with weight, the smaller the child. To appreciate this point, consider a cube of

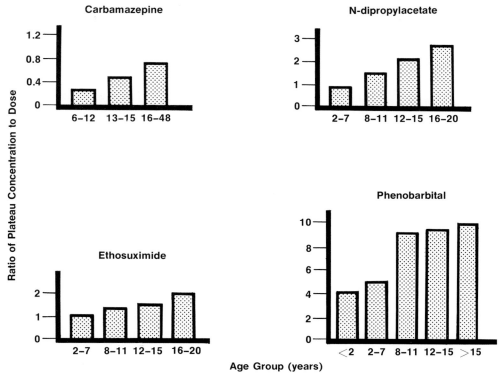

Figure 15-5. *The plateau plasma drug concentrations of several antiepileptic drugs were measured after chronic oral medication in children. An increased clearance per kg body weight explains the lower ratio of concentration to dose per kg in the youngest children. (Adapted from the data of Morselli, P.L.: Antiepileptic drugs.* In *Drug Disposition During Development. Edited by P.L. Morselli. Spectrum Publications, New York, 1977, Chap. 11, pp. 311–360.)*

length L. The area of each face is L^2 and having 6 sides the total surface area is therefore $6\,L^2$. The weight is proportional to volume, that is L^3. Thus, since the ratio of surface area to volume is $6/L$, diminishing the size by decreasing L increases the surface-area-to-volume ratio. The need for a higher maintenance dose per kilogram body weight, the smaller and hence usually the younger the child, is seen in Figure 15-2 for children between the ages of 6 months and 12 years. Note the complementary decrease in the half-life with decreasing size and age. Thus, not only may a child of one require a larger maintenance dose per kilogram body weight than an adult, but also, because of a shorter half-life, the drug may need to be given more frequently, especially if the drug has a low therapeutic index and if large fluctuations around the plateau concentration are to be avoided.

In addition to the need to correct dosage for surface area, with creatinine, and perhaps with predominantly excreted drugs, there is the need to correct for the approximately 25 percent decrease in renal function in adults between 25 and 55 years of age. The correction needed for drugs that are predominantly metabolized is not well established. The clearance of diazepam (Fig. 15-4) does not appear to change within this 30-year span, but the metabolic clearance of antipyrine does (Fig. 15-7). However, the variability in the antipyrine clearance is large, and age captures only about 6 percent of the total variance.

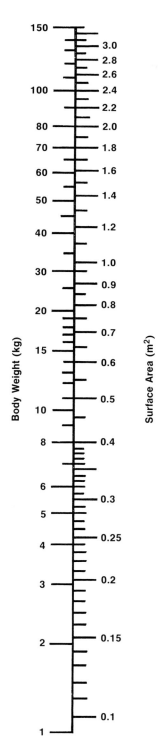

Figure 15-6. *Nomogram relating body surface area to body weight for children and adults of average height for weight.*

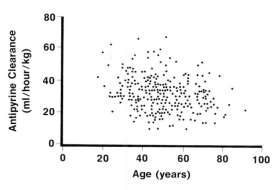

Figure 15-7. *The clearance of antipyrine, an extensively metabolized drug, declines but marginally with age, when studied in 307 healthy subjects, each of whom received 1 gram antipyrine intravenously. Age accounts for little of the variability in clearance within this population. (Adapted from Vestal, R.E., Norris, A.H., Tobin, J.D., Cohen, B.H., Shock, N.W., and Andres, R.: Antipyrine metabolism in man: Influence of age, alcohol, caffeine, and smoking. Clin. Pharmacol. Ther., 18: 425–432, 1975.)*

The Elderly. A decrease in the metabolic clearance in the elderly has been established for a few drugs. Old age is accompanied by a decrease in weight and by an increased incidence of previous hepatic and other diseases, so that any generalization at present is difficult.

The marked and progressive decrease in renal function implies that the dosage regimens of drugs that are predominantly excreted unchanged, should be reduced in the geriatric population. For example, an 80-year-old patient requires, on the average, only 70 percent of the usual adult dosage expressed on a body weight basis; the actual dose required would be even less because the geriatric patient is lighter. Despite the apparent need for dosage adjustment, none appears to be made in practice. Perhaps it is a therapeutic oversight; a depressed clearance may explain, in part, the increased frequency and degree of adverse drug effects often noted in the elderly.

General Equations. To return to the example of creatinine and similarly handled drugs, from 6 months to 20 years of age, the relationship between renal clearance and age is expressed in Equations 3 and 4, while beyond 20 years, this relationship is expressed in Equation 1. These equations can now be combined to give the general equations:

declines, note that there are pairs of age values in which the same rate of administration is required. For example, on the average, a 4-year-old child (16 kg) requires the same rate of drug administration as an 86-year-old person (60 kg).

$$\frac{\text{Maintenance}}{\text{dosage}} = \frac{[140 - \text{Age (years)}] \times [\text{Surface area (m}^2)]}{153} \times \frac{\text{Usual adult}}{\text{maintenance dosage}} \qquad 5$$

$$\frac{\text{Maintenance}}{\text{dosage}} = \frac{[140 - \text{Age (years)}] \times [\text{Weight (kg)}]^{0.7}}{1660} \times \frac{\text{Usual adult}}{\text{maintenance dosage}} \qquad 6$$

that permit the calculation of a maintenance dosage for a patient of any age, except the neonate. The value of the numerator, 153, in Equation 5, is the product of the age-related decline in renal function for a 55-year-old, 85 (140 − 55), and 1.8, the surface area, in square meters, of an average 70-kg adult. The value of the numerator, 1660, in Equation 6, is the product of the age-related decline in renal clearance, 85, and $70^{0.7}$ or 19.5. Because renal clearance increases up to 20 years and then

The relationships expressed in the last two equations have been incorporated into a generalized nomogram (Fig. 16-4). Hopefully, the nomogram will serve to facilitate and to improve the initial estimate of the dosage regimen needed for a patient of any age beyond 6 months. In general, a correction in the usual adult dosage is worthwhile when administering drugs to the very young, to the child, and to the aged. A correction is also worthwhile in emaciated and obese patients.

Study Problems

(Answers to Study Problems can be found in Appendix G.)

1. Calculate a dosage regimen of gentamicin to treat a severe infection caused by *Pseudomonas aeruginosa,* in a child, age 4 years, weight 15 kg, with normal renal function. The usually recommended adult dose of gentamicin is 1 mg/kg administered intramuscularly every 8 hours. This antibiotic is almost completely renally excreted unchanged.

2. Digoxin is frequently administered orally in a daily maintenance dose of 0.25 mg for the treatment of congestive heart failure. Listed in Table 15-3 are average digoxin pharmacokinetic data obtained in hospitalized patients of different ages.

Table 15-3.[a]

Age of Patient	6 days	6 months	4 years	Adult (55 years)
Wt. (kg)	3.5	7.5	16	70
$t_{1/2}$ (hours)	54	18	32	44
Cl (ml/min/kg)	1.8	6.4	4.0	1.73
V (liters/kg)	8	10	11	7

[a]Abstracted from Iisalo, E.: Clinical pharmacokinetics of digoxin. Clin. Pharmacokinet., 2: 1–16, 1977, and from Wettrell, G., and Anderson, K.E.: Clinical pharmacokinetics of digoxin in infants, Clin. Pharmacokinet., 2: 17–31, 1977.

(a) Using the information in Table 15-3 and the appropriate equations or nomograms complete Table 15-4. Assume that the availability of digoxin is independent of age.
(b) Discuss briefly the differences observed in the calculated doses in the table.
(c) Estimate the required daily oral maintenance for an 80-year-old patient weighing 51 kg. Assume that, like creatinine, digoxin elimination varies with age.

Table 15-4. Calculated Daily Oral Maintenance Digoxin Dose (μg/kg body weight) Based on Weight, Surface Area, and Observed Clearance Values

Age:	6 days	6 months	4 years	Adult (55 years)
1. Based on weight	4	4	4	4
2. Based on surface area (adult = 1.8 m²)				4
3. Based on observed clearance				4

16

renal function impairment

Objectives

The reader will be able to:

1. **Make a judgement, using pharmacokinetic principles, on when alteration of drug administration should be considered in renal failure.**

2. **Either calculate or use a nomogram to estimate how much the elimination of a drug is changed in a patient with known renal function impairment.**

3. **Estimate the creatinine clearance of a patient from the patient's age, weight, sex, and serum creatinine.**

4. **From pharmacokinetic considerations establish a dosage regimen for a drug in a patient with known renal function impairment.**

5. **Sketch the amount in the body with time following a dosage regimen recommended for a patient with renal function impairment.**

6. **Estimate steady-state levels of drug and active metabolite(s) in a patient with renal failure, given the appropriate pharmacokinetic information.**

7. **List the assumptions that underlie the application of kidney function tests to dosage regimen adjustment in renal failure.**

THE usual dosage regimen in patients with impaired renal function may result in excessive accumulation of drug to levels potentially producing undesirable side effects and toxicity. To avoid toxic reactions the clinician needs information on which drugs accumulate excessively in renal failure and, more importantly, he needs to know how to adjust drug administration to achieve an optimal therapeutic response. Accumulation occurs for a drug whose major route of elimination is renal excretion. Serious consideration must be given to decreasing the rate of administration of such a drug, particularly if it has a low therapeutic index;

but by how much is a difficult question. The answer requires an estimate of both kidney function and the contribution of the renal route to total elimination. The when and how to individualize a regimen in patients with impaired renal function is the substance of this chapter.

Change in Drug Elimination

The effect of renal failure on the disposition of a drug is readily described using the concept of clearance based on *unbound* drug. Renal failure causes a decrease in total clearance. The magnitude of the change depends on the reduction in renal clearance and on the fraction that renal clearance is of total clearance. Defining kidney function, *KF*, as the ratio of the renal clearance of a drug in renal failure, $Clu_R(f)$, to that in the fully functioning normal kidney, $Clu_R(n)$, then

$$Clu_R(f) = KF \cdot Clu_R(n) \qquad 1$$

Under conditions of normal renal function, renal clearance is a fraction, *fe*, of the total clearance, that is,

$$Clu_R(n) = fe \cdot Clu(n) \qquad 2$$

The clearance by extrarenal routes is therefore,

$$\frac{\text{Extrarenal}}{\text{clearance}} = (1 - fe) \cdot Clu(n) \qquad 3$$

Under any condition,

$$\frac{\text{Total}}{\text{clearance}} = \frac{\text{Renal}}{\text{clearance}} + \frac{\text{Extrarenal}}{\text{clearance}} \qquad 4$$

If it is assumed that extrarenal, usually metabolic, clearance based on unbound drug does not change in renal failure, then on substituting Equations 1 to 3 in Equation 4 the following useful relationship is derived for the unbound clearance in renal failure.

$$Clu(f) = Clu(n) \cdot [1 - fe(1 - KF)] \qquad 5$$

From this relationship one can readily calculate the change expected in the unbound clearance. For a drug with a value of zero for *fe*, no change in clearance would be expected. If *fe* is 1.0 then the clearance varies in direct proportion to kidney function.

Recall that $t_{1/2} = 0.7\ Vu/Clu$. The value of the half-life of a drug in a patient with renal failure, $t_{1/2}(f)$, compared to the value in a patient with a fully functioning normal kidney, $t_{1/2}(n)$, is then

$$\frac{t_{1/2}(f)}{t_{1/2}(n)} = \frac{Vu(f) \cdot Clu(n)}{Vu(n) \cdot Clu(f)} \qquad 6$$

where $Vu(f)$ and $Vu(n)$ are the unbound

volumes of distribution in renal failure and in the normal situation, respectively. If the unbound volume of distribution is unchanged in renal failure, then

$$t_{1/2}(f) = \frac{t_{1/2}(n)}{1 - fe(1 - KF)} \qquad 7$$

and since $k = 0.7/t_{1/2}$

$$k(f) = k(n)\,[1 - fe(1 - KF)] \qquad 8$$

Thus,

$$\frac{Clu(f)}{Clu(n)} = \frac{k(f)}{k(n)} = \frac{t_{1/2}(n)}{t_{1/2}(f)} \qquad 9$$

The unbound volume of distribution is sometimes altered in renal failure; for example, the tissue binding of digoxin is decreased. In this case, Equations 7 to 9 are not valid.

Adjustment of Dosage Regimens

The simplest way of conceiving the adjustment of a dosage regimen in renal failure is in terms of the steady-state unbound concentration. At steady state:

$$F \cdot \frac{D_M}{\tau} = Clu \cdot Cu_{av} \qquad 10$$

If the objective is to maintain the same average unbound concentration, Cu_{av}, then the rate of administration of a drug in renal failure, $(D_M/\tau)(f)$, compared to the normal rate of administration, $(D_M/\tau)(n)$, is

$$\frac{(D_M/\tau)(f)}{(D_M/\tau)(n)} = \frac{Clu(f)}{Clu(n)} \cdot \frac{F(n)}{F(f)} \qquad 11$$

where $F(f)$, $F(n)$ are the availabilities of drug in renal failure and in patients with normal renal function, respectively. Assuming that the availability does not change, the rate of administration in renal failure is

$$(D_M/\tau)(f) = (D_M/\tau)(n) \cdot [1 - fe(1 - KF)] \qquad 12$$

With the two preceding assumptions, the only information required to establish a dosage regimen for a patient with renal failure is (1) the *normal* dosage regimen for the patient, (2) the kidney function as a fraction of the *normal,* and (3) the fraction of the total elimination of the unchanged drug that occurs by renal excretion in the absence of hepatic or renal dysfunction.

The *normal* dosage regimen is that determined to be appropriate for the individual without renal or hepatic function impairment. The *normal* dosing schedule is determined by the patient's age, height and weight or surface area, and the condition being treated (Chap. 15). The individual, therefore, might be an infant, a child, an adult, or a geriatric patient.

The kidney function is expressed in terms of the fraction of that which is normal for the individual. Again, the kidney function varies with the age and weight of the patient. However, the information required is simply the kidney function as a fraction of the normal for a patient of his age, height, and weight. The kidney function is assumed to remain stable during treatment.

The third piece of information that is needed is the fraction of the total elimination of a drug that normally occurs by renal excretion. This value, too, should be that for a normal individual of the same age, height, and weight as the patient. Of the three kinds of information, this is probably the most difficult to determine accurately. The percentage of a dose excreted unchanged is given in many texts; however, one has to be careful in interpreting the value because the figure quoted is sometimes that obtained after an oral dose, in which case the fraction of the dose absorbed is unknown. Sometimes the assay techniques used do not distinguish between drug and metabolite(s). Also, it is not uncommon for the urine collection to be incomplete either because of a missed sample or because the urine was not collected until virtually all the drug had been eliminated.

In general, the loading dose is not changed; the same amount of drug in the body is needed for therapeutic response.

The adjustment of a maintenance regimen may be made by a decrease in the maintenance dose, a decrease in the frequency of administration, or a combination of both. These approaches are not identical. As an example of the use of Equation 12, consider how the dosage regimen of amikacin sulfate, a drug that is virtually completely eliminated by excretion, should be altered in renal function impairment. The suggested dosage regimen for adult, average-sized patients with normal renal function is 7.5 mg/kg intramuscularly every 12 hours. For a 23-year-old patient weighing 68 kg who has an endogenous creatinine clearance of 20 ml/min/1.8 m², the following information is derived:

1. *Normal* dosage regimen:
   7.5 mg/kg × 68 kg = 500 mg to be administered intramuscularly every 12 hours.
2. Kidney function—120 ml/min/1.8 m² is assumed to be the normal kidney function:

$$\frac{20 \text{ ml/min}}{120 \text{ ml/min}} = 0.17$$

Using Equation 12 or the nomogram of Figure 16-1, it is apparent that the maintenance dosing rate of amikacin sulfate should be decreased by a factor of 6 in this patient. Thus, the dosage regimen might be one of the following: (1) The dosing interval may be increased by a factor of 6. Dosage regimen: 500 mg every 72 hours. (2) The maintenance dose may be decreased by a factor of 6. Dosage regimen: 500 mg initially, then 83 mg every 12 hours. (3) Both the dosing interval and the maintenance dose may be adjusted to decrease the average rate of administration by a factor of 6. Dosage regimen: 500 mg initially, then 167 mg every 24 hours. The package insert for amikacin sulfate suggests reducing the maintenance dose.

To appreciate adjustment of dosage regimens in renal failure, it is often helpful to

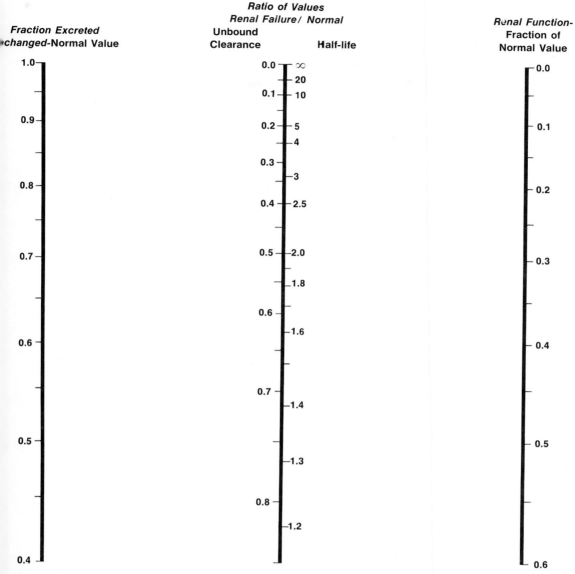

Figure 16-1. *Estimation of dosage regimens in patients with renal function impairment. To be used to determine how to change a normal dosage regimen. The normal dosage regimen depends upon age, weight, and condition being treated. Activity and toxicity of metabolites are not taken into consideration.*

How to use nomogram: *With a ruler, connect the fraction of drug normally excreted unchanged and the patient's kidney function, expressed as a fraction of normal value in a person of the same age. Read off from the center line the unbound clearance and the half-life relative to their normal values in a patient of the same age.*

Modification of Dosage Regimen

I. Initial dose—no change (see text)

II. Adjustment of rate of administration for maintenance of drug in body.

   A. Change in dosing interval, τ, only.

$$\tau(failure) = \frac{t_\frac{1}{2}\ (failure)}{t_\frac{1}{2}\ (normal)} \cdot \tau(normal)$$

   B. Change in maintenance dose, D_M, only.

$$D_M(failure) = \frac{Cl_u(failure)}{Cl_u(normal)} \cdot D_M(normal)$$

   C. Change in rate of administration D_M/τ

$$(D_M/\tau)(failure) = \frac{Cl_u(failure)}{Cl_u(normal)} \cdot [(D_M/\tau)(normal)]$$

prepare a sketch of the amount of drug in the body with time. Using the previous example with amikacin a sketch may be prepared if one additional piece of information is known, the normal half-life, which for amikacin is approximately 2 hours. Figure 16-2 is a sketch of the drug in the body on a regimen of 500 mg every 12 hours. An individual with normal renal function (curve A) and the patient above (curve B) with renal function 17 percent of normal are shown. From Equation 7 it is seen that the half-life would be about 12 hours in the patient above. For graphic purposes, absorption from the intramuscular site is assumed to be instantaneous.

To avoid unwanted accumulation, three regimens were suggested, all of which resulted in a sixfold decrease in the average rate of administration and produced the same average steady-state amount in the body. Figure 16-3 is a sketch of the drug in the body from each of the three regimens. Clearly, changing the interval only (curve A) results in much greater fluctuation with many hours at high levels and many hours at low levels. The desirability of this is dif-

ficult to support, except in terms of convenience to the patient. The intramuscular dose need only be given every three days. Changing the maintenance dose only (curve B) reduces fluctuation but still suffers from the inconvenience of frequent intramuscular injections. Changing both the maintenance dose and the dosing interval reduces both fluctuation and inconvenience to the patient and as such may be preferred for many drugs.

In this example, the administration of the usual dosage regimen to the patient with renal dysfunction resulted in a twofold increase in the maximum amount in the body and a sixfold increase in the average amount at plateau. It is important, however, to consider whether the maximum amount (or concentration) or the average amount is more closely related to the efficacy and toxicity of the drug. Only a twofold reduction in the maintenance dosing rate would be required if the former were true. An argument can be made for wanting to attain high concentrations of this antimicrobial drug intermittently in order to optimize efficacy. However, chronic toxicity of the aminoglycosides has been shown to be related to the total exposure to the drug. Thus, elevation of the average level by a factor of three, when the maintenance dose is decreased by only one-half, may be undesirable. Which adjustment is the most appropriate for amikacin, as well as for other aminoglycosides, is not settled at this time.

An additional point should be made. Since the normal regimen is one in which the dosing interval is much greater than the half-life, the average steady-state amount of drug in the body is much less than the dose. Consequently, adjusting the dosage regimen to maintain the same average amount in the body produces a situation in which the loading dose may be too large. This is seen in curves B and C in Figure 16-3. One could argue for decreasing the loading dose in addition to the rate of administration under these circumstances.

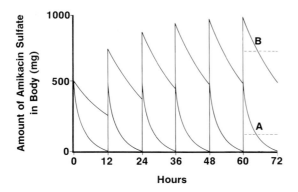

Figure 16-2. *Sketch of the amount of amikacin sulfate in the body with time following a regimen of 500 mg every 12 hours in a patient whose kidney function is normal, curve A, and in a patient whose age and weight are the same but whose kidney function is 17 percent of normal, curve B. Intravenous bolus administration is simulated. The normal half-life is assumed to be 2 hours. The dashed lines are the average plateau values.*

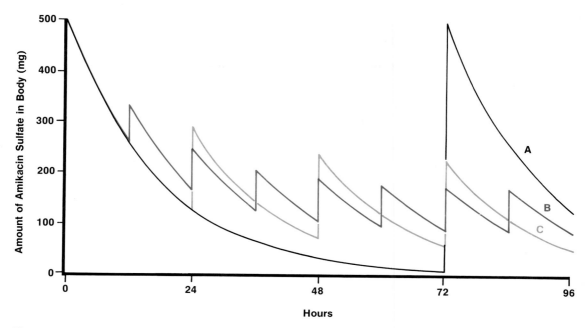

Figure 16-3. *Sketch of the amount of amikacin sulfate in the body with time in a patient whose kidney function is 17 percent of normal. Intravenous administration is simulated. The dosage regimens are: curve A, 500 mg every 72 hours; curve B, 500 mg initially, 83 mg every 12 hours; curve C, 500 mg initially, 167 mg every 24 hours.*

Estimation of Renal Function

Measurement of endogenous creatinine clearance is a good means of determining a patient's renal function. However, because the measurement is made by relating the total amount of creatinine in the urine to the serum creatinine, an incomplete urine collection can lead to an underestimate of creatinine clearance.

In adult patients who are neither obese nor emaciated the 24-hour output of creatinine in the urine per kilogram body weight is fairly constant. Hence, a check of the 24-hour urinary creatinine is a quick means of roughly assessing the reliability of a measured creatinine clearance value (Table 16-1). Diet contributes little (20-35%).

In contrast to a measurement of creatinine clearance, a serum creatinine concentration (usually expressed in units of mg percent, or mg/dl) is routinely measured in the hospital setting; because its estimation does not include errors in urine collection or

in urine creatinine concentration measurement, it is often a more reliable estimate of kidney function. Table 16-1 summarizes some of the relationships currently found to approximate creatinine clearance from serum creatinine values. These relationships include corrections for both age and weight. It should be emphasized that they are most accurate for individuals with an average muscle mass (source of creatinine) for their age, weight, and height. For both the emaciated and the obese adult patient, poor estimates are obtained.

Creatinine is constantly produced and is almost entirely excreted unchanged in the urine. Consequently,

$$\begin{matrix} \text{Rate of} \\ \text{creatinine} \\ \text{production} \end{matrix} = \begin{matrix} \text{Creatinine} \\ \text{clearance} \end{matrix} \times \begin{matrix} \text{Serum} \\ \text{creatinine} \end{matrix} \quad 13$$

The rate of production of creatinine and that of creatinine clearance both tend to decline with age. Consequently, the serum

Table 16-1. Estimation of Both Creatinine Clearance and the 24-Hour Urinary Excretion of Creatinine in Adults[a]

Population	Creatinine Clearance (ml/min)	24-hour Urinary Excretion (mg/24 hours)
Males	$\dfrac{98 - 0.8\,(\text{Age} - 20)^{b}}{\text{Serum creatinine}}$	$(29 - 0.2 \times \text{Age}) \times (\text{Body weight})^{d}$
	$\dfrac{(140 - \text{Age}) \times (\text{Body weight})^{c}}{72 \times \text{Serum creatinine}}$	
Females	$\dfrac{88 - 0.7\,(\text{Age} - 20)}{\text{Serum creatinine}}$	$(25 - 0.18 \times \text{Age}) \times (\text{Body weight})$
	$\dfrac{(140 - \text{Age}) \times (\text{Body weight})}{85 \times \text{Serum creatinine}}$	

[a] Adults 20 years of age and older. Poor estimates are obtained for obese and emaciated patients. Adapted from the review by Lott, R.S., and Hayton, W.L.: Estimation of creatinine clearance from serum creatinine concentration. Drug Intel. Clin. Pharmacol. *12*: 140–150, 1978.
[b] Age in years, serum creatinine concentration in mg/dl. Applicable to adults whose body surface area is close to 1.8 m². Otherwise, correction for body surface area may be appropriate.
[c] Age in years, body weight in kilograms, serum creatinine concentration in mg/dl.
[d] Age in years, body weight in kilograms.

creatinine tends to remain constant (about 0.9 mg/dl) from age 20 on for normal renal function. Thus, although renal function decreases with age, kidney function in the individual patient may be expressed as a fraction of the normal for his or her age group, as follows:

$$\text{Kidney function } (KF) = \frac{0.9}{\text{Serum creatinine (mg/dl)}} \qquad 14$$

A Nomogram—A Unifying Approach

Figure 16-4 is a nomogram that may be used for several purposes.

1. *Estimation of loading dose* in any age group when the dose in the adult is known. This estimation is based on the assumption that the volume of distribution per kilogram is constant.

2. *Estimation of maintenance doses in children* when the dosage regimen for a young adult is known. As discussed in Chapter 15 the usual dosage regimen is often determined for an older patient population. To use the nomogram for estimat-

ing pediatric maintenance dosages the regimen in the young adult must be obtained. The adjustment assumes that the dosing rate should be changed on the basis of body surface area. A shorter half-life in the child or infant must also be considered, that is, both D_M and τ may need to be decreased by the same proportion.

3. *Estimation of kidney function* when a creatinine clearance measurement is made. The kidney function as a percent of normal may be estimated in the child, in the adult, or in the geriatric patient. This estimate can be used in Figure 16-1 or in Equation 12 to determine how much the maintenance dosing rate should be changed.

4. *Estimation of normal creatinine clearance values for adults and geriatric patients,* when the age and weight are known. Furthermore, for drugs eliminated primarily by the renal route or when the total clearance decreases as does renal function with age, the adjustment in the maintenance dosage required for the geriatric patient may be approximated when the dosage in the young adult is known.

When the usual dosage regimen is given for an older population, the dosage at other adult or geriatric ages can be approx-imated from estimating the creatinine clearance in the patient and relating it to the creatinine clearance of the age group commonly receiving the drug. For example, consider the dosage requirement of an 80-kg, 25-year-old individual when the dosage regimen given is for a 70-kg, 55-year-old patient. The estimated creatinine clearance of the 25-year-old is 130 ml/min, the calcu-lated value for the 55-year-old is 83 ml/min. The ratio of clearance estimates is 1.6. Thus, the dose needed in the 25-year-old is 1.6 times the usual dosage regimen.

The nomogram of Figure 16-4 can be useful, but its assumptions and limitations must be kept fully in mind.

General Guidelines and Limitations

Except for drugs with very low therapeu-tic indices, a reduction of less than 33 per-cent in the dosing rate based on a change in kidney function alone, is probably unwar-ranted. Variability in the absorption, distri-bution, and extrarenal elimination of drugs for a variety of reasons is usually at least of this magnitude and the therapeutic range is often sufficiently large to make adjustment here unnecessary. Consequently, as long as the fraction excreted unchanged is 0.33 or less and the metabolites are inactive, no change in a regimen is called for, based on kidney function, regardless of the function. Similarly, regardless of the contribution of the renal route, if the kidney function is 0.67 of normal or greater, no change is needed (see Eq. 12).

When the fraction excreted unchanged approaches one and the kidney function approaches zero, there is little elimination, and the dosing rate must be drastically re-duced. Two particularly difficult problems are encountered here. One is the large change in the chronic requirements for a drug with only a small change in renal function, e.g., a change of 0.05 to 0.20 in KF gives a quadrupling in the required rate of

administration. The second problem is as-sociated with the accuracy of measurements of renal function and the stability of the function itself. Administration of drugs with an fe approaching one to a patient with severe renal failure requires great caution. The plasma concentration and the thera-peutic and toxic effects should be closely monitored in this situation. The use of the nomogram in Figure 16-1 or of Equation 12 should never take the place of monitoring, especially in these circumstances. The methods do, however, serve as a useful guide to modify dosage regimens in renal function impairment. Table 16-2 lists the half-lives and fraction excreted unchanged for selected drugs. The values for additional drugs are given in Table 7-1.

There are, of course, a number of as-sumptions upon which the preceding ad-justments are based. The methods falter if (1) availability changes in renal failure; (2) metabolites are either therapeutically active or toxic, or both; (3) failure in renal function alters the ability to metabolize the drug; or (4) the metabolism or renal excre-tion exhibits concentration-dependent ki-netics. Also, the renal function is assumed to be constant with time, and the renal clearance of the drug is assumed to be di-rectly proportional to the renal clearance of the compound used to determine renal function.

A note of caution should be emphasized on the last qualification. It is assumed that, regardless of whether the compound is eliminated primarily by glomerular filtra-tion or by active secretion, the clearance of the compound decreases in proportion to the clearance of the compound used to de-termine renal function. This assumption appears to be valid to a first approximation. Para-aminohippuric acid, procainamide, carbenicillin, and penicillin are examples of actively secreted compounds whose renal clearances are apparently proportional to endogenous creatinine clearance and inulin clearance, regardless of the cause of renal function impairment.

Furthermore, no consideration has been

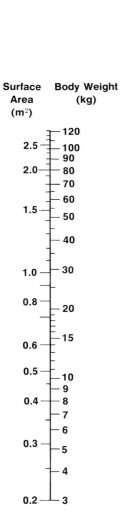

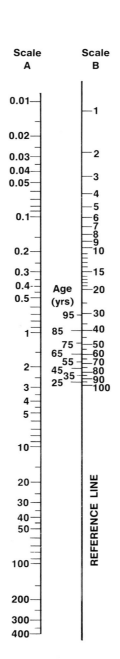

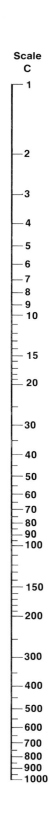

Figure 16-4. *Estimation of dosages and renal function in all but the neonate.*

1. **Estimation of loading dose,** *when the usual loading dose/kg body weight is known. With a ruler, join patient's body weight with loading dose/kg body weight on* Scale A *and read off the appropriate dose on* Scale C.

    Example: *Q. What is the loading dose for a 25-kg child when the usual adult dose is 1.5 mg/kg?*
        A. 38 mg.

2. **Estimation of loading dose,** *when the usual adult loading dose is known. With a ruler, join 70 kg weight with the usual adult loading dose on* Scale C. *Keeping ruler at point of intersection on* Scale A, *move the left-hand side of rule to patient's body weight and read off the appropriate dose on* Scale C.

    Example: *Q. What is the loading dose for a 15-kg child when the usual adult loading dose is 200 mg?*
        A. 43 mg.

3. **Estimation of pediatric dosages,** *when the dosage for a 25-year-old patient is known. With a ruler, join 70 kg body weight with the daily adult dosage on* Scale C. *Keeping ruler at point of intersection on the* Reference Line, *move the left-hand side of ruler to patient's body weight and read off the appropriate dosage on* Scale C. *Alternatively, given the adult dosage/kg body weight, the corresponding pediatric dosage is estimated as follows: With a ruler, join 70 kg weight with the adult dosage/kg body weight on* Scale A. *Keeping the ruler at the point of intersection on the* Reference Line, *move the left-hand side of the ruler to the patient's weight and read off the appropriate dosage/kg body weight on* Scale A.

    Example: *Q. What is the daily dosage for a 20-kg child when the usual adult daily dose is 50 mg/day?*
        A. 20 mg/day.
        Q. What is the hourly dosage for a 15-kg child when the usual adult dosage is 1 mg/kg/day?
        A. 1.6 mg/kg/hour or 24 mg/hour.

Note: The dosing interval depends on the half-life and the therapeutic index of the drug; a daily dose may have to be given in divided doses.

4. **Estimation of kidney function remaining in children or young adults** *when creatinine clearance is known. With a ruler, join the patient's weight to the patient's creatinine clearance (ml/min) on* Scale C. *Read off kidney function, as a percent of the normal value in a subject of the same weight, from the point of intersection with* Scale B.

    Example: *Q. What percent of normal kidney function has a 40-kg child with a creatinine clearance of 30 ml/min?*
        A. 37 percent.

5. **Estimation of usual creatinine clearance and dosage in adults or geriatric patients.** *With a ruler, join the patient's weight with age and read off the anticipated creatinine clearance (ml/min) on* Scale C. *Keeping the ruler on the intersection point on* Scale C, *move the left-hand side of the ruler to 70 kg body weight and read off the dosage, expressed as a percent of that in a 70 kg, 25-year-old individual,* Scale B.

    Example: *Q. What is the estimated creatinine clearance and the dosage needed in a 65-year-old patient, weighing 55 kg, when the usual daily dosage in a 70-kg, 25-year-old is 100 mg/day?*
        A. 62 ml/min; 50 percent of the young adult dose, or 50 mg/day.

Note: The estimation of geriatric dosage assumes that total clearance decreases in direct proportion to creatinine clearance.

6. **Estimation of renal function remaining in adults or geriatric patients** *when creatinine clearance is known. With a ruler, join the patient's weight with age and read off the anticipated creatinine clearance (ml/min) on* Scale C. *Keeping the ruler at this point on* Scale C *move the left-hand side of the ruler to meet the 100 percent value on* Scale B. *Now, keeping ruler on the corresponding point of intersection on the body weight line, move the right-hand side of the ruler to the patient's observed creatinine clearance (ml/min) on* Scale C *and read off the degree of kidney function remaining, expressed as a percent of the value expected for the patient's age and weight, on* Scale B.

    Example: *Q. What is the degree of kidney function of a 60-kg, 75-year-old patient with a creatinine clearance of 30 ml/min?*
        A. 55 percent.

Note: The same answer is obtained by dividing the observed clearance by the expected creatinine clearance, estimated using Procedure 5.

This nomogram incorporates the geriatric creatinine clearance data of Siersbaek-Nielsen (Siersbaek-Nielsen, K., Hansen, J., Kampermann, J., and Kristensen, M.: Rapid evaluation of creatinine clearance. Lancet, 1: 1133–1134, 1971.)

Table 16-2. Approximate Half-Lives and Fraction Excreted Unchanged of Selected Drugs[a]

Drug	$t_{1/2}$ (hours)	fe	Drug	$t_{1/2}$ (hours)	fe
Ampicillin	0.8	0.88	Kanamycin	2	0.97
Carbenicillin	1.1	0.9	Lincomycin	5	0.7
Cephaloridine	1.7	0.92	Methicillin	0.5	0.88
Cephalexin	1.0	0.95	Minocycline	10–12	0.11
Cephazolin	2.0	0.95	Oxacillin	0.5	0.8
Chloramphenicol	2.3	0.0	Ouabain	14	0.8
Chlortetracycline	7	0.18	Penicillin G	0.5	0.9
Cyclacillin	0.7	0.9	Polymyxin B	4	0.87
Colistin	2	0.93	Rifampicin	3	0.0
Doxycycline	23	0.51	Rolitetracycline	10	0.7
Digitoxin	170	0.3	Streptomycin	3	0.96
Digoxin	40	0.71	Sulfadiazine	10	0.6
Erythromycin	1.4	0.8	Tetracycline	8–9	0.50
5-Fluorocytosine	3	0.97	Tobramycin	2	0.99
Gentamicin	2	0.98	Trimethoprim	10–12	0.7
Isoniazid			Vancomycin	6	0.98
Fast acetylators	1.5	0.3			
Slow acetylators	3	0.5			

[a]Modified from Dettli, L.: Drug dosage in renal disease. Clin. Pharmacokinet., *1*: 126–134, 1976.

given to intersubject differences in: absorption, distribution and metabolism, the response to a given plasma concentration, or disease state and physiologic functions. Renal function is only one of several sources of variability. Adjustment of drug administration based on renal function must be put into perspective.

Further Considerations

Renal disease often affects more than just renal clearance. Furthermore, other diseases that may alter dosage requirements are sometimes concurrently present. Digoxin, as previously mentioned, binds much less to tissues in uremia, resulting in a smaller volume of distribution and a shorter half-life than that predicted from the loss of renal function. This decreased tissue binding reduces the loading dose required, but has little or no effect on the maintenance dose of the drug. However, the presence of severe congestive heart failure, the condition for which the drug is most often used, is associated with decreased metabolic

clearance and with a daily maintenance dosage requirement reduced beyond that expected for renal function impairment alone. Phenytoin and many other acidic drugs are two to three times less well-bound to plasma proteins in uremia. Part of this change is due to a decreased concentration of plasma albumin. The mechanism accounting for the rest of the change is uncertain, although displacement by an endogenous compound(s) that accumulates in renal failure has been suggested. The unbound values of both clearance and volume of distribution of these principally metabolized drugs remain essentially unchanged, and no change in dosage regimen is anticipated in renal function impairment. The total plasma clearance, however, increases two- to threefold, giving rise to a corresponding drop in the steady-state plasma concentration. This change must be carefully considered when interpreting plasma concentrations of these drugs in patients with renal disease.

Perhaps, the *most* commonly invalid assumption is that metabolites are pharmacologically and toxicologically inactive. For example, the metabolite of procainamide, N-acetylprocainamide, is essentially equipotent, but perhaps less toxic than the drug itself. Prediction of the total activity of the drug and of the dosage adjustment needed in renal failure is therefore much more complex. There are ways of treating such situations. The most useful is by the steady-state approach. There is insufficient information to date on the kinetics of N-acetylprocainamide. Accordingly, a hypothetic drug, similar to procainamide, is used to illustrate the use of the steady-state approach.

Figure 16-5 shows the input and disposition of a drug and its active metabolite under normal renal function conditions. Table 16-3 lists the normal average values for several pharmacokinetic parameters of this drug and its active metabolite.

Assume that the drug and its active metabolite are equipotent and equitoxic in terms of plasma concentration. Further,

assume that the rate of administration of the drug is 100 mg/hour.

At steady state the plasma concentration of the drug may be calculated from the average rate of absorption and the total clearance,

$$C_{av} = \frac{0.8 \times 100 \text{ mg/hour}}{20 \text{ liters/hour}} = 4 \text{ mg/liter}$$

The rate of formation of the active metabolite is 0.3 times the rate of absorption of the drug; therefore,

$$Cm_{av} = \frac{0.3 \times 0.8 \times 100 \text{ mg/hour}}{20 \text{ liters/hour}}$$
$$= 1.2 \text{ mg/liter}$$

In an anuric patient the total clearance is the extrarenal clearance. For this drug, the extrarenal clearance is 10 liters/hour; for the metabolite, it is 4 liters/hour. The predicted steady-state concentration of the drug in the anuric patient is, therefore,

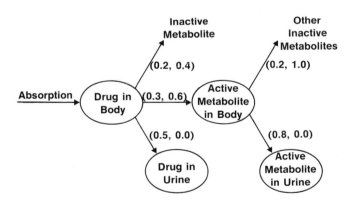

Figure 16-5. *Model for the absorption and disposition of a drug and for the disposition of an active metabolite. The first number in parentheses refers to the fraction of the elimination of the drug or metabolite that normally occurs by the pathway shown with an arrow. The second number refers to the same fraction when there is no kidney function.*

Table 16-3. Normal Average Pharmacokinetic Parameters of a Drug and Its Active Metabolite

Parameter	Drug	Active Metabolite
Total clearance	20 liters/hour	20 liters/hour
Renal clearance	10 liters/hour	16 liters/hour
Fraction excreted unchanged	0.5	0.8
Availability	0.8	0.3[a]

[a] Fraction of drug converted to active metabolite.

$$C_{av}(f) = \frac{0.8 \times 100 \text{ mg/hour}}{10 \text{ liters/hour}} = 8 \text{ mg/liter}$$

Because 0.6 of the total elimination goes to the active metabolite in the anuric patient, the steady-state concentration of the metabolite is

$$Cm_{av}(f) = \frac{0.6 \times 0.8 \times 100 \text{ mg/hour}}{4 \text{ liters/hour}}$$
$$= 12 \text{ mg/liter}$$

Note that the average drug concentration is two times as great in the anuric patient, while the active metabolite concentration is increased ten times. If the drug and the active metabolite are equipotent and additive in their activities, then in the anuric patient the rate of administration should be $(4 + 1.2)/(8 + 12)$ or 0.26 that of normal. Thus, the anuric patient would require only 26 mg/hour. Although the metabolite makes a minor contribution to the total activity in patients with normal renal function, in the anuric patient it is primarily responsible for the activity.

Study Problems

(Answers to Study Problems can be found in Appendix G.)

1. (a) Rank the conditions in Table 16-4 from most important to least important for considering a change in a dosage regimen in adult patients with varying degrees of renal function impairment.
   (b) Name the conditions below for which you would recommend a change in the usual dosage regimen.
   (c) List the assumptions you must make to arrive at your answer to (b).

Table 16-4.

Condition	Drug	Percent of Dose Normally Excreted Unchanged	Kidney Function (percent of normal)
a	A	20	10
b	B	90	5
c	C	90	50
d	D	10	70
e	E	70	10

2. Vancomycin is chosen for the therapy of a 3-year-old boy with staphylococcal pneumonia. The organism has been found to be refractory to other antibiotics. Unfortunately, the child has reduced renal function (endogenous creatinine clearance of 7 ml/min—uncorrected for body surface area). A usual intravenous dose for a child is 20 mg/kg every 12 hours.

Approximately 98 percent of a dose of vancomycin is normally excreted unchanged, and the normal elimination half-life is 6 hours. The normal creatinine clearance of a child of this age is 124 ml/min/1.8m². Based on the height and weight of the patient, his surface area is 0.60 m².

(a) Determine a dosage regimen that would attain and maintain the amount of drug in the body within, what would appear to be, the usual therapeutic range, thus decreasing the chances of developing ototoxicity and further impairment of renal function, problems known to occur with the drug.

(b) Sketch the anticipated amount of vancomycin in the body (mg/kilogram body weight) for a child with normal renal function who receives the normal dosage schedule, and in the child with renal impairment who receives the dosage schedule that you have calculated in (a).

3. Although controversial, it has been asserted that 8 percent of digitoxin is normally metabolized to digoxin in the body. Assume the following normal values for two drugs.

(a) What steady-state plasma concentrations would you expect for both compounds in a normal patient taking 0.1 mg digitoxin per day?

(b) What are the expected steady-state concentrations of the two drugs in an anuric patient taking 0.1 mg digitoxin per day?

(c) Comment on the degree to which you think the active metabolite, digoxin, contributes to the therapeutic effect in the anuric patient.

Table 16-5.

	Availability	Clearance (ml/min)	Fraction Excreted Unchanged	Usual Therapeutic Concentration (micrograms/liter)
Digitoxin	1.0	6	0.3	10–20
Digoxin	0.6	150	0.7	1–2

Unifying Problems

(Answers to Unifying Problems can be found in Appendix G.)

1. Lithium salts are administered orally for prevention and treatment of recurrent manic depressive disorders. For optimal therapy the lithium ion plasma concentration must be kept within fairly narrow limits because the drug has a low therapeutic index. Therapeutic concentrations are approximately 0.6 to 1.6 mEq (milliequivalent/liter). Concentrations of 2 mEq/liter and higher are associated with toxicity. Renal excretion is the only route of elimination. The renal excretion of lithium is dependent on sodium excretion. The renal clearance of lithium relative to the clearance of creatinine in an individual patient is shown in Figure 16-6 as a function of the output of sodium in the urine.

For further considerations, assume the following values:

Patient's weight $= 70$ kg.
C_{av} (desired) $= 1.2$ mEq/liter.
Absorption complete and virtually instantaneous.
Apparent volume of distribution of lithium ion $= 0.70$ liters/kg.
Molecular weight of lithium carbonate (Li_2CO_3) $= 74$.

(a) Estimate this patient's daily dosage requirement for lithium carbonate (creatinine clearance $= 120 \text{ ml/min/1.8 m}^2$):
   (*i*) When the patient's sodium intake and output are 175 mEq/day.
   (*ii*) When the patient is on a severely salt-restricted diet (assume a sodium output of 25 mEq/day).
(b) Sketch the anticipated amount of drug in the body with time if one-half of the daily dose that you calculated in (a)(*i*) above were given every 12 hours (no loading dose).
(c) This patient developed renal disease subsequent to initiation of lithium therapy. The patient's renal function stabilized with a creatinine clearance of $21 \text{ ml/min/1.8 m}^2$. The patient had a urinary sodium output of 175 mEq/day.
   (*i*) Estimate the dose required every 12 hours under this new condition to maintain a C_{av} of 1.2 mEq/liter. Assume that the ratio of the clearances of lithium to creatinine remained as shown in Fig. 16-6 and that the volume of distribution did not change.
   (*ii*) If this patient were taken off the drug while having reduced renal function, approximately how long (in days) would it take for the plasma lithium concentration to fall below the therapeutic range, i.e., 0.6 mEq/liter.

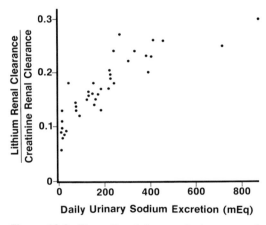

Figure 16-6. *The ratio of the renal clearance of lithium to that of creatinine varies with the urinary sodium output, which is a function of the dietary intake of sodium. (Redrawn from Thomsen, K., and Schou, M.: Renal lithium excretion in man. Am. J. Physiol., 215: 823–827, 1968.)*

2. Table 16-6 contains the usual values for several pharmacokinetic parameters and the usual route and schedule of administration for Drugs A, B, C, and D.
   (a) Sketch the expected blood concentration of drug (C_b) as a function of time following the usual regimen for *Drug B* in
      (*i*) An average patient with normal renal function.
      (*ii*) The same patient when anuric (no urine production).
      Assume complete and rapid absorption (relative to elimination) and instantaneous distribution that do not change in renal failure. *Scale axes* appropriately.
   (b) Assume, in turn, that each of the drugs listed in the table is essential to the therapeutic management of an anephric patient.

(i) What dosage regimen would you suggest for each drug?

(ii) What assumptions have you made about these drugs?

(c) If *Drug D* were given orally in a single 90-mg dose, what is the maximum blood drug concentration that you would anticipate?

Table 16-6. Usual Values

Drug	Half-life (hours)	Volume of Distribution (based on blood) (liters)	Fraction Excreted Unchanged	Route	Dosage Regimen	
					Initial Dose (mg)	Maintenance Regimen (mg/dosing interval)
A	38	500	0.6	P.O.	1	0.25 mg/day
B	24	12	0.8	P.O.	240	120 mg/day
C	12	30	0.0	I.V.	—	60 mg/12 hours
D	8	900	0.1	I.M.	—	90 mg/8 hours

17

drug interactions

Objectives

The reader will be able to:

1. **List reasons why drug interactions are graded phenomena.**

2. **Ascertain whether either the pharmacokinetics or the pharmacodynamics of a drug, or both, are altered by another drug, given unbound drug concentration-time data.**

3. **Show graphically the consequence of a pharmacokinetic drug interaction when the mechanism of the interaction and the circumstances of its occurrence are given.**

4. **Anticipate the likely changes in the plasma and unbound concentration of a drug with time when its pharmacokinetics is altered by concurrent drug therapy.**

5. **Suggest an approach to the modification in the dosage regimen of a drug when its pharmacokinetics is altered by concurrent drug administration.**

A *drug interaction* occurs when either the pharmacokinetics or the pharmacodynamics of one drug is altered by another. A *therapeutic drug interaction* occurs when one drug significantly alters the degree of response of another drug. Drug interactions are a concern because, occasionally, the outcome of concurrent drug administration is diminished therapeutic efficacy or increased toxicity of one or more of the administered drugs. Drug interactions frequently arise because multiple drug therapy is the rule rather than the exception. Patients commonly receive two or more drugs concurrently; indeed, an inpatient on the average receives five drugs during a hospitalization. The reasons for multiple drug therapy are many. One reason is that combination drug therapy has been found to be beneficial in the treatment of some conditions, including a variety of cardiovascular diseases, infections, and cancer. Another reason is that patients frequently suffer from several diseases or conditions, and each may require the use of one or more drugs. Furthermore, drugs are prescribed by different clinicians, and each clinician may be unaware of the others' therapeutic maneuvers. Even when a patient's total drug regimen is known, the undesirable consequences of drug interaction may arise from a lack of understanding of or a failure to recall the mode of action and the pharmacokinetics of each drug; many undesirable interactions are therefore potentially avoidable.

The possibilities of interactions between drugs within the body are almost limitless. Yet few of these interactions are of a type or of a sufficient magnitude to be clinically important. Many interactions between drugs within the body take place without affecting either the unbound drug concentration or the therapeutic activity of the drugs involved. Also, the dosage of many drugs needed to demonstrate a clinically significant drug interaction exceeds the median lethal dose. Moreover, many affected processes and pathways of drug elimination are too minor to be of concern.

Implicit in the definition of a drug interaction is the concept that, like essentially all responses of the body, they are graded. The degree of interaction depends upon the concentration of the interacting species and hence on dose and on time. Thus, not only are drug interactions a source of variability in drug response, but they are a cause of additional variability within a patient population receiving the interacting drugs. This last point is well illustrated by the data in Table 17-1. Chloral hydrate is thought to

Table 17-1. Prospective Study of 237 Warfarin-Treated Patients for Detection of Interaction Between Warfarin and Chloral Hydrate[a]

Received chloral hydrate during warfarin therapy	237
During warfarin therapy received chloral hydrate for at least 3 consecutive days and did not receive chloral hydrate for at least 3 consecutive days before or after this period	69
Impossible to evaluate interaction (clinically unstable or multiple drug changes)	28
Potentiation of hypoprothrombinemic action of warfarin	22
No demonstrable interaction	19

[a]Abstracted from Koch-Weser, J.: Hemorrhagic reactions and drug interactions in 500 warfarin-treated patients. Clin. Pharmacol. Ther., *14*: 139–146, 1973.

potentiate transiently the anticoagulant effects of warfarin. Yet in only 22 of 237 patients who were studied prospectively and who received chloral hydrate during warfarin therapy, was potentiation of warfarin's effect unambiguously demonstrated. The reasons for these differences in response are many. Included are individual differences in the dosage regimen and duration of administration of each drug, in the sequence of drug administration, and in patient compliance. Pharmacodynamics and pharmacokinetic differences due to genetics, to concurrent disease states, and to many other factors also contribute. Thus, the circumstances associated with a clinically significant interaction in an individual should always be carefully documented.

Classification

One system of classifying drug interactions is to note whether drug response is increased or decreased. While perhaps clinically useful, this classification does not help to define the mechanism of the interaction. In this book interactions are classified on the basis of whether the pharmacokinetics or pharmacodynamics of a drug is altered; occasionally, both are changed. Distinction between the two is best made by relating response to the unbound concentration of the pharmacologically active species. No change in the unbound concentration-response curve implies a pharmacokinetic drug interaction, which can arise either through a physical interaction, such as competition for protein binding sites, or through altered physiology, such as altered blood flow at an absorption site. The result is a change in one or more of the primary pharmacokinetic parameters, ka, F, fu, V, Cl_R, Cl_H, which in turn, alter the secondary pharmacokinetic parameters, such as half-life.

Before proceeding, a discussion of what is meant by the word *interaction* is worthwhile. Strictly speaking, this word implies a *mutual effect*. The interaction between two drugs, A and B, might thus be denoted by A ↔ B. An example of a mutual interaction is the competition between two drugs for a common binding site on albumin: One drug displaces but is also displaced by the other. Another less common type of a mutual interaction is where each drug affects the other, but through different mechanisms. For example, phenobarbital appears to reduce the absorption of the diuretic, furosemide, but the renal clearance of phenobarbital is increased by diuresis. Clearly,

Table 17-2. Classification and Examples of Drug Interactions

Pharmacodynamic Interactions

Response	Example	Comment
↑	Digoxin $\overset{a}{\leftarrow}$ Chlorothiazide	By inducing hypokalemia chlorothiazide enhances digoxin cardiotoxicity.
	Chlorpheniramine $\overset{b}{\leftrightarrow}$ Alcohol	Mutual sedative effects.
↓	Guanethidine ← Chlorpromazine	Chlorpromazine blocks uptake of guanethidine at postganglionic adrenergic neuron.
	Warfarin ↔ Vitamin K_1	Each lowers the effectiveness of the other.

Pharmacokinetic Interactions

Parameter	Response	Example	Comment
Absorption Rate	↑	Acetaminophen ← Metoclopramide	Metoclopramide hastens stomach emptying.
	↓	Acetaminophen ← Propantheline	Propantheline slows stomach emptying.
Availability	↑	Digoxin ← Propantheline	Propantheline enhances availability of slowly dissolving digoxin tablets.
	↓	Lincomycin ← Kaolin	Mechanism unknown—possibly kaolin adsorbs lincomycin.
Volume of distribution	↑	Salicylic acid ↔ Phenylbutazone	Competitive displacement from plasma (and tissue) binding sites.
	↓	Benzylpenicillin ← Probenecid	Mechanism uncertain
Hepatic clearance	↑	Warfarin ← Phenobarbital	Phenobarbital induces microsomal enzymes.
	↓	Tolbutamide ← Phenylbutazone	Phenylbutazone inhibits tolbutamide oxidation.
Renal clearance	↑	Salicylic acid ← Bicarbonate	Elevated urine pH by bicarbonate diminishes tubular reabsorption of salicylate.
	↓	Benzylpenicillin ← Probenecid	Probenecid inhibits the secretion of penicillin.

[a] Denotes a unidirectional interaction; the arrow points to affected drug.
[b] Denotes a mutual (bidirectional) interaction.

in the case of a mutual interaction, the measured response of one drug cannot be considered without also defining the level of the other.

When given in sufficient quantities, two drugs almost always mutually affect each other; this may not be the case, however, at concentrations achieved in therapy. For example, the carbonic anhydrase inhibitor, acetazolamide, by raising urinary pH, decreases the renal clearance of amphetamine, but amphetamine, at doses normally given, does not affect the response or the pharmacokinetics of acetazolamide. This interaction is *unidirectional* and may be denoted by A → B. In a unidirectional interaction, the unaffected drug, A, can be considered independently, but the change in response of the affected drug, B, cannot be adequately defined without also considering the concentration-response curve of the effect of drug A on drug B.

The material in Chapter 11 forms the basis for discussing many aspects of pharmacokinetic drug interactions. For convenience, in this chapter, the effect of one drug on another is examined under the separate headings of altered absorption, displacement, and altered clearance. However, it should be borne in mind that several pharmacokinetic parameters can be altered simultaneously. Examples of drug interactions are listed in Table 17-2.

Altered Absorption

It was stated in Chapters 9 and 13 that the more rapid the absorption process the higher and earlier is the peak plasma drug concentration and that neither the total area under the concentration-time curve after a single dose nor the area within a dosing interval at the plateau after chronic dosing, changes unless the availability of the drug is altered. Therapeutic consequences of a change in either the rate or the extent of drug absorption were discussed in Chapter 13. Events that are likely to prevail during drug interaction are now considered.

These events are illustrated in Figure 17-1.

Figure 17-1A depicts the situation in which a patient is stabilized on drug A and receives drug B, which reduces the availability of drug A. It is apparent that if no steps are taken to change the dosing rate of drug A, its level will fall to a lower plateau, the time being determined by the elimination half-life of this drug. Suppose that it was then noticed that the patient was no longer being treated effectively with drug A, and that, having recognized the problem, the offending drug was withdrawn. The concentration of drug A would then return, in 3.3 of its elimination half-lives, to the previous plateau value. Therapeutic control would again be restored. Alternatively, on another occasion, in anticipation of the problem but desiring to give the two drugs together, the dosing rate of drug A is appropriately increased at the time that drug B is introduced. As long as drug B continues to be administered, therapeutic control is satisfactory. A problem arises, however, if drug B is subsequently withdrawn but the dosing rate of drug A is not correspondingly reduced. Then, in 3.3 of its elimination half-lives, the level of drug A in the body reaches a higher plateau and toxicity may result.

Another possible situation is one in which drug A is added to the regimen of a patient stabilized on drug B (Fig. 17-1B). Here, as before, optimal therapy with drug A in the presence of drug B is achieved only if the usual dosing rate is appropriately increased. However, the danger of the concentration of drug A rising too high, if the dosing rate of drug A is not readjusted when drug B is withdrawn, must always be kept in mind.

Displacement

The most common explanation for altered distribution in a drug interaction is displacement. Displacement is the reduction in the binding of a drug to a macromolecule, usually a protein, caused by competition of another drug, the *displacer,*

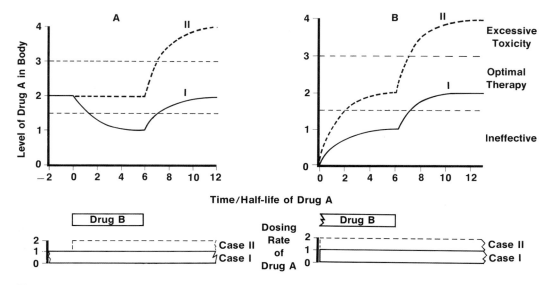

Figure 17-1. Altered absorption. *As long as drug B is administered, the availability of drug A is reduced by one-half. For simplicity, drug A is assumed to be given at a constant rate; intermittent administration will produce fluctuations, but the general shape of the curve will not be altered. The therapeutic concentration range is assumed to lie between 1.5 and 3 units for drug A.*

A, Patient stabilized on drug A. The level of drug A will fall by one-half (case I), unless the dosing rate is doubled (case II), when drug B is concurrently administered. A problem potentially arises if administration of drug A is not reduced to its preexisting rate, when drug B is removed (case II).

B, Patient stabilized on drug B. Adequate levels of drug A will not be achieved (case I) unless the usual dosing rate of this drug is doubled (case II). When drug B is withdrawn, there is a potential problem similar to that considered in A.

for the common binding site(s). The result is a rise in the fraction of drug unbound in plasma or tissue, or both. Sometimes, drug binding is diminished through an allosteric effect. The second drug, binding at another site, induces a conformational change in the protein, thereby reducing the affinity of the first drug for the protein. Occasionally, an allosteric effect causes an enhanced affinity between drug and protein; drug binding is then increased. Although the effects of allosteric interactions may be similar, the term displacement should be restricted to the competitive interaction at the common binding site.

Conditions Favoring Displacement

Two conditions must be met before substantial displacement occurs in plasma. First, most of the drug must be bound to a protein,

that is, the value of fu must be low. Obviously, if the drug is not bound it cannot be displaced. From Equation 12, Chapter 4, restated here,

$$fu = \frac{1}{[1 + K \cdot (P)]} \qquad 1$$

the value of fu is low when the protein has a high affinity for the drug (K high) and when the molar concentration of the drug is much lower than that of the binding protein. The concentration of unbound binding sites, (P), is the difference between the concentrations of total and occupied sites. Second, the displacer must occupy most of the binding sites, thereby substantially lowering the number of sites available to bind the drug. This second condition is most likely to be met when the displacer also has a high affinity for the binding site and when its concentration approaches or exceeds the molar concentration of the protein binding sites. Let us look at the condition for displacement in greater detail.

Table 17-3 lists two groups of acidic drugs that bind to albumin, a protein that exists abundantly in plasma (120 grams/3 liter; 0.6 mM) and in the interstitial fluids (150 grams). Not all of the drugs bind to and hence compete for the same primary binding site on albumin. Albumin, and other proteins, have many binding sites, each exhibiting some degree of specificity; possessing an acidic function is not a sufficient criterion for predicting the ability of one drug to displace another acidic drug. Moreover, even though almost all those drugs that compete for the same site have a high affinity for albumin, only a few are generally listed as displacers, such as salicylic acid, phenylbutazone, and some sulfonamides. This list is limited, because the plasma concentration, achieved during therapy, must approach or exceed 0.6 mM, the concentration of plasma albumin. For a substance with a molecular weight of 250, this concentration corresponds to 150 mg/liter. This concentration is achieved during salicylate and sulfonamide therapy, because these drugs are commonly given in doses approaching 1 gram and because they possess relatively small volumes of distribution, 10 to 20 liters. With phenylbutazone the plasma concentration achieved with the

usual dose, 100 mg ($V = 10$ liters), is only 10 mg/liter, but because its clearance is low and half-life is long (3 days), the plateau concentration ultimately achieved is high when administered every 6 to 8 hours.

Displacers share an expected common property, that is, their value of fu changes with plasma concentration. This follows from Equation 1. The number of available binding sites, (P), being the difference between the total and the occupied sites, is sensitive to a change in the concentration of displacer. Therefore, displacers must be drugs that show concentration-dependent disposition kinetics.

So far, distinction has been made between displacers and the displaced drug, but it should be apparent that this classification is arbitrary. Phenylbutazone is said to displace warfarin from albumin, but only because the plasma concentration of phenylbutazone (100 mg/liter) approaches the molar concentration of albumin, whereas that of warfarin (1–4 mg/liter) does not. Both drugs have approximately the same affinity for the same site on albumin and if the concentrations were reversed, warfarin would be called the displacer (Fig. 17-2). Thus, displacement is a matter of the point of reference.

The conclusions drawn from the interactions between acidic drugs and albumin are generally applicable to all drug-protein in-

Table 17-3. Binding of Selected Acidic Drugs to Albumin[a]

Drugs That Bind to and Compete for One of Two Sites, Designated A and B, on Albumin

Site A	Site B
Iophenoxic acid	Ethacrynic acid
Oxyphenbutazone	Flufenamic acid
Phenylbutazone	p-Chlorophenoxyisobutyric acid
Sulfadimethoxine	
Sulfinpyrazone	
Warfarin	

[a]Abstracted from Sudlow, G., Birkett, D.J., and Wade, D.N.: The characterization of two specific binding sites on human serum albumin. Mol. Pharmacol., *11*: 824–832, 1975.

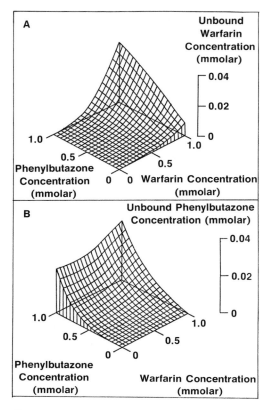

Figure 17-2. *Phenylbutazone displaces and is displaced by warfarin from common binding sites on albumin. The three-dimensional surfaces show how unbound concentrations of warfarin, A, and phenylbutazone, B, depend upon the total concentration of both drugs. (From Aarons, L., Schary, W.L., and Rowland, M.: An* in vitro *study of drug displacement interactions: Warfarin-salicylate, warfarin-phenylbutazone. J. Pharm. Pharmacol., 31: 322–330, 1979.)*

teractions. Displacement interactions appear to be much less common between basic drugs than between acidic drugs, perhaps because in general the former have larger volumes of distribution and are given in smaller doses and therefore their concentrations are lower. Basic drugs, however, often tend to bind more to glycoproteins and lipoproteins than to albumin, and because both of these classes of proteins are in much lower molar concentrations than albumin in plasma, a displacement interaction between some basic drugs is antici-

pated. The molar concentration of the specialized transport proteins, which avidly bind many hormones, is also very low, and displacement interactions between steroids, for example, occur despite a low plasma concentration of these substances.

Equilibrium Considerations

Displacement interactions in plasma have been studied primarily *in vitro*. The drugs of interest are added to a sample of plasma and the changes in binding are measured. The data displayed in Figure 17-2 were obtained in this manner. Substantial displacement from plasma proteins can frequently be demonstrated *in vitro;* yet this may be of little therapeutic consequence. Indeed, as the following calculation shows, drug displacement is unlikely to be clinically significant unless drug is substantially bound to and displaced from both plasma and tissue binding sites.

Suppose that the body contained 42 mg of a drug with the following characteristics: $V = 42$ liters, $fu = 0.1$, $fu_T = 0.1$, unbound drug distributes evenly throughout the total body water. At equilibrium, 7.1 percent of the dose resides in plasma (Equation 6, Chap. 4), the plasma concentration is 1 mg/liter, and the unbound concentration throughout the body is 0.1 mg/liter. This situation is depicted schematically in Figure 17-3A.

Imagine now that it is possible to displace instantly and completely the drug from the plasma proteins. The unbound plasma drug concentration would then rise to 1 mg/liter, but only momentarily, because displaced drug would rapidly move down the newly created unbound concentration gradient into the large tissue water space. At the new equilibrium (Fig. 17-3B), the displaced 6.4 percent would only increase the unbound drug concentration by $6.4/(100 - 6.4)$ or 6.8 percent, to 0.107 mg/liter. This is a trivial increase compared to the normal fluctuation in concentration.

The volume of distribution increases

when displacement from plasma proteins produces a net movement of drug from plasma into tissues; fu/fu_T increases (Eq. 20, Chap. 4). Conversely, net movement of drug from tissue into plasma decreases the volume of distribution. In practice, the former occurs much more frequently. It should be borne in mind, however, that tissue displacement may still and indeed often does occur; the change in the volume of distribution reflects a relative, not an absolute, change in binding. Occasionally, the volume of distribution shows no change even though displacement in plasma occurs. This necessarily implies an equivalent change in the degree of binding within tissues and an increase in the unbound concentration for a given amount of drug in the body. Taking the warfarin-phenylbutazone interaction as an example, the volume of distribution of warfarin is hardly changed, yet its value of fu (0.005–0.010), and its unbound concentration, almost double in

the presence of approximately 1 gram of phenylbutazone.

Clearance and Half-life

The points made here summarize those made in Chapters 4, 5, and 11. Because clearance of a drug with a high extraction ratio is unaffected by binding, but the volume of distribution is generally increased, displacement results in a prolonged half-life. In contrast, for a drug with a low extraction ratio, the half-life tends to shorten, but perhaps only slightly, since clearance and volume of distribution tend to increase to the same extent.

The Plateau

The preceding comments refer to equilibrium situations in which the drug is given only once in the absence or in the presence of a displacer. In drug therapy it is more

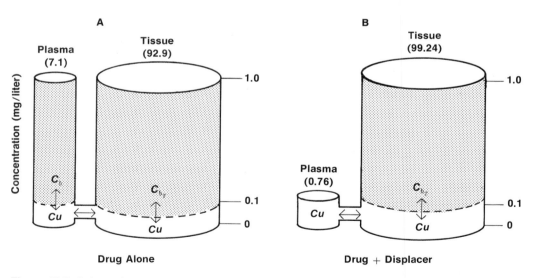

Figure 17-3. *Schematic representation of the consequences at equilibrium of drug displacement from plasma proteins only. Each reservoir is characterized by its volume, proportional to the amount of drug, and its height, proportional to concentration. Drug Alone: In this example the bound (shaded) and unbound (clear) concentrations of drug in both plasma and tissue are equal. Drug plus Displacer: Even though all drug bound to plasma proteins is displaced, upon reequilibration, the amount is too small to significantly affect the unbound drug concentration, which increases by only 7 percent. The calculations were made from the following information: Dose, 42 mg; plasma volume, 3 liters; tissue volume, 39 liters; fu = fu_T = 0.1; after displacement fu = 1, fu_T = 0.1. Unbound drug is assumed to distribute evenly throughout the 42 liters of total body water. Values in parentheses refer to percent of drug in body.*

common to give both drug and displacer on a multiple dose regimen. The influence of displacement on the unbound concentration at steady state (Cu_{ss}) depends on the extraction ratio of the drug and perhaps on the route of administration.

Consider a drug with a low extraction ratio. Recall the following facts: Clearance depends on fu, but unbound clearance (Cl_u) does not; the rate of drug elimination is directly proportional to the unbound concentration, Cu. Recall also the equality (Eq. 18, Chap. 6)

$$\text{Rate of elimination} = Cl_u \cdot Cu = Cl \cdot C \quad 2$$

When drug is infused at a constant rate, R_{inf}, and steady state is achieved,

$$R_{inf} = Cl_u \cdot Cu_{ss} = Cl \cdot C_{ss} \quad 3$$

However, since unbound clearance, e.g., that of a glomerularly filtered drug, is unaffected by displacement, the same is true of the value of Cu_{ss}. Thus, although displacement by increasing fu increases clearance (and hence causes the total plasma concentration to fall), no change in response and therefore in dose is anticipated at steady state. Neither is any change anticipated, following displacement, in the average unbound concentration at plateau, Cu_{av}, upon chronic oral dosing. Also with the half-life tending to be shorter, displacement results in a slightly greater fluctuation of the unbound drug concentration around the average value.

Now consider a drug with a high extraction ratio. Since clearance is unaffected by displacement, the steady-state blood concentration is also unaffected following a constant-rate intravenous infusion. However, as binding is diminished, the value of Cu_{ss} and therefore the response to the drug must be increased. The maintenance dose of the drug may need to be reduced. Furthermore, as displacement prolongs the half-life, a smaller fluctuation around the average plateau concentration is anticipated.

Prediction of the outcome when a drug with a high extraction ratio is given orally and when elimination occurs predominantly in the liver, is more difficult. In the presence of the displacer, both unbound drug clearance and availability decrease but which, if either, predominates to affect the unbound drug concentration at plateau is presently not well understood. Irrespective of the effect of displacement, however, the unbound concentration at the plateau is always lower than that achieved following an equivalent intravenous dosing rate.

Kinetic Consequences

The consequences of displacement on the total and unbound concentration, for drugs with either a high or a low extraction ratio, after various modes and routes of administration were discussed in Chapter 11 (Figs. 11-1 and 11-2). The kinetic consequences of displacement under the more usual clinical situation, in which both drug and displacer are given chronically, remain for discussion. Unfortunately, experimental data under these situations are sparse. Accordingly, the following discussion is centered around simulated, but probably reasonably realistic, situations. Although there are many possible combinations of events, only three situations are presented. In each case the displacer is added to the regimen of a patient already stabilized on the drug; both drug and displacer are administered intravenously by constant infusion, and both are assumed to be always at distribution equilibrium. While these conditions are somewhat restrictive, the situations chosen do illustrate the importance of both kinetics and the manner of drug administration on the likely therapeutic outcome.

The first situation involves displacement from both plasma and tissue binding sites of a drug with a low extraction ratio. Displacement is assumed to increase fu fourfold and fu_T twofold. Accordingly, clearance is increased fourfold, the volume of distribution twofold, and hence the half-life is reduced by one-half. The unbound volume of distribution correspondingly decreases approximately twofold, so that the unbound concentration doubles for a given amount in the body. Also the concentration of displacer is assumed to be constant as soon as administered (loading dose plus infusion) and to fall almost immediately to zero when withdrawn. The scenario that follows is depicted in Figure 17-4; this and the subsequent two figures are semilogarithmic plots, so that changes in unbound and total concentrations can be visualized simultaneously.

It can be seen in Figure 17-4 that although the unbound concentration at steady state is independent of binding (Equation 3), as expected, significant changes in this concentration, and presumably the effect, may occur. The initial rise in the unbound concentration and the sharp fall in the plasma concentration upon the sudden introduction of the displacer reflect the new distribution equilibrium condition.

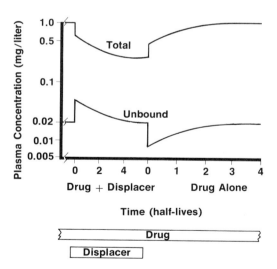

Figure 17-4. *When constantly infused, the unbound concentration of a drug with a low extraction ratio eventually returns to the preexisting value if a displacer is infused or withdrawn. As a consequence of decreased tissue binding, the half-life is shorter and the time required to go from one steady state to another is less in the presence of the displacer.*

The unbound concentration subsequently falls because the rate of elimination ($Cl_u \cdot Cu$) now exceeds the rate of infusion, ($Cl_u \cdot Cu_{ss}$). Eventually, it returns to the predisplacer steady-state value, but the time required to do so depends upon the half-life of the drug *in the presence of the displacer.* For example, if the half-life, although shortened by displacement, is still one day, then 3 to 4 days will elapse before the unbound concentration returns to the predisplacer value. The validity of this last statement can be appreciated by imagining that the rise in unbound concentration results not from displacement but rather from the administration of a bolus dose of drug and that the disposition kinetics of the drug changes to that in the presence of the constant amount of displacer. The situation is then analogous to that which occurs to the concentration as it falls from one plateau to a lower one upon reducing the rate of infusion (see Fig. 8-2).

The sharp fall in the unbound concentration when the displacer is removed results from increased binding in both the tissues and plasma. The total plasma concentration rises initially because the increase in plasma protein binding is greater than the increase in tissue binding. Both the unbound and total plasma concentrations subsequently rise because the rate of elimination ($Cl_u \cdot Cu$) is less than the rate of infusion. Eventually the level returns to the predisplacer value, but now the time to do so depends upon the half-life of the drug *in the absence of the displacer.* Because this half-life is longer than the half-life in the presence of the displacer, it will take longer than when the displacer was coadministered.

After distribution equilibrium, the changes in the plasma concentration parallel those of the unbound drug. This follows since the value of *fu*, although different in magnitude, is constant within each period that the concentration is rising or falling. However, it is apparent that the plasma concentration is a poor measure of the un-

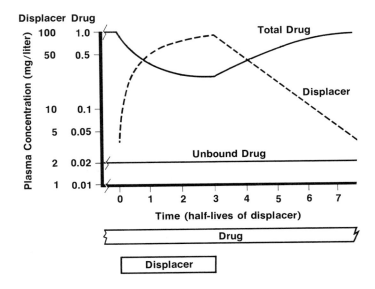

Figure 17-5. *When constantly infused, the unbound concentration of a drug with a low extraction ratio remains virtually unchanged if a displacer with a long half-life, relative to the drug, is either infused or withdrawn. The changes in plasma drug concentration reflect the displacement.*

bound drug and hence of the response when displacement occurs.

The importance of both the mode of administration of the displacer and its pharmacokinetics on the therapeutic outcome is illustrated in Figure 17-5. The displacer is again infused, but without a loading dose, and it has a longer half-life than that of the drug. This situation is more likely to prevail in practice than that depicted in Figure 17-4 for two reasons. First, because of potential risks, administration of a loading dose of the displacer is less common. Second, because the high concentration required for significant displacement is, in general, more likely to be achieved with a drug that has a long half-life; one with a short half-life would have to be given either in a large dose or frequently, both unlikely events.

In contrast to the first situation, slow accumulation and correspondingly slow elimination of the displacer result in insignificant changes in the unbound drug concentration and therefore response. This is a consequence of the kinetics of the displacer being the rate-limiting step. The concentration of displacer is changing so slowly relative to that of the drug, that at all times the

drug is at a virtual steady state, with rate out $(Cl_u \cdot Cu_{ss})$ matching the rate of infusion. The plasma drug concentration changes with the concentration of the displacer.

In the case just discussed no change in the effect and hence in the dosage regimen of the drug is anticipated even though displacement had occurred. Indeed, if only response were monitored, no displacement would have been suspected. A rise in unbound drug concentration and perhaps an increase in response would occur initially were a loading dose of displacer given.

The last example, depicted in Figure 17-6, deals with a drug having a high extraction ratio given by constant intravenous infusion. Now, if a loading dose followed by a constant infusion of displacer is given, displacement not only initially increases but also causes a sustained rise in the unbound drug concentration, to a new steady state. The total blood drug concentration, however, approaches its previous steady-state value as a consequence of no change in blood clearance. Since the half-life of the drug is prolonged as a result of an increase in the volume of distribution, the time required to reach steady state is longer in the presence than in the absence of the displacer. A reduced rate of administration might be required in this situation.

Diminished Unbound Clearance

A reduction of the unbound clearance of a drug is potentially the most dangerous type of drug interaction. The unbound drug concentration rises perhaps to a toxic level, unless an adjustment in dosage is made. Consequently, it is extremely important to be able to identify, to characterize, and, where possible, to avoid this type of interaction. Inhibition of drug metabolism is the major cause of reduced unbound clearance.

An Equilibrium Consideration

The phenylbutazone→warfarin interaction, whereby phenylbutazone produces a sustained enhancement in the anticoagulant effect of warfarin and sometimes causes serious bleeding episodes, is well documented. Warfarin is highly bound in plasma to albumin. Phenylbutazone, devoid of inherent anticoagulant activity, displaces warfarin. Consequently, displacement has been advocated as the primary mechanism for this interaction.

Figure 17-7 shows the temporal effects of phenylbutazone administration on the plasma and unbound concentrations of warfarin in a subject who ingested 10 mg warfarin daily for one month. The half-life of warfarin is approximately 2 days and therefore, as anticipated, a steady state for this drug was reached within the first 12 days when warfarin alone was administered. At that time the warfarin plasma concentration was 4 mg/liter and only 0.5 percent (0.02 mg/liter) was unbound, that is, $fu = 0.005$. Warfarin is completely absorbed, and therefore its clearance, estimated by dividing the daily dosing rate by the steady-state plasma concentration was 0.1 liter/hour. Thus, warfarin is a highly bound drug with a low extraction ratio.

Phenylbutazone is also poorly extracted,

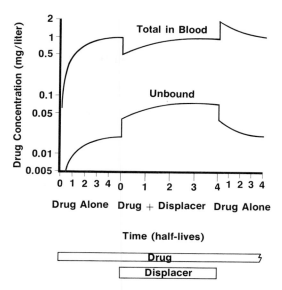

Figure 17-6. *Displacement of a drug with a high extraction ratio from its binding sites in blood, markedly elevates the unbound concentration during constant infusion. The half-life of the drug being prolonged, the time required to go from one steady state to another is longer in the presence than in the absence of the displacer. The concentration of displacer is assumed to be constant when administered and to fall immediately to zero when withdrawn.*

is highly bound ($fu = 0.004$–0.010), and has a half-life (approximately 3 days) even longer than that of warfarin. Accordingly, when on day 13 the subject commenced the usually recommended dosage regimen of phenylbutazone, 100 mg 3 times a day, the plasma concentration of this drug rose and eventually reached a plateau of approximately 100 mg/liter, after approximately 8 days. During this period, the plasma warfarin fell steadily in half, to 2.0 mg/liter, and the value of fu for warfarin rose approximately threefold.

At this point, the situation and the events appear remarkably similar to those depicted in Figure 17-5: a pure displacement interaction. However, there is one important difference: The unbound warfarin concentration rose and remained elevated during phenylbutazone administration. Because the effect of warfarin is related to its

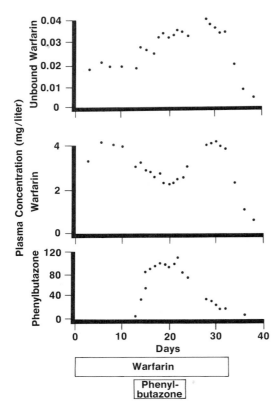

Figure 17-7. *Warfarin–phenylbutazone interaction. A subject received 10 mg warfarin orally each day and phenylbutazone, 100 mg three times a day, on days 13 to 22. As the phenylbutazone concentration rose, bound warfarin was displaced and the plasma warfarin concentration fell. The sustained elevation in the unbound warfarin during phenylbutazone administration implies inhibition of warfarin elimination. (Modified from Schary, W.L., Lewis, R.J., and Rowland, M.: Warfarin–Phenylbutazone interaction in man: A long term multiple dose study. Res. Commun. Chem. Pathol. Pharmacol., 10: 663–672, 1975.)*

unbound concentration, this sustained elevation is in accord with the observed sustained augmentation of the effect as long as phenylbutazone is coadministered. Examination of Equation 3 indicates that to account for the elevated values of unbound drug, either the rate of entry of drug into the body is increased or the value of Cl_u is decreased. Since the dosage regimen of warfarin was unaltered and warfarin is fully available, Cl_u must have decreased.

Warfarin is almost exclusively metabolized in the liver to either weakly active or inactive metabolites. Thus, a lower value for Cl_u implies a decrease in the ability of the liver to metabolize warfarin. Analysis of several metabolites of warfarin in both plasma and urine subsequently confirmed that, indeed, phenylbutazone inhibits warfarin elimination and that it is this inhibition and not displacement that probably accounts for the clinical picture.

The interaction between phenylbutazone and warfarin is even more complex than portrayed above. Commercial warfarin is a racemate, and the S($-$) isomer is five times more active than the R($+$) isomer. Phenylbutazone inhibits the formation of 7-hydroxywarfarin, a major metabolite of only the more active isomer. Phenylbutazone also induces many drug-metabolizing enzymes including the ones responsible for the metabolism of the R($+$) isomer. However, being the less potent isomer, induction is of little therapeutic importance. Nonetheless the lesson is clear: Drug interactions may be complex; careful observations are required to unravel the facts.

A Graded Response

The pharmacokinetics of warfarin is independent of dose because the plasma concentration, C, is below the value for the Michaelis-Menten constant, Km. Thus, for each metabolic pathway

$$\text{Rate of metabolite formation} = \frac{Vm \cdot C}{Km} \qquad 4$$

or expressed in terms of the clearance associated with the metabolite formation, Cl_m

Rate of metabolite formation
$$= Cl_m \cdot C = fm \cdot Cl \cdot C \qquad 5$$

where fm is the fraction of the dose of drug that is converted to the metabolite. In the presence of an inhibitor the rate of metabolite formation is slowed, the value of the new rate being given by the expression

Rate of metabolite formation $= \dfrac{Cl_m \cdot C}{1 + C_I/K_I}$ 6

where C_I is the concentration of the inhibitor and K_I is the inhibition constant, given by the concentration of inhibitor that decreases the clearance associated with the metabolite formation twofold. According to this relationship, the degree of inhibition of warfarin 7-hydroxylation should vary with the plasma concentration of phenylbutazone. Unfortunately, such data are not presently available but they are for the interaction between the sulfonamide, sulfaphenazole, and the oral hypoglycemic agent, tolbutamide.

Sulfaphenazole is no longer prescribed. One reason is that it inhibits the metabolism of a number of drugs and thereby causes excessive drug accumulation and toxicity. For example, hypoglycemic crises have been reported when patients, stabilized on tolbutamide, have had sulfaphenazole added to their drug therapy; the half-life of tolbutamide, usually 4 to 8 hours, was prolonged to values ranging from 24 to 70 hours. Tolbutamide, like warfarin, undergoes dose-independent pharmacokinetics and, moreover, oxidation to hydroxytolbutamide is the obligatory pathway of tolbutamide elimination, that is, $Cl_m = Cl$ and $fm = 1$. If it is assumed that sulfaphenazole does not substantially affect the volume of distribution of tolbutamide and its volume of distribution is constant, then Equation 6 can be written for tolbutamide in the simple form:

Rate of tolbutamide elimination $= \dfrac{k \cdot Ab}{(1 + I/K_I)}$ 7

where Ab and I are the amounts of tolbutamide and sulfaphenazole in the body, and K_I may now be defined as the amount of inhibitor that diminishes the apparent elimination rate constant, $k/(1 + I/K_I)$, of tolbutamide by one-half, or doubles the half-life of tolbutamide. For sulfaphenazole, the K_I value is 200 mg. This value is small

compared to the 1 to 2 gram daily dose of the sulfonamide that was usually recommended.

Given the preceding information it is now possible to appreciate why a hypoglycemic crisis did not usually occur until many days after sulfaphenazole had been added to the patient's regimen and why treatment of the crisis often had to be continued for several days, even though the administration of both drugs was stopped.

The likely events following oral administration of 0.5 gram tolbutamide and 1.0 gram sulfaphenazole twice daily are portrayed in Figure 17-8. Initially, when only tolbutamide is given, the expected plateau is reached within 3 to 4 half-lives or by 30 hours. When sulfaphenazole is also given, it accumulates and blocks tolbutamide oxidation, ultimately causing a rise in the level of the sulfonylurea to approximately seven times its usual value. Also a period of 2 to 3 days is required before this elevated level of tolbutamide falls to the level observed in the absence of sulfaphenazole or falls to zero if both drugs are stopped.

A more exact quantitative picture of the events may be gained from two equations. One, previously examined (Eq. 7, Chap. 13), defines the average amount of drug at the plateau

$$Ab_{av} = \dfrac{1.44 \times \text{Dose} \times \text{Half-life}}{\text{Dosing interval}} \quad 8$$

The other follows from Equation 7. The term $k/(1 + I/K_I)$ can be considered as the new (and smaller) elimination rate constant of tolbutamide in the presence of the inhibitor. It follows therefore that the new half-life of tolbutamide ($t_{1/2,\text{inhibited}}$) is related to the normal half-life ($t_{1/2,\text{normal}}$) by

$$t_{1/2,\text{inhibited}} = t_{1/2,\text{inhibited}} \cdot [1 + (I/K_I)] \quad 9$$

Obviously, the value of the half-life changes continuously with changes in the amount of inhibitor in the body, but once sulfaphenazole reaches a plateau, the half-life of tolbutamide becomes constant. For example,

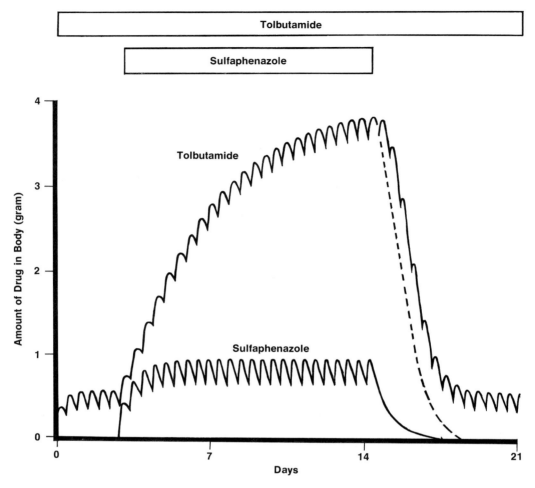

Figure 17-8. *Tolbutamide–sulfaphenazole interaction kinetics simulation when tolbutamide (0.5 gram, twice daily) is given in the absence and in the presence of sulfaphenazole (1 gram, twice daily). The bars denote the duration of each drug regimen. In the presence of sulfaphenazole, an inhibitor of tolbutamide oxidation, the amount of tolbutamide rises from one plateau to another, when output once again equals input. Upon cessation of sulfaphenazole, the decline of tolbutamide, whether continued (solid line) or stopped at the same time as sulfaphenazole (dotted line), is primarily controlled by the rate of removal of sulfaphenazole. Consequently, several days transpire before the level of tolbutamide once again falls into the accepted therapeutic range. (From Rowland, M., and Matin, S.B.: Kinetics of drug-drug interactions. J. Pharmacokin. Biopharm. 1: 553–567, 1973.)*

when 1 gram of sulfaphenazole ($t_{1/2} = 12$ hours) is given twice daily, the average amount of inhibitor in the body at plateau, according to Equation 8, is 1.4 grams. This plateau is reached within two days. Substituting this amount of inhibitor into Equation 9 indicates that the new half-life of tolbutamide is eight times (1 + 1.4 gram/ 0.2 gram) longer than normal, that is, 32 to

64 hours. Accordingly, it takes approximately one week to reach a new plateau; the average amount of tolbutamide in the body is now eight times the average plateau level in the absence of the inhibitor (Eq. 8).

These data suggest that if tolbutamide and sulfaphenazole had to be given together, the dosing rate of tolbutamide would have to be reduced by one-eighth to maintain the normal amount of tolbutamide in the body. These data also explain why stopping tolbutamide at the same time as sulfaphenazole would not resolve a toxicity problem much quicker than stopping sulfaphenazole alone; the rate of decline of tolbutamide is determined by its half-life and that in turn is controlled by the rate of removal of sulfaphenazole. Interestingly, tolbutamide has no demonstrable effect on sulfaphenazole elimination; this sulfonamide is eliminated primarily by glucuronidation.

The influence of inhibition on tolbutamide kinetics is dramatic because this drug is eliminated by only one pathway, $fm = 1$, instead of by several, the more usual situation. Commonly, one pathway may only account for 50 percent ($fm = 0.5$) or less of drug elimination. Then, even if this pathway is completely inhibited, the half-life of the drug increases no more than twofold. Because the average amount of drug in the body would also not be raised more than twofold, no change in the dosage regimen of the drug may be warranted, unless the therapeutic index of the drug is small.

Inhibition of metabolism and secretion are examples of a chemically mediated pharmacokinetic interaction. The lower hepatic clearance of lidocaine when given together with propranolol, a β-adrenergic blocking drug, is an example of a physiologically mediated pharmacokinetic interaction. Propranolol diminishes cardiac output and hence hepatic blood flow, which, in turn, reduces the clearance of lidocaine, a drug highly extracted by the liver. Presumably, since the degree of β-adrenergic blockade is a graded response, the interaction with lidocaine is dependent on the plasma concentration of propranolol.

Beneficial Interactions

Penicillin-probenecid combination therapy is an example of the successful use of a drug interaction. Probenecid competitively inhibits the renal secretion of penicillin thereby substantially reducing its renal clearance, the major component of total clearance. Consequently, in the presence of probenecid, higher than usual plasma concentrations of penicillin are achieved following a normal dosage regimen of the antibiotic. Occasionally a large single dose or a high dose regimen of penicillin is needed to ensure effective treatment of an infection. Probenecid is then of little extra value, because the high concentration of antibiotic now overcomes the probenecid blockade of its secretion. Being a competitive interaction, the degree of inhibition by probenecid might be restored by raising its dose in proportion to the dose of penicillin. However, cost and potential toxicity, associated with the high concentration of probenecid, probably make this an impractical measure. Of note is the lack of a major effect of penicillin on probenecid elimination. Although actively secreted into the kidney tubule, being lipophilic, unlike penicillin, probenecid is mostly reabsorbed. Consequently, the renal clearance of probenecid is low; metabolism is the major route of its elimination.

Elevated Unbound Clearance

The unbound clearance of a drug can be increased in numerous ways. Raising urine pH by giving acetazolamide or sodium bicarbonate increases the renal clearance of salicylic acid and other acids whose renal clearance is pH sensitive. Giving ammonium chloride or ascorbic acid to make the urine more acidic, increases the renal clearance of pH-sensitive basic drugs. Some drugs increase the metabolic clearance of other drugs. They do so most commonly by inducing the drug-metabolizing enzymes, but they may also activate enzymes or retard enzyme degradation. Occasionally, like glucagon, they increase liver blood flow and thereby increase the hepatic clearance of drugs that are highly extracted by that organ.

The resulting changes in the pharmacokinetic parameters and the kinetic conse-

Study Problems

*(**Answers to Study Problems can be found in Appendix G.**)*

1. The usual dosage regimen of a drug (half-life of 13 hours) is 100 mg every 8 hours. Eighty percent is oxidized to a single inactive metabolite; the remainder is excreted unchanged. It is necessary to give the drug to a patient who is also taking another drug that is an inhibitor of this drug's oxidation pathway. Knowing that the oxidation proceeds at 20 percent of the normal value in the presence of the other drug (level is constant with time), suggest how the dosage regimen of the affected drug should be adjusted to maintain the usual average amount of drug in the body.

2. Drug B is a known plasma protein displacer and enzyme inducer of Drug A. A single intravenous dose of Drug A is administered alone and again several weeks later after Drug B is repeatedly administered and steady state is achieved. The clearance, half-life, fraction unbound, and fraction excreted unchanged of Drug A when given alone are 1.2 liters/hour, 26 hours, 0.05, and 0.1, respectively. In the presence of Drug B the enzyme activity and the fraction unbound are approximately doubled. Prepare separate semi-logarithmic graphs to illustrate the salient features of the effect of Drug B on the total and unbound concentrations and the urinary excretion rate of Drug A. On each graph show the time course of Drug A in the presence as well as in the absence of Drug B.

3. A drug (A) is given by infusion at a rate of 25 mg/hour to maintain a constant plasma concentration. The data in Table 17-4 are obtained in a subject who is infused at this rate in the absence and presence of another drug (B) (assume that it is at steady state when present). Given this information and the observation that the creatinine clearance in this subject is 120 ml/min,

Table 17-4.

Plateau Plasma Concentration of Drug B (mg/liter)	Data for Drug A			
	Plateau Plasma Concentration (mg/liter)	Urinary Excretion Rate at Steady State (mg/hour)	Fraction Unbound in Plasma	Half-life (hours)
0	10.0	15	0.1	12
20.0	6.7	4	0.3	8

(a) Determine if there is evidence for Drug A being secreted and/or reabsorbed in the kidney.
(b) Determine the mechanism(s) by which Drug B interacts with Drug A.
(c) Discuss the therapeutic implications of coadministering these drugs.

Unifying Problem

(Answer to Unifying Problem can be found in Appendix G.)

Normal values for the pharmacokinetic parameters, clearance, fraction unbound and fraction excreted unchanged are listed in Table 17-5 for drugs A through G. Situations are presented which alter the kinetics of each of these drugs. On the right indicate whether the value of each parameter would be observed to increase (↑), decrease (↓), or show little or no change (↔). All drugs are administered orally and have volumes of distribution greater than 50 liters.

Table 17-5.

Drug	Normal Values				Observations				
	Clearance[a] (ml/min)	Fraction[a] Unbound	Fraction Excreted Unchanged	Situations	Clearance[a]	Volume of Distribution[a]	Half-life	Availability	Fraction Excreted Unchanged
A	280	0.9	0.7	Simultaneous administration of a competitive inhibitor of renal secretion.					
B (acid, renal clearance pH sensitive)	200	0.1	1.0	Urine pH increased by another drug					
C	1200	0.5	0.99	Simultaneous administration of a competitive inhibitor of metabolism					
D	1200	0.05	0.01	Simultaneous administration of a drug that displaces drug D from plasma proteins					
E	50	0.4	0.5	Simultaneous administration of a drug that displaces drug E from tissue binding sites					
F	10	0.1	0.01	Simultaneous administration of a drug that displaces drug F from plasma proteins					
G	1300	0.7	0.95	Simultaneous administration of an enzyme inducer for several days					

[a]Based on measurement of drug concentration in blood.

18

monitoring drug therapy

Objectives

The reader will be able to:

1. **Define and describe what is meant by target concentration strategy.**

2. **List the criteria for determining when monitoring plasma drug concentrations and applying target concentration strategy are appropriate.**

3. **Interpret plasma concentration data under both steady-state and nonsteady-state conditions.**

4. **Estimate the pharmacokinetic parameters of a drug in an individual patient when provided with the plasma concentration and other appropriate data.**

5. **Evaluate a pharmacokinetic problem observed during chronic drug therapy and ascribe the problem to a change in availability, compliance, clearance, volume of distribution, or a combination of these.**

DRUGS are administered to achieve a therapeutic objective. Once this objective is defined, a drug and its dosage regimen are chosen for the patient. Drug therapy is subsequently managed as shown schematically in Figure 18-1. Traditionally, this management has been accomplished by monitoring the incidence and intensity of both the desired therapeutic effects and the undesired side and toxic effects. Examples of this method of individualizing drug therapy are shown in Table 18-1.

Although clearly preferable, it is not always possible to use a direct measure of the desired effect as a therapeutic end point. Thus, of the examples of monitoring of drug therapy listed in Table 18-1, only with thiopental is the dosage clearly titrated to the therapeutic effect. Sometimes, signs of toxicity are used as a dosing guide. The

dose of salicylates, for example, when used in the treatment of rheumatic diseases, is often increased until tinnitus or nausea and vomiting intervene. In moderate to severe asthmatic cases, theophylline too is frequently titrated to a toxic end point. Excessive dryness of the mouth is a common measure of the upper dosage of atropine when used as a spasmolytic agent.

The therapeutic effects of salicylates, theophylline, and atropine, although often subjective and vague, can be assessed and hence can be used in judging the success of therapy. This is not so readily accomplished with the antiepileptic drugs; the therapeutic effect is the nonoccurrence of fits. A fit may be infrequent and, as a result, delays and difficulties exist in assessing therapeutic success. Toxic effects that can be readily measured, for example, nystagmus and

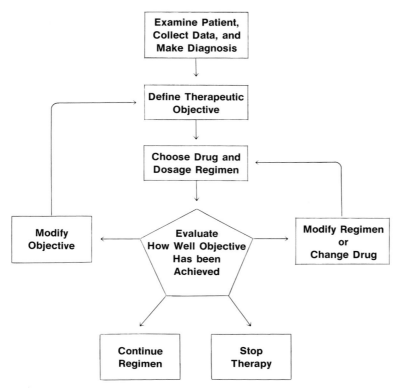

Figure 18-1. *General scheme for initiation and management of drug therapy. The major tasks are: defining the therapeutic objective, choosing the drug and its dosage regimen, and evaluating how well the objective has been achieved. Monitoring the plasma drug concentration often may assist in accomplishing the last two tasks.*

ataxia, have therefore been used to assist in titrating the upper limit of an epileptic patient's requirements. A similar situation arises in the use of oral anticoagulants; the therapeutic objective is the prevention of emboli. Here again the therapeutic response cannot readily be assessed, and therefore an alternative, simple, and rapid laboratory test, prothrombin time, is substituted as the therapeutic objective. Likewise, for immunosuppressive, hypoglycemic, and uricosuric agents, clinical laboratory tests are employed as alternative therapeutic end points. Clearly, to be useful, any alternative test must be graded and must always be closely related to the true therapeutic effect.

The seriousness of the first toxic effect observed is a major determinant of its use as an end point. The titration of young

persons on salicylate therapy to the occurrence of tinnitus is safe, as tinnitus is an easily measured mild toxicity, although it does not always occur before the advent of more serious toxicity; its presence may be particularly difficult to assess in young children and in patients with impaired hearing. In contrast, titrating the dosage of digoxin and related glycosides to cardiac toxicity is always unsafe.

Another approach is to monitor the plasma concentration. It may be especially useful if the concentration is closely related to the probability and severity of toxicity and if the therapeutic effect is hard to evaluate as with antiepileptic drugs, for which the desired response is the nonoccurrence of fits. In this way, the plasma concentration serves as an intermediate therapeutic end point and as a prophylactic of toxicity. At a minimum, the plasma concentration can serve as an additional piece of information to guide and assess drug therapy.

The application of the plasma concentration of a drug as an alternative therapeutic objective is known as *target concentration strategy*. The basic idea is to apply a strategy to achieve and maintain a target concentration or a range of concentrations.

Target Concentration Strategy

This strategy is useful as an adjunct in initiating and monitoring drug therapy when a number of criteria listed below are satisfied. Some of the criteria are absolute in nature, others are relative. Most of them, however, must be met for the strategy to be routinely effective.

Direct Concentration-Effect Relationship

The plasma concentration of a drug must quantitatively correlate with both the intensity and the probability of therapeutic and toxic effects. The data in Figure 18-2 suggest that this is so for the therapeutic effect of quinidine. Every time the concentration dropped below a critical value, about 4 mg/liter in this patient, the attacks of paroxysmal ventricular tachycardia reappeared. Additional doses of quinidine increased the concentration and caused the restoration of normal sinus rhythm, an all-or-none response. The data for procainamide in Figure 18-3 suggest that the frequency of premature ventricular contractions, a graded response, is directly related to the plasma concentration of procainamide in a patient with coronary artery disease. The probability of the responses of

Table 18-1. Examples of Monitoring Drug Therapy by the Effects Produced or by Alternative Tests

Drug	Condition	Observation Suggesting Increased Dosage	Observation Suggesting Holding or Decreasing Dosage	Severe Toxic Signs
Group I. Drugs Monitored by Effects				
1. Salicylates	Rheumatoid arthritis or rheumatic fever	Inadequate reduction of inflammation and pain	Tinnitus, nausea, vomiting	Metabolic acidosis
2. Theophylline	Constrictive airway disease	Insufficient broncho-dilation	Nausea, vomiting	CNS stimulation
3. Atropine	GIT spasms	Inadequate control	Dryness of mouth	Palpitations
4. Phenytoin	Convulsive disorders	Inadequate reduction of frequency of epileptic fits	Nystagmus	Ataxia and lethargy
5. Thiopental	Induction of anesthesia	Insufficient anesthesia	Anesthesia too deep	Respiratory failure
Group II. Drugs Monitored by Effects and Alternative Tests				
6. Warfarin	Thromboembolic disease	Prothrombin time too short	Prothrombin time too long	Hemorrhage
7. Immuno-suppressive agents	Renal transplantation	Rosette inhibition test; antibodies too high	Antibodies too low	Infection
8. Tolbutamide	Adult onset diabetes	Glucose in urine	No glucose in urine	Hypoglycemic shock
9. Uricosurics	Gout	Elevated serum uric acid	Decreased serum uric acid	

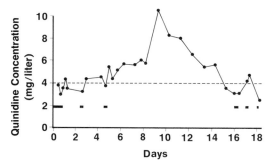

Figure 18-2. *The recurrence of ventricular tachycardia (━) appears to be associated with a drop in the plasma quinidine concentration below about 4 mg/liter (dashed line) in a patient with coronary heart disease. (Redrawn by permission from Sokolow, M., and Edger, R.: Blood quinidine concentration as a guide in the treatment of cardiac arrhythmias. Circulation, 1: 576–592, 1950.)*

each of these drugs should be obtainable from an adequate sample of the patient population.

A direct relationship between concentration and effect is insufficient grounds for plasma concentration monitoring of antiarrhythmic drugs; the effect itself is easily monitored. Maintenance of "therapeutic" concentrations of quinidine and procainamide does, however, appear to be useful in protecting against potentially lethal arrhythmias, independent of the degree of the effectiveness of these drugs in suppressing advanced chronic arrhythmias and in reducing toxicity.

Lack of Other Dosing Guides

The strategy becomes particularly attractive when other end points either are difficult to quantitate, as with the nonoccurrence of epileptic fits, or are lacking, as in the prophylactic use of drugs.

Nature of the Therapeutic Regimen

The strategy is best considered when the objective is to maintain the therapeutic effect. The strategy most often then involves the maintenance of a steady-state concen-

tration within the range required for optimizing utility (Chap. 12). Drugs for which acute or intermittent effects are desired, such as certain hypnotics (induction of sleep), aspirin (headache), and nitroglycerin (angina), are best monitored by their acute effects. Obviously, the occurrence of tolerance also diminishes the potential for application of the strategy.

Therapeutic Problem Anticipated

Target concentration strategy is also indicated when there is a high probability of encountering a therapeutic failure, that is, either a lack of effect or the occurrence of undue toxicity. A therapeutic failure is most likely to arise if the drug has a low therapeutic index (see Table 12-1) and a great variability in its pharmacokinetics, or if the patient is at particular risk due to concurrent disease (Chaps. 14, 16) or to multiple drug therapy (Chap. 17). A higher frequency of therapeutic failures is also antici-

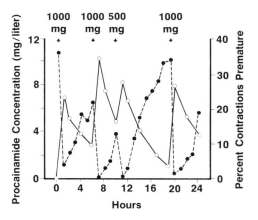

Figure 18-3. *Inverse relationship between the frequency of premature ventricular contractions (●---●) and serum procainamide concentrations (○—○) in a patient who has coronary artery disease. (Redrawn from figure in Koch-Weser, J.: Correlation of serum concentrations and pharmacologic effects of antiarrhythmic drugs. In Pharmacology and the Future of Man, Proc. 5th Int. Congr. Pharmacol., San Francisco, 1972. S. Karger, Basel, 1973, Vol. 3.)*

pated when noncompliance or erratic absorption is likely.

Presentation of a Problem

For some drugs the strategy is applied only when a problem arises. The problem may be a lack of response, at usual or even larger dosages, due to one or more of the following conditions: noncompliance, poor availability, unusually rapid elimination, or a pharmacodynamic resistance to the drug. Measurement of the plasma concentration permits a distinction to be made between these pharmacokinetic and pharmacodynamic causes of the problem. Similarly, the cause of a toxic or unusual response at customary or low dosages may be ascertained.

Present State of Knowledge

Efficient use of the strategy requires prior knowledge of the following: the target concentration, the pharmacokinetic parameters of the drug, and the conditions in which this concentration and these parameters are likely to be altered, and, if so, the extent of the change. The last two requirements are relative in that, by monitoring the concentration, adjustments in dosage can be made for altered pharmacokinetics. The target concentration, however, must be known.

Analytical Considerations

A sensitive, accurate, and specific assay for the drug must be available. In addition, to be useful, the results must be available before the next therapeutic decision is to be made, often by the time the next dose is to be given. The half-life is a useful index of this "turn-around" time, because it is the time frame in which accumulation on multiple dosing and disappearance on discontinuing a drug occur. For example, reporting a result three or more half-lives after a sample is taken may not have prevented a patient, with an unduly low clearance, from developing excessive toxicity.

Interrelationships

The relationship between the effect of a drug and the dose administered was discussed in Chapter 12. One of the principal reasons for plasma concentration monitoring is to adjust for the pharmacokinetic source of variation in the response to drugs. The unbound drug concentration at the active site is undoubtedly a much better correlate of response than is the plasma concentration. Since the "active site" concentration can rarely be measured, the unbound concentration in plasma would appear to be next best. However, its measurement is difficult and often inaccurate; therefore, the plasma concentration must be relied upon. Unfortunately, the plasma concentration does not always bear a constant relationship to the concentration at the active site. There are two reasons for this. Both are a consequence of the specific distribution of drug to the active site. One concerns the time required for drug to distribute to the site of action; the other concerns the binding to plasma proteins. Both can contribute toward variability in the relationship between the plasma concentration and the concentration at the active site. In addition, the response to a given drug concentration at the active site may be altered by a number of factors, e.g., the presence of physiologic or pharmacologic antagonists or synergists, genetic factors, severity of an illness, development of tachyphylaxis or tolerance, or the presence of active metabolites (Chap. 12).

The Target Concentration

The target concentration initially chosen is the value or range of values with the greatest probability of therapeutic success (Chap. 12), bearing in mind that the population value may be inappropriate for an individual. Higher concentrations may be appropriate when the condition is severe, and the converse may be true when the condition is mild. If altered protein binding is anticipated, such as in uremia, in stress, or when displacing drugs are also being administered, then the target concentration should be adjusted to attain the same unbound concentration.

The principles for establishing a dosage regimen to achieve a desired concentration or to keep within concentration limits were presented in Chapter 13. Adjustment in the usual dosage regimen can often be anticipated based on the patient's age, weight, and clinical status, especially renal, hepatic, and cardiovascular functions. Yet, even after taking these factors into account, sufficient unpredictability in the kinetics of the drug in the individual patient may remain to warrant monitoring the plasma concentration. From such observations, the patient's current pharmacokinetic parameters can be estimated, and a new dosage regimen can be designed to more closely achieve the target value.

The frequency of monitoring is a function of the presumed change in the factors that influence drug response. For example, the plasma phenytoin concentration in epileptic patients, whose state of health and drug therapy may remain stable, may only need to be monitored several times a year; more frequent monitoring may be indicated if the patient's health deteriorates or if therapy with other drugs is altered. Daily or even more frequent monitoring of plasma theophylline concentrations may be needed for optimal use of the drug in the treatment of an asthmatic patient in an intensive care unit, especially if congestive heart failure, pneumonia, severe constrictive airway disease, and smoking concurrently coexist. These conditions alter theophylline metabolism, which is likely to be quite variable in this situation.

Evaluating the Measured Concentration

Several kinds of information are needed to evaluate efficiently a measured plasma concentration. A history of drug administration, which includes the doses and times of dosing, and the time of sampling are mandatory. So too are the patient's age and weight. The importance of knowing other factors, such as concurrent disease states; concurrent drug therapy; renal, hepatic, and cardiovascular functions; serum protein concentrations; active metabolites; and assay methods, varies with the drug under consideration. Examples are given in Table 18-2.

Data Interpretation

After collecting the necessary information, including the present and previous, if any, plasma concentration measurements, two approaches may be taken to evaluate the data. One approach, comparison of the observed value with that predicted from known information, is helpful in identifying the cause of any problem. The other approach, estimation of the pharmacokinetic parameters of the drug in the individual, is particularly useful in determining the patient's dosage requirement. Data treatment is similar, irrespective of the approach. One must first establish, from the dosing history and the time of sampling, whether the measured value is a good estimate of the maximum, average, or minimum concentration at steady state on a fixed regimen or of a nonsteady-state value obtained either shortly after starting the drug or following an erratic dosage schedule.

Steady State. The most readily handled value, an estimate of average steady-state concentration, is only obtained after dosing for at least 3 half-lives (in the patient), and when the fluctuation of the concentration within a dosing interval is small. The second condition, small fluctuations, probably prevails when the dosing interval is less than one-half of the half-life in the patient.

The observed concentration is compared with that expected in the individual; the latter value is calculated from the expected

Table 18-2. Information Pertinent to the Plasma Concentration Monitoring
of Selected Drugs

Drug	Concurrent Disease States	Plasma-Protein Binding	Concurrent Drug Therapy	Active Metabolites	Other Pertinent Information
Digoxin	Renal disease, congestive heart failure, thyroid disease	—[a]	Diuretics	—	Distribution characteristics
Gentamicin	Renal disease	—	Some penicillins	—	Composed of three isomers
Phenytoin	Renal disease, chronic hepatic disease	Strongly bound to albumin	Dicumarol, isoniazid, phenylbutazone, some sulfa drugs	—	Saturable metabolism
Procainamide	Renal and hepatic diseases	—	—	N-acetyl procainamide	Acetylation polymorphism
Theophylline	Pneumonia, chronic obstructive lung disease, congestive heart failure, hepatic cirrhosis, acute pulmonary edema	Moderately bound to albumin	Triacetyl-oleandomycin, erythromycin, phenobarbital?	3-methyl xanthine?	Available in many dosage and salt forms

[a] Therapeutically unimportant.

values of availability and clearance and from the rate of administration.

$$C_{av}(\text{expected}) = \frac{F}{Cl}(\text{expected}) \cdot \frac{D}{\tau} \quad 1$$

If the ratio of observed to predicted concentrations is greater than 1.0, either the input is greater or the elimination is slower than expected, or both. The converse applies to a ratio less than 1. Thus, a set of explanations exists that is consistent with each observation.

Perhaps the most common cause of an altered input is noncompliance, a problem of patient education. Availability is a factor that only needs to be considered for drugs whose availability is low or variable. Renal and hepatic clearances are each valid considerations for altered elimination, depend-

ing on the major route of elimination of the drug.

The dosage regimens of many drugs are often such that there is considerable fluctuation in the plasma concentration. The dosing interval may be fixed, with its value comparable to or greater than the half-life, or the drug may be taken every 4 hours for four doses, but not again for 12 hours, a common dosing schedule when prescribed (four times a day). In both cases, the fluctuation must be considered to evaluate a measurement properly.

When considerable fluctuation is anticipated, the preferred time of sampling is often just before the next dose. The concentration observed from a sample obtained soon after an intravenous dose or at the peak time after an oral dose, is often unreliable. Either absorption or distribution, or both, may take some time to be essentially complete, and both these processes vary from time to time and among patients. Variability in the rates of these processes has less effect on the minimum concentration. Sometimes, however, the observation may be closer to a peak or an average than to a trough concentration. In either event, proper evaluation requires knowing the time of sampling within the dosing interval, the dosing interval relative to the half-life expected in the patient, and the absorption and distribution characteristics of the drug. For a fixed-dose and dosing-interval regimen, assuming instantaneous absorption, the concentration expected at time t within a dosing interval τ under steady-state conditions is given by the product of the maximum concentration at steady state (see Table 13-8) times the fraction remaining at time t, e^{-kt}, that is,

$$C = \frac{F \cdot D \cdot e^{-kt}}{V(1 - e^{-k\tau})} \qquad 2$$

or, since $k = Cl/V$

$$C = \frac{F \cdot D \cdot e^{-\left(\frac{Cl}{V}\right)t}}{V(1 - e^{-\left(\frac{Cl}{V}\right)\tau})} \qquad 3$$

Again, the observed concentration may be compared to the predicted value; where it differs, probable causes can be proposed, based upon knowledge of the variability usually observed in the compliance, availability, clearance, and volume of distribution of the drug.

Fluctuation may be viewed in absolute terms or relative to the peak concentration. Assuming instantaneous absorption, it should be recalled that the difference between peak, $C_{ss,max}$, and trough, $C_{ss,min}$, concentrations at steady state is

$$C_{ss,max} - C_{ss,min} = \frac{F \cdot D}{V} \qquad 4$$

Thus, the maximal value at the peak can be estimated from the trough value. One of the two concentrations, and occasionally both,

may be out of the therapeutic range and perhaps dictate the need to adjust dosage. The same conclusion may be drawn from considerations of the fluctuation relative to the peak concentration. The maximum value of this ratio is (from relationships in Table 13-8)

$$\frac{C_{ss,max} - C_{ss,min}}{C_{ss,max}} = 1 - e^{-k\tau} \qquad 5$$

For a patient with a higher than usual clearance and therefore a shorter than usual half-life, the relative fluctuation may be unusually large and a larger than usual maintenance dose may be required. In this case a shorter dosing interval may be preferred to minimize the degree of fluctuation.

For a regular daily dosage regimen of either unequal dosing intervals or unequal doses, or both, the expected steady-state concentration may be calculated from the dosing history as subsequently shown in the section on the estimation of parameter values.

Nonsteady State. A plasma sample may be taken before a plateau has been achieved or following an erratic pattern of administration. Although steady-state principles obviously cannot be applied in these circumstances, other methods are available to evaluate the data obtained. Consider, for example, the case of sampling while drug accumulates during a constant-rate intravenous infusion. A plasma concentration obtained during such an infusion is a function of the rate of administration, the clearance, and the volume of distribution (Chap. 8).

$$C = \frac{R_{inf}}{Cl}(1 - e^{-\left(\frac{Cl}{V}\right)t}) \qquad 6$$

The values of C, R_{inf}, and t are known; the clearance and volume are unknown. Evaluation of a plasma concentration requires knowing whether clearance or the volume of distribution is the more variable, and appreciating upon which of these two parameters the concentration is the more dependent. The latter may be considered from the events depicted in Figure 18-4 during the infusion of a drug in three separate situations. In case A, the values of the clearance and volume parameters are those anticipated, the average values. In the other two situations the half-life is threefold greater than the average value, in case B due to a threefold reduction in clearance, in case C due to a corresponding increase in the volume of distribution.

In any situation, with little drug having been eliminated, the initial concentration is primarily a function of infusion rate and volume of distribution. Accordingly, there is little virtue in taking a sample before the usual half-life to estimate dosage require-

ments to achieve therapeutic concentrations. The steady-state concentration depends only upon the rate of administration and the value of clearance (Chap. 8). Accordingly, sampling at this time provides the most confidence in estimating dosage requirements.

Sampling between the time of initiating the infusion and steady state often leads to inconclusive information. At two usual half-lives, a decreased clearance, case B, can hardly be detected. Furthermore, the observation at this time of a low concentration, case C, cannot be distinguished from that resulting from a clearance that is greater than usual. However, the observation of a concentration greater than the usual steady-state value at this time is a clear indication that clearance is less than usual. Indeed, the greater the difference between the observed and predicted values, the lower is the probable value of clearance and the greater is the need to reduce the rate of administration to avoid toxicity.

In the region of 2 to 6 usual half-lives, the major consideration in interpreting a single observation is whether the clearance or the volume parameter is the more variable. For example, the clearance (in units of liter/hour/kg) of theophylline varies over an eightfold range or more, particularly if age and disease state are considered. The range of values for the volumes of distribution (liter/kg) is only about twofold. Thus, estimates of the clearance of theophylline can be made from nonsteady-state values obtained at 2 to 4 usual half-lives.

Although the preceding concepts were developed for administration by infusion, they also apply to multiple oral dose therapy, provided that availability and fluctuation are also considered.

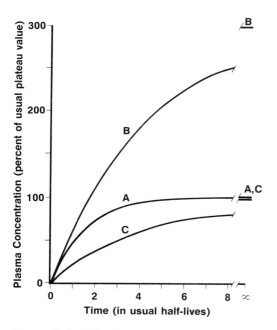

Figure 18-4. *Following a constant-rate infusion, monitoring the concentration at one usual half-life does little to distinguish between a patient with average values of clearance and volume,* **case A** *and one with a threefold reduction in clearance and an average volume of distribution,* **case B.** *Distinguishing between these patients, without producing undue toxicity, is probably best done by monitoring at four usual half-lives. Although a threefold increase in volume of distribution,* **case C,** *is readily detected at one usual half-life, this observation provides little information on the final plateau concentration to be achieved.*

Estimation of Parameter Values

The preceding discussion was oriented toward evaluating a plasma concentration by comparing the observed value with that expected in the patient. Another approach

Table 18-3. Dosing History of Aminophylline

Date	Time	Time Since Dose (hours)	Oral Dose (mg)
June 1	6:00 P.M.	24	400
	10:00 P.M.	20	200
June 2	8:00 A.M.	10	300
	12:00 noon	6	300
	6:00 P.M.	Blood sample drawn	

is to use the observation to estimate the pharmacokinetic parameters of the drug in the individual patient. This information is required to adjust a dosage regimen.

Clearance. When a value is a good estimate of an average steady-state concentration, the availability is not variable, compliance is assured, and the patient is on a fixed-dose, fixed-interval dosage regimen, then the clearance is readily estimated from

$$Cl = \frac{F \cdot D/\tau}{C_{av}} \qquad 7$$

If the availability of the drug is questionable, an estimate of Cl/F is obtained.

The clearance and half-life may also be estimated under conditions of unequal dose and unequal dosing interval. Consider the aminophylline dosing history (Table 18-3) of a 70-kg, 26-year-old male asthmatic patient who concurrently has pneumonia.

The availability of theophylline is 1.0, but aminophylline is only 85 percent theophylline. The volume of distribution of theophylline is relatively constant at 0.5 liter/kg. The amount of drug in the body is that remaining from the previous doses, thus,

$$C(\text{observed}) = \frac{F}{V}(D_1 \cdot e^{-kt_1} + D_2 \cdot e^{-kt_2}$$

$$+ D_3 \cdot e^{-kt_3} + D_4 \cdot e^{-kt_4}) \qquad 8$$

where t_1 to t_4 are the times since the doses D_1 to D_4 were administered.

In the preceding case, a plasma concentration of 18 mg/liter was measured. There is a value of k consistent with this observation. The value of k can be obtained by

iteratively solving the right side of the equation with different values of k. A value of 0.04 for k gives 16.5; a value of 0.03 gives 18.9. Therefore, k must be about 0.034 hours^{-1}, which corresponds to a half-life of 20 hours $(0.7/k)$. The clearance must then be 1.2 liters/hour $(k \cdot V)$.

When two concentrations are obtained during the decline phase within a dosing interval or after discontinuing the drug, the value of the elimination rate constant or half-life can be readily calculated, since

$$k = \frac{\ln(C_1/C_2)}{t} \qquad 9$$

One's confidence in the estimate depends upon the error in the ratio of the two values, including errors in the assay. Generally, if the values differ by a factor of 2 or more, the estimate is reliable. Again, clearance may be estimated from the product $k \cdot V$. When three or more values are available, the estimate of half-life is best obtained from a fit of the data plotted on semilogarithmic graph paper.

Volume of Distribution. An estimate of this parameter may be made from a plasma concentration obtained following a loading dose, provided that the blood sample is taken just after absorption and distribution are complete and when little drug has been eliminated.

$$V = \frac{F \cdot D_L}{C} \qquad 10$$

Obviously, for some drugs the two conditions may be mutually exclusive. Also if availability is not 1, only the ratio V/F is estimated.

When the concentrations just before and just after a dose are measured on multiple dose therapy, the volume of distribution may be estimated from the relationship

$$V = \frac{F \cdot \text{Dose}}{(C_2 - C_1)} \qquad 11$$

The precision of this estimate depends upon the confidence one has in the difference between the two values as well as upon considerations of the values of F and the postdosing concentration, C_2, as stated previously.

Compliance and Availability. Compliance is frequently a question in evaluating a plasma level. Assuming that clearance and availability have not changed, compliance can often be evaluated by carefully controlling drug administration.

Availability can be evaluated by changing the dosage form or by administering the drug intravenously and appropriately monitoring the plasma concentration (see Chap. 13). In this case, clearance is assumed to be constant; furthermore, compliance must be maintained.

Assessment Using Target Concentration Strategy

A dosage regimen is initially chosen which, on the average, is expected to produce the target concentration, usually a steady-state average value in the middle of the therapeutic concentration window. A plasma concentration is then measured to assess how successful the regimen has been. If successful and if the therapeutic response is adequate, the regimen is maintained until treatment is complete or a problem arises. If unsuccessful, the cause of the failure must be identified and, where possible, remedied. The approach adopted to solve a problem systematically can be appreciated by considering two case histories with theophylline.

CASE 1. A severely asthmatic, 65-kg male patient was admitted to the hospital with an exacerbation of his condition. For several weeks the patient had been on a regimen of 3 100-mg aminophylline tablets (255 mg theophylline) every 6 hours. A plasma sample, taken at the time of admission and just before the next dose, had a theophylline concentration of 4 mg/liter.

The lack of response in the patient and the low plasma concentration are consistent in that the usual therapeutic window is 10 to 20 mg/liter. Using the average pharmacokinetic parameter values ($F = 1.0$, $V = 0.5$ liter/kg, $Cl = 0.045$ liter/hour/kg), the calculated value for the trough concentration at steady state (Eq. 3) is 11 mg/liter. Since absorption is not a source of problem with this drug, noncompliance or an unusually high clearance is the suspected explanation.

To rapidly restore the drug effect and to clarify the situation, it was decided to give 500 mg of aminophylline intravenously to bring the concentration into the therapeutic region. Plasma samples were obtained just before and 3 and 6 hours after the dose. The usual 300 mg oral dose of aminophylline was given 6 hours before the test dose.

Figure 18-5 is a semilogarithmic plot of the resulting data. Clearance, readily estimated in this situation, as shown from the area under the corresponding plasma concentration-time curve, is 3.6 liters/hour, a value within the usual range. The half-life, 5.5 hours, is also within the usual range. Since availability is usually close to 1, noncompliance therefore appears to have been the primary problem. The solution is patient education, although a slight increase in dose may be needed. For clearance to have been the explanation, the half-life would have to have been about 3 hours or less.

CASE 2. Mrs. D. H., a 64-year-old, 64-kg patient in an intensive care unit, had been receiving, for several days, 300 mg of aminophylline every 6 hours for her asthmatic problem. She had a number of concurrent diseases including congestive heart failure. A theophylline concentration of 32 mg/liter was measured in a plasma

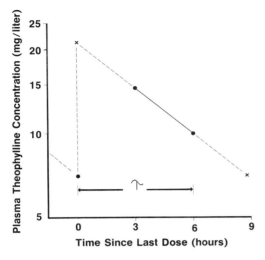

Figure 18-5. *Assessment of theophylline pharmacokinetic parameters in an apparently unresponsive patient, case 1. The points (●) are the concentrations of theophylline following an intravenous test bolus dose; the patient had previously been taking the drug orally. The concentrations (X), just after the bolus and at the time when the value has returned to the predose concentration, are estimated by extrapolating the observed decline in concentration on a semilogarithmic plot. Clearance may be estimated either by dividing the intravenous dose by the area under the curve be-between the X values, or from $Cl = 0.7 \times V/t_{\frac{1}{2}}$, where V = dose divided by the initial increase in concentration.*

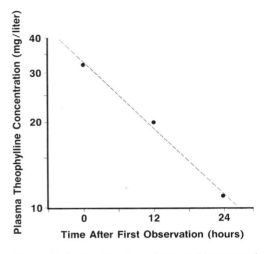

Figure 18-6. *Identification of the problem associated with theophylline administration in a patient showing toxicity, case 2. The half-life of theophylline (16 hours), observed after discontinuing the usual regimen, is two to three times the usual value. Assuming a usual volume of distribution, the clearance must be unusually low, explaining excessive drug accumulation and the signs of toxicity.*

sample obtained subsequent to a period of nausea and vomiting. The next dose was withheld, and a plasma sample, obtained 12 hours after the last dose, was found to contain 20 mg/liter of theophylline. Based on this observation, the drug was again withheld for another 12 hours at which time the concentration in plasma was 11 mg/liter.

A semilogarithmic plot of all the data (Fig. 18-6) reveals a half-life of about 16 hours. Assuming a normal volume of distribution, 32 liters, the clearance in this pa-

tient is calculated to be 1.4 liters/hour, a low value. A reduced rate of theophylline administration is clearly needed in this patient.

Arguably, in both of the preceding examples, dosage could have been adjusted solely by titrating to the effects observed. A point in favor of concentration measurement is that an assessment could be made of why toxicity and a lack of effect occurred. These measurements also permitted facile and rapid estimation of the patient's dosage requirement which otherwise might have required a considerable degree of readjusting from observing the effects alone. The fineness of the adjustment was also much greater with plasma concentration data.

Study Problems

(Answers to Study Problems can be found in Appendix G.)

1. List and briefly describe the criteria for performing drug concentration monitoring and applying target concentration strategy.

2. (a) Determine an appropriate oral dosage regimen of aminophylline for Mrs. D.H. (refer to case 2 in text) to maintain an average theophylline concentration of 15 mg/liter.
    (b) Following recovery from the acute problems for which Mrs. D.H. was placed in the intensive care unit, her asthma problem recurred while on the new regimen recommended in part (a). A plasma concentration (a minimum steady-state value) of 5 mg/liter was then measured, suggesting that the kinetics of the drug in the patient had changed. Prior to her discharge from the hospital an adjustment in her theophylline therapy is apparently needed. What dosage regimen would you now suggest to maintain an average theophylline concentration of 15 mg/liter?

3. Had a concentration of 6 mg/liter been obtained at 6 P.M. on June 2 for the 70-kg, 26-year-old male asthmatic patient whose dosing history is given in Table 18-3, what values would you estimate for the clearance and the half-life of theophylline?

4. Given the usual parameter values: $F = 0.85$ (theophylline in aminophylline), $V = 0.5$ liters/kg, and $Cl = 0.05$ liters/hour per kg, pharmacokinetically interpret each of the following theophylline concentrations obtained in 3 different patients following the infusion of aminophylline at a constant rate of 0.8 mg/hour/kg in each of the patients. No theophylline was present at the start of the infusions. In your interpretations include both a comparison of observed and predicted plasma concentrations and an estimation of the values of Cl and $t_{1/2}$ in the patient. Assume that the volume of distribution (liters/kg) is the same in all the patients.

Patient	Time of Sampling (hours into infusion)	Plasma Theophylline Theophylline Concentration (mg/liter)
1	3	3.5
2	16	18
3	30	6

Definitions of Symbols*

Aa — Amount of drug at absorption site remaining to be absorbed, mg.

Ab — Amount of drug in body, mg.

Ab_{av} — Average amount of drug in body during a dosing interval at plateau, mg.

$Ab(m)$ — Amount of metabolite in body, mg.

Ab_{min} — The minimum amount of drug in the body required to obtain a predetermined level of response, mg.

$Ab_{N,max}$, $Ab_{N,min}$ — Maximum and minimum amounts of drug in body after the Nth intravenous bolus dose of fixed size and given at a fixed dosing interval, mg.

Ab_{ss} — Amount of drug in body at steady state during constant intravenous infusion, mg.

$Ab_{ss,max}$, $Ab_{ss,min}$ — Maximum and minimum amounts of drug in body during a dosing interval at steady state on administering a fixed dose at a fixed dosing interval, mg.

Ae — Cumulative amount of drug excreted unchanged in the urine, mg.

$Ae_{\tau,ss}$ — Cumulative amount of drug excreted unchanged in the urine during a dosing interval at steady state, mg.

Ae_{∞} — Cumulative amount of drug excreted unchanged in the urine to time infinity after a single dose, mg.

ARE — Amount of drug remaining to be excreted in the urine, mg.

Area — Total area under the plasma drug concentration-time curve, mg-hour/liter.

$Area_b$ — Total area under the blood drug concentration-time curve, mg-hour/liter.

C — Concentration of drug in plasma, mg/liter.

C_a — Concentration of drug in the fluids at the absorption site, mg/liter.

C_A — Concentration of drug in arterial blood, mg/liter.

C_{av} — Average drug concentration in plasma during a dosing interval at plateau on administering a dosage regimen of a fixed dose at equal dosing intervals, mg/liter.

C_b — Concentration of drug in blood, mg/liter.

C_I — Concentration of inhibitor of metabolism, mg/liter.

Cm — Concentration of a metabolite in plasma, mg/liter.

Cm_{ss} — Concentration of a metabolite at steady state during a constant rate intravenous infusion of a drug, mg/liter.

$C_{N,max}$, $C_{N,min}$ — Maximum and minimum concentrations of drug in plasma after the Nth dose on administering a regimen of fixed dose at equal dosing intervals, mg/liter.

C_{max}, C_{min} — Maximum and minimum plasma drug concentrations desired, mg/liter.

C_o — Dose divided by the volume of distribution (apparent), mg/liter.

*Usual units are given.

280

C_{ss}	Concentration of drug in plasma at steady state during a constant rate intravenous infusion, mg/liter.	F_H	Fraction of drug entering the liver that escapes elimination in that organ, no units.
$C_{ss,max}$. $C_{ss,min}$	Maximum and minimum concentrations of drug in plasma at steady state on administering a regimen of fixed dose at equal dosing intervals, mg/liter.	fm	Fraction of drug absorbed that is converted to a metabolite, no units.
		fu	Ratio of unbound to total drug concentrations in plasma, no units.
Cl	Total clearance of drug from plasma, liters/hour.	fu_b	Ratio of unbound concentration in plasma to total drug concentration in blood, no units.
Cl_b	Total clearance of drug from blood, liters/hour.		
Cl_H	Hepatic clearance of drug from plasma, liters/hour.	fu_T	Ratio of unbound to total drug in tissues (outside plasma), no units.
Cl_m	Clearance of drug from plasma to a metabolite, liters/hour.	GFR	Glomerular filtration rate, ml/min.
$Cl(m)$	Total clearance of a metabolite, liters/hour.	k	Elimination rate constant, $hour^{-1}$.
Cl_R	Renal clearance of drug, liters/hour.	K	Association constant for the binding of drug to protein, liter/mole.
Cl_u	Clearance of unbound drug, liters/hour.	ka	Absorption rate constant, $hour^{-1}$.
Cu or (D)	Concentration of drug unbound, mg/liter.	ke	Urinary excretion rate constant, $hour^{-1}$.
D_L	Loading dose, mg.	KF	Kidney function as a fraction of normal kidney function, no units.
D_M	Maintenance dose of a fixed dose regimen, mg.		
$D_{M,max}$	Maximum maintenance dose to remain within C_{max} and C_{min}, mg.	km	Rate constant associated with the formation of a metabolite, $hour^{-1}$.
(DP)	Concentration of bound drug in plasma, mg/liter.	K_I	Inhibition constant, mg/liter.
E	Extraction ratio, no units.	$k(m)$	Rate constant for the elimination of a metabolite, $hour^{-1}$.
E_H	Hepatic extraction ratio, no units.		
E_R	Renal extraction ratio, no units.	Km	Michaelis-Menten constant, mg/liter.
F	Availability of drug, no units.	Kp	Equilibrium distribution ratio of drug between a tissue and blood, no units.
fb	Ratio of bound to total drug concentrations in plasma, no units.	n	A unitless number.
		N	Number of doses, no units.
fe	Fraction of drug absorbed that is excreted unchanged in the urine, no units.	(P)	Concentration of binding sites on protein that are unoccupied by drug, moles/liter.

P_t — Total concentration of sites on protein available for binding drug, moles/liter.

Q — Blood flow, liters/min.

Q_H — Hepatic blood flow (portal vein plus hepatic artery), liters/min.

R_{AC} — Accumulation ratio (index), no units.

R_{inf} — Rate of constant intravenous infusion, mg/hour.

t_D — Duration of effect, hours.

$t_{1/2}$ — Elimination half-life, hours.

T_M — Maximum rate of drug transport (secretion) into renal tubule, mg/hour.

V — Volume of distribution (apparent) based on drug concentration in plasma, liters.

V_b — Volume of distribution (apparent) based on drug concentration in blood, liters.

V_B — Blood volume, liters.

Vm — Maximum rate of metabolism by an enzymatically mediated reaction, mg/hour.

V_P — Plasma volume, liters.

V_T — Physiologic volume outside plasma into which a drug distributes (extracellular to total body water minus plasma volume), liters.

V_u — Volume of distribution (apparent) based on unbound drug concentration in plasma, liters.

ϵ — Ratio of dosing interval to half-life, no units.

τ — Dosing interval, hours.

τ_{max} — Maximum dosing interval to remain within C_{max} and C_{min}, hours.

Selected Reading

General

GIBALDI, M.: Biopharmaceutics and Clinical Pharmacokinetics. Lea & Febiger, Philadelphia, 1977.

GILLETTE, J. R., and MITCHELL, J. R. (eds): Concepts in Biochemical Pharmacology. Handbook of Experimental Pharmacology. Springer-Verlag, Berlin, 1975, Vol. XXVIII. Part 3.

GOLDSTEIN, A., ARONOW, L., and KALMAN, S.M.: Principles of Drug Action: The Basis of Pharmacology. 2nd ed. John Wiley & Sons, Inc., New York, 1974.

LA DU, B. N., MANDEL, H. G., and WAY, E. L. (eds): Fundamentals of Drug Metabolism and Drug Disposition. Williams & Wilkins, Baltimore, 1971.

LEVINE, R. R.: Pharmacology—Drug Actions and Reactions. Little, Brown and Co., Boston, 1973.

SWARBRICK, J.: Current Concepts in the Pharmaceutical Sciences: Biopharmaceutics. Lea & Febiger, Philadelphia, 1970.

WAGNER, J. G.: Fundamentals of Clinical Pharmacokinetics. Drug Intelligence Publications, Hamilton, Illinois, 1975.

Concepts

ANTON, A. H., and SOLOMON, H. M. (eds): Symposium. Drug Protein Binding. Ann. N. Y. Acad. Sci., 226: 1–362, 1973.

AZARNOFF, D. L., and HUFFMAN, D. H.: Therapeutic implications of bioavailability. Annu. Rev. Pharmacol. Toxicol., 16: 53–66, 1976.

BENET, L. Z.: Biopharmaceutics as the basis for the design of drug products. In Drug Design. Edited by E. J. Ariens. Academic Press, Inc., New York, Vol. IV. 1973, pp. 24–29.

BLANCHARD, J., SAWCHUK, R., and BRODIE, B. B. (eds): Principles and Perspectives in Drug Bioavailability. S. Karger, New York, 1979.

CONNEY, A. H.: Drug metabolism and therapeutics. N. Engl. J. Med., 280: 653–660, 1969.

GOLDSTEIN, A.: The interaction of drugs and plasma proteins. Pharmacol. Rev., 1: 102–65, 1949.

JUSKO, W. J., and GRETCH, M.: Plasma and tissue protein binding of drugs in pharmacokinetics. Drug Metab. Rev., 5: 43–140, 1976.

NIES, A. S., SHAND, D. G., and WILKINSON, G. R.: Altered hepatic blood flow and drug disposition. Clin. Pharmacokinet., 1: 135–155, 1976.

NIMMO, W. S.: Drugs, disease and altered gastric emptying. Clin. Pharmacokinet., 1: 189–203, 1976.

OLDENDORF, W. H.: Blood-brain barrier permeability to drugs. Annu. Rev. Pharmacol., 14: 239–48, 1974.

TESTA, B., and JENNER, P. (eds): Drug Metabolism: Chemical and Biochemical Aspects. Marcel Dekker, New York, 1978.

ROWLAND, M.: Effect of some physiologic factors on bio-availability of oral dosage forms. In Current Concepts in the Pharmaceutical Sciences: Dosage Form Design and Bioavailability. Edited by J. Swarbrick. Lea & Febiger, Philadelphia, 1973, pp. 181–222.

ROWLAND, M., BENET, L. Z., and GRAHAM, G. G.: Clearance concepts in pharmacokinetics. J. Pharmacokinet. Biopharm., 1: 123–136, 1973.

STOWE, C. M., and PLAA, G. L.: Extrarenal excretion of drugs and chemicals. Annu. Rev. Pharmacol., 8: 337–356, 1968.

VESSELL, E. S. (ed): Symposium. Drug Metabolism in Man. Ann. N. Y. Acad. Sci., 1971, Vol. 179.

WEINER, I. M.: Transport of weak acids and bases. *In* Handbook of Physiology. Section 8. Renal Physiology. Edited by J. Urloff and R. W. Berliner. American Physiological Society, The Williams and Wilkins Company, Baltimore, 1973, pp. 521–554.

WILKINSON, G. R.: Pharmacokinetics of drug disposition: Hemodynamic considerations. Annu. Rev. Pharmacol., *15*: 11–27, 1975.

WILKINSON, G. R., and SHAND, D. G.: A physiological approach to hepatic drug clearance. Clin. Pharmacol. Ther., *18*: 377–390, 1975.

WILLIAMS, R. T.: Detoxication Mechanisms: The Mechanisms and Detoxication of Drugs, Toxic Substances and Other Organic Compounds. 2nd ed. John Wiley & Sons, New York, 1959.

Kinetics

ARIENS, E. J.: Modulation of pharmacokinetics by molecular manipulation. *In* Drug Design. Edited by E. J. Ariens, Academic Press, New York, 1971, Vol. 2.

EGER, E. I. (ed): Anesthetic Uptake and Action. Williams and Wilkins, Baltimore, 1974.

GIBALDI, M., and PERRIER, D.: Pharmacokinetics, Marcel Dekker, New York, 1975.

RIGGS, D. S.: The Mathematical Approach to Physiological Problems. Williams and Wilkins, Baltimore, 1963.

PAGLIARO, L. A., and BENET, L. Z.: Critical compilation of terminal half-lives, percent excreted unchanged, and changes of half-life in renal and hepatic dysfunction for studies in humans with references. J. Pharmacokin. Biopharm., *3*: 333–384, 1975.

TEORELL, T., DEDRICK, R. L., AND CONDLIFFE, P. G. (eds): Pharmacology and Pharmacokinetics. Plenum Press, New York, 1974.

WAGNER, J. G.: Biopharmaceutics and Relevant Pharmacokinetics, Drug Intelligence Publications, Hamilton, Illinois, 1971.

Therapeutic Regimens

ARIENS, E. J. (ed): Molecular Pharmacology: The Mode of Action of Biologically Active Compounds. Academic Press, Inc., New York, 1964, Vol. I.

BALLARD, B. E., and NELSON, E.: Prolonged action pharmaceuticals. *In* Remington's Pharmaceutical Sciences. 15th ed. Edited by J. E. Hoover. Mack Publishing Co., Easton, Pa., 1975., pp. 1618–1643.

DAVIES, D. S., and PRICHARD, B. N. C. (eds): Biological Effects of Drugs in Relation to their Plasma Concentrations. Macmillan Publishing Co., London, 1973.

GOODMAN, L. S., and GILMAN, A.: The Pharmacological Basis of Therapeutics. 6th ed. Macmillan Publishing Co., Inc., New York, 1980.

KRÜGER-THIEMER, E.: Formal theory of drug dosage regimens. Part I. J. Theor. Biol., *13:* 212–235, 1966.

KRÜGER-THIEMER, E.: Formal theory of drug dosage regimens. II. The exact plateau effect. J. Theor. Biol., *23*: 169–190, 1969.

LEVY, G., and GIBALDI, M.: Pharmacokinetics of drug action. Annu. Rev. Pharmacol., *12*: 85–98, 1972.

ROBINSON, J. R. (ed): Sustained and Controlled Release Drug Delivery Systems. Marcel Dekker, New York, 1978.

ROWLAND, M.: Drug administration and regimens. *In* Clinical Pharmacology. 2nd ed. Edited by K. L. Melmon and H. F. Morelli. Macmillan Publishing Co., Inc., New York, 1978, Chap. 2.

Individualization

General

ALVAN, G.: Individual differences in the disposition of drugs metabolized in the body. Clin. Pharmacokinet., *3*: 155–175, 1978.

LEVY, G. (ed): Clinical pharmacokinetics, A symposium. American Pharmaceutical Assoc., Washington, D.C., 1974.

REIDENBERG, M. M.: Individualization of drug therapy. A symposium. Med. Clin. North Am., *58*: 905–1159, 1974.

SMITH, S. E., and RAWLINS, M. D.: Variability in Human Drug Response. Butterworths, London, 1973.

Genetics

KALOW, W.: Pharmacogenetics: Heredity and the Response to Drugs. W. B. Saunders, Philadelphia, 1962.

LA DU, B. N., and KALOW, W.: Symposium on Pharmacogenetics. Ann. N. Y. Acad. Sci., *151*: 1–691, 1968.

Age

CROOKS, J., O'MALLEY, K., and STEVENSON, I. H.: Pharmacokinetics in the elderly. Clin. Pharmacokinet., *1*: 280–296, 1976.

JUSKO, W. J.: Pharmacokinetic principles in pediatric pharmacology. Pediatr. Clin. North Am. *19*: 81, 1972.

KITANI, K. (ed): Liver and Ageing—1978. Elsevier, Northern Holland, 1978.

MORSELLI, P. L.: Clinical pharmacokinetics in neonates. Clin. Pharmacokinet., *1*: 81–98, 1976.

MORSELLI, P. L. (ed): Drug Disposition during Development. Spectrum Publications, New York, 1977.

RANE, A., and WILSON, J. T.: Clinical Pharmacokinetics in infants and children. Clin. Pharmacokinet., *1*: 2–24, 1976.

SHIRKEY, H. C.: Dosage (posology). *In* Pediatric Therapy. Edited by H. C. Shirkey. The C. V. Mosby Co., St. Louis, 1972, pp. 32–46.

TRIGGS, E. J., and NATION, R. L.: Pharmacokinetics in the aged: A review. J. Pharmacokin. Biopharm., *3*: 387–418, 1975.

Disease

ANDERSON, R. J., GAMBERTOGLIO, J. G., and SHRIER, R. W.: Clinical Use of Drugs in Renal Failure. Charles C Thomas, Springfield, Illinois, 1975.

BENET, L. Z. (ed): The Effect of Disease States on Drug Pharmacokinetics. American Pharmaceutical Association, Washington, D. C., 1976.

BLASCHKE, T. F.: Protein binding and kinetics of drugs in liver diseases. Clin. Pharmacokinet., *2*: 32–44, 1977.

DETTLI, L.: Drug dosage in renal disease. Clin. Pharmacokinet., *1*: 126–134, 1976.

DU SOUICH, P., MCLEAN, A. J., LALKA, D., ERILL, S., and GIBALDI, M.: Pulmonary disease and drug kinetics. Clin. Pharmacokinet., *3*: 257–266, 1978.

PARSONS, R. L.: Drug absorption in gastrointestinal disease with particular reference to malabsorption syndromes. Clin. Pharmacokinet., *2*: 45–60, 1977.

REIDENBERG, M. M.: The binding of drugs to plasma proteins from patients with poor renal function. Clin. Pharmacokinet., *1*: 121–125, 1976.

THOMSON, P. D., MELMON, K. L., RICHARDSON, J. A., COHEN, K., STEINBRUNN, W., CUDIHEE, R., and ROWLAND, M.: Lidocaine pharmacokinetics in advanced heart failure, liver disease, and renal failure in humans. Ann. Intern. Med., *78*: 499–507, 1973.

TILLEMENT, J. P., L'HOSTE, F., and GIUDICELLI, J. F.: Diseases and drug protein binding. Clin. Pharmacokinet. *3*: 144–154, 1978.

WELLING, P. G., CRAIG, W. A., and KUNIN, C. M.: Prediction of drug dosage in patients with renal failure using data derived from normal subjects. Clin. Pharmacol. Ther., *18*: 45–52, 1975.

Drug Interactions

AMERICAN PHARMACEUTICAL ASSOCIATION. Evaluation of Drug Interactions. 2nd ed. The Association, Washington, D. C., 1977.

CLUFF, L. E., and PETRIE, J. C. (eds): Clinical Effects of Interaction Between Drugs. American Elsevier Publishing Co., Inc., New York, 1974.

COHEN, S. N., and ARMSTRONG, M. F.: Drug Interactions. A Handbook for Clinical Use. Williams and Wilkins, Baltimore, 1974.

KRISTENSEN, M. B.: Drug interactions and clinical pharmacokinetics. Clin. Pharmacokinet., *1*: 351–372, 1976.

MORSELLI, P., GARATTINI, S., and COHEN, S. N. (eds): Drug Interactions, Raven Press, New York, 1974.

ROWLAND, M., and MATIN, S. B.: Kinetics of drug-drug interactions. J. Pharmacokinet. Biopharm., *1*: 553–567, 1973.

Monitoring

AZARNOFF, D. L.: Implications of blood level assays of therapeutic agents. Proceedings of the 2nd Deer Lodge Conference on Clinical Pharmacology. Clin. Pharmacol. Ther., *16*: 129–288, 1974.

KOCH-WESER, J.: The serum level approach to individualization of drug dosage. Eur. J. Clin. Pharmacol., *9*: 1–8, 1975.

SADÉE, W., and BEELEN, G. C. M.: Drug Level Monitoring. Wiley-Interscience, New York, 1980.

SHEINER, L., and TOZER, T. N.: Clinical pharmacokinetics: The use of plasma concentration of drugs. *In* Clinical Pharmacology. Edited by K. L. Melmon and H. F. Morelli. 2nd ed. Macmillan Publishing Co., Inc., New York, 1978.

appendices

Appendix A. Blood to Plasma Concentration Ratio

The interrelationships among extraction ratio, blood flow, and blood clearance of drugs require the measurement of drug concentration in whole blood. Because plasma is the usual site of measurement, knowledge of how the blood concentration and plasma concentration are related can be useful.

At equilibrium the ratio of blood to plasma concentrations is dependent on plasma protein binding, partitioning into the blood cells and the volume of the blood cells. This dependence is, perhaps, most readily appreciated from mass balance considerations as follows:

$$C_b \cdot V_B = C \cdot V_P + C_{bc} \cdot V_{bc}$$

| Amount in blood | Amount in plasma | Amount in blood cells | 1 |

where C_b = blood concentration of drug

V_B = blood volume

C = plasma concentration of drug

V_P = plasma volume

C_{bc} = blood cell concentration of drug

V_{bc} = volume of blood cells

The ratio of the concentration in the blood cell to that unbound in plasma, Cu, is a measure of the affinity of the blood cell for the drug. Using γ for this ratio and since $Cu = fu \cdot C$,

$$C_{bc} = \gamma \cdot Cu = \gamma \cdot fu \cdot C \qquad 2$$

The volume of blood cells is a function of the hematocrit, H, and the blood volume, that is,

$$V_{bc} = H \cdot V_B \qquad 3$$

The plasma volume is related to the hematocrit by

$$V_P = (1 - H)V_B \qquad 4$$

Substituting Equations 2 to 4 in Equation 1

$$C_b \cdot V_B = (1 - H) \cdot V_B \cdot C + fu \cdot \gamma \cdot H \cdot V_B \cdot C \qquad 5$$

Dividing by $V_B \cdot C$,

$$\frac{C_b}{C} = 1 + H[fu \cdot \gamma - 1] \qquad 6$$

This relationship clearly shows how the ratio of concentrations, blood/plasma, varies with the hematocrit, the protein binding, and the affinity of the drug for the blood cells. The ratio can be calculated if these parameters are known. If the hematocrit and the affinity are constant, a plot of the ratio against fu gives a straight line with an intercept of $1 - H$ and with a slope of $H \cdot \gamma$. This correlation is useful in situations in which the plasma protein binding is variable, such as for certain drugs in uremia, in hypo- and hyperalbuminemic states, and in displacement interactions. In situations in which the plot is not linear, the affinity of the blood cells or the hematocrit is also changing.

If Equation 6 is rearranged to solve for γ, a useful means of determining the affinity of the blood cells for the drug is obtained, namely,

$$\gamma = \frac{H - 1 + (C_b/C)}{fu \cdot H} \qquad 7$$

Determination of γ requires measurement of the hematocrit, the concentration ratio, and the fraction of drug in plasma unbound to plasma proteins.

Appendix B. Assessment of Area

Several methods exist for measuring the area under a concentration-time curve. One method, to be discussed here, is the simple numerical estimation of area by the *trapezoidal rule*. The advantage of this method is that it only requires a simple extension of a table of experimental data. Other methods include the use of a planimeter, comparing the weight of a paper corresponding to the area under the experimental curve to the weight of a paper of known area, and the use of digital computers.

General Case: Consider the blood concentration data, first two columns of Table B-1, obtained following the oral administration

of 50 mg of a drug. What is the total area under the curve?

Figure B-1 is a plot of the concentration against time after drug administration. If a perpendicular line is drawn from the concentration at 1 hour (7 mg/liter) down to the time-axis, then the area bounded between zero time and 1 hour is a trapezoid whose area is given by the product of the average concentration and the time interval. The average concentration is obtained by adding the concentration at the beginning and end of the time interval and dividing by 2. Since, in the first interval, the respective concentrations are 0 and 7 mg/liter and the time interval is 1 hour, it follows that:

$$\underset{\substack{\text{Area of trapezoid} \\ \text{within the} \\ \text{first time interval}}}{\text{Area}_1} = \underset{\substack{\text{Average concentration} \\ \text{over the first interval}}}{\frac{0 + 7}{2} \text{ mg/liter}} \times \underset{\substack{\text{First time} \\ \text{interval}}}{1 \text{ hour}}$$

Table B-1. Calculation of the Total Area Using the Trapezoidal Rule

Time (hours)	Blood Concentration (mg/liter)	Time Interval (hours)	Average Concentration (mg/liter)	Area (mg × hours/liter)
0	0			
1	7	1	3.5	3.5
2	10	1	8.5	8.5
3	5	1	7.5	7.5
4	2.5	1	3.75	3.75
5	1.25	1	1.88	1.88
6	0.6	1	0.93	0.93
7	0.2	1	0.4	0.4
8	0	1	0.1	0.1
			Total Area =	26.60

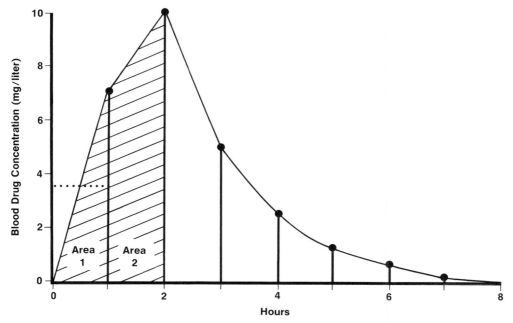

Figure B-1. *Plot of concentration-time data of Table B-1. The dotted line is the average concentration in the first interval.*

or,

$$\text{Area}_1 = 3.5 \text{ mg} \times \text{hours/liter}$$

In this example, the concentration at zero time is zero. Had the drug been given as an intravenous bolus, the concentration at zero time might have been the extrapolated value, C_0 (see page 82).

The area under each time interval can be obtained in an analogous manner to that outlined above. The total area under the concentration-time curve over all times is then simply given by

Total area = Sum of the individual areas

Usually, *total* area means the area under the curve from zero time to infinity. In practice, infinite time is taken as the time beyond which the area is insignificant.

The calculations used to obtain the total area under the curve, displayed in Figure B-1, are shown in Table B-1. In this example the total area is 26.6 mg × hours/liter.

Special Case—An Intravenous Bolus: When a drug is given as an intravenous bolus and the decline is exponential, the total area under the curve is calculated most rapidly by dividing the extrapolated zero time concentration (C_0) by the elimination rate constant, k. For example, if C_0 is 100 mg/liter and k is 0.1 hour^{-1}, then the total area is 1000 mg × hours/liter.

Proof: The total area under the curve is given by

$$\text{Total area} = \int_0^\infty C \cdot dt$$

But $C = C_0 \cdot e^{-kt}$, and since C_0 is a constant it follows that

$$\text{Total area} = C_0 \int_0^\infty e^{-kt} \cdot dt$$

which upon integrating between time zero and infinity yields

$$\text{Total area} = \frac{C_0}{-k}[e^{-kt}]_0^\infty = \frac{C_0}{-k}[0 - 1] = \frac{C_0}{k}$$

Study Problems

1. The following data (Table B-2) were obtained following the ingestion of 50 mg of a drug:

Table B-2.

Time (hours)	0	0.5	1	1.5	2	3	4	6	8	12
Plasma concentration (mg/liter)	0	0.38	0.6	0.73	0.85	0.95	0.94	0.87	0.66	0.37

Estimate the total area under the concentration-time curve. It should be noted that the last sample was taken before the concentration had fallen off to an insignificant value. (Hint: To estimate the area beyond the last observation, imagine that this last measurement was the zero-time concentration following an intravenous bolus. Assume that the disposition kinetics of the drug does not change beyond the last observation.)

2. The set of data displayed in Figure B-1 is unusual in that the time between collection of blood samples is constant: in this case, 1 hour. Prove in this special case that

$$\text{Total area} = \frac{\text{Time}}{\text{interval}} \times \left[\left(\frac{\text{First + last concentration}}{2} \right) + \left(\begin{array}{c} \text{Sum of all other} \\ \text{concentrations} \end{array} \right) \right]$$

Use the data in Table B-1 to confirm that this simple method works satisfactorily.

Answers to Study Problems

1. *10.93 mg × hours/liter.* Using the trapezoidal rule, the area up to 12 hours is 8.21 mg × hours/liter. The elimination rate constant, obtained from a semilogarithmic plot of the concentration-time data, is 0.136 hour^{-1}. Assuming that the last concentration (0.37 mg/liter) is the zero-time concentration following an intravenous bolus dose, the area beyond this last observation (C_0/k) is 2.72 mg × hours/liter.

2. Consider a set of n concentration-time values. Let C_o, C_1, C_{n-1}, C_n be the concentrations at zero time, the first time, the $(n-1)$th time, and the nth time, respectively. Let Δt be the constant interval of time. Using the trapezoidal rule, the total area under the curve is given by

$$\text{Total area} = \text{area}_1 + \text{area}_2 + \cdots \cdots \text{area}_{n-1} + \text{area}_n$$

or,

Total area

$$= \Delta t \left(\frac{C_o + C_1}{2} \right) + \Delta t \left(\frac{C_1 + C_2}{2} \right) \cdots \cdots + \Delta t \left(\frac{C_{n-2} + C_{n-1}}{2} \right) + \Delta t \left(\frac{C_{n-1} + C_n}{2} \right)$$

which upon expansion and collecting terms reduces to

$$\text{Total area} = \Delta t \left(\frac{C_0}{2} + C1 + C_2 + \cdots \cdot C_{n+1} + \frac{C_n}{2} \right)$$

or,

$$\text{Total area} = \Delta t \left[\frac{(C_0 + C_n)}{2} + (C_1 + C_2 + \cdots \cdot C_{n+1}) \right]$$

Appendix C. Estimation of the Elimination Half-Life from Cumulative Urine Data

Consider the urine data in Table C-1 obtained following a 50-mg intravenous bolus dose of a drug. These are the same data as presented in Table 7-2. The cumulative amount excreted up to any time t, Ae_t, is obtained by summing the amount excreted unchanged in each time interval up to that time. For example, by 8 hours, 34.0 mg have been excreted. Initially, large amounts are excreted, but as the amount of drug in the body falls, so does the excretion rate of drug, and by 24 hours, a limiting amount (39.1 mg) has been excreted (Fig. C-1). Small amounts continue to be excreted beyond 24 hours, since, theoretically, the amount of drug in the body approaches, but never falls to, zero. However, these additional amounts do not substantially alter the 24-hour value. Accordingly, 39.1 mg can be taken to be a reasonable estimate of the total amount of drug to be excreted unchanged (Ae_∞). Half this amount (approximately 20 mg) is excreted by 2.6 hours (Fig. C-1). Interestingly, this is the value for the half-life of this drug, estimated from plasma concentration and urinary excretion rate data (pp. 88–89). As the following analysis shows, this is more than a mere coincidence.

The rate of excretion at any time is given by:

$$\frac{dAe}{dt} = ke \cdot Ab \qquad 1$$

The amount excreted up to time t is obtained by integrating the rate equation:

$$Ae_t = ke \int_0^t Ab \cdot dt \qquad 2$$

Since the drug was given as an intravenous bolus, $Ab = \text{Dose} \cdot e^{-kt}$, so that

$$Ae_t = ke \int_0^t \text{Dose} \cdot e^{-kt} \cdot dt \qquad 3$$

or

Table C-1. Urine Data Obtained Following an Intravenous Bolus Dose of Drug

	Observation			Treatment of Data		
Sample	Time of Collection (hours)	Volume of Urine (ml)	Concentration of Unchanged Drug in Urine (μg/ml)	Amount Excreted in Time Interval (mg)	Cumulative Amount Excreted (mg)	Amount Remaining to Be Excreted (mg)
0	0	—	—	—	0	39.1
1	0–2	120	133	16.0	16.0	23.1
2	2–4	180	50	9.0	25.0	14.1
3	4–6	89	63	5.6	30.6	8.5
4	6–8	340	10	3.4	34.0	5.1
5	8–12	178	18	3.2	37.2	1.9
6	12–24	950	2	1.0	39.1	—

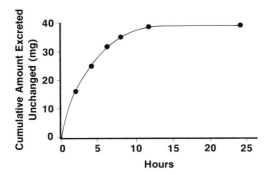

Figure C-1. *The amount of drug excreted unchanged in the urine accumulates asymptotically toward a limiting value, Ae_∞, following an intravenous bolus dose. Half that limiting amount is excreted in one half-life.*

$$Ae_t = ke \cdot \text{Dose} \left| \frac{e^{-kt}}{-k} \right|_o^t \qquad 4$$

Remembering that $e^{-o} = 1$, the preceding equation reduces to

$$Ae_t = \frac{ke \cdot \text{Dose}}{k} [1 - e^{-kt}] \qquad 5$$

but since $e^{-\infty} = 0$, the amount excreted by infinite time (Ae_∞) must be given by

$$Ae_\infty = \frac{ke \cdot \text{Dose}}{k} \qquad 6$$

which when substituted into the preceding equation yields

$$Ae_t = Ae_\infty (1 - e^{-kt}) \qquad 7$$

This last equation is analogous to the plasma concentration-time profile seen during the constant intravenous infusion of a drug (cf. p. 98). At one elimination half-life, e^{-kt} ($e^{-0.70}$) is 0.5, so that

$$Ae_{t_{1/2}} = Ae_\infty/2 \qquad 8$$

Hence, a simple way of estimating the elimination half-life is to find the time required to excrete half the total amount to be excreted. In practice this is most often obtained by interpolating between points on the cumulative excretion plot and consequently can only be regarded as a rough

estimate of the half-life. A graphic solution of the half-life and ke, utilizing all the data, is obtained by rearranging Equation 7

$$Ae_\infty - Ae_t = Ae_\infty \cdot e^{-kt} \qquad 9$$

and taking logarithms

$$\log (Ae_\infty - Ae_t) = \log Ae_\infty - \frac{k}{2.3} t$$

Thus, a plot of $Ae_\infty - Ae_t$ against time on semilogarithmic paper should give a straight line of slope $-k/2.3$.

As the difference, $Ae_\infty - Ae_t$, is the amount remaining to be excreted (ARE), the resulting plot is sometimes called the ARE plot. In practice, the value of ARE at each time is obtained by subtracting the cumulative amount excreted up to that time from the total amount excreted. These values are presented in the last column of Table C-1 and the corresponding semilogarithmic plot of ARE versus time is shown in Figure C-2. The elimination half-life, taken as the time for the ARE to fall by one-half, is 2.8 hours. Hence, $k = 0.25$ hours^{-1}, and since $fe = 0.78$ (39.1 mg/50 mg), the excretion rate constant, ke is 0.20 hours^{-1} ($fe \cdot k$).

Several points should be noted. First, at zero time the value for ARE is Ae_∞. Second, the value of ARE is plotted against the actual time of urine collection, e.g., the time at which 5.1 mg remains to be excreted is 8 hours (Table C-1). In this last respect, the ARE plot has a distinct advantage over the excretion rate plot, in which the excretion rate is plotted against the midpoint of the urine collection interval. Recall that the use of the midpoint time was necessary because the excretion rate is an average value over the period of collection.

Although the ARE plot tends to smooth out the data, it is not used as frequently as the excretion rate plot for four reasons: (1) It requires an accurate estimate of Ae_∞, since an underestimation of Ae_∞ tends to underestimate grossly the true ARE values as Ae_t approaches Ae_∞. This means that

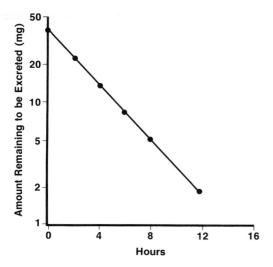

Figure C-2. *The amount remaining to be excreted (ARE), following an intravenous bolus dose of drug, declines exponentially with time. In one half-life, the ARE falls by one-half.*

there has to be complete urine collection for at least four half-lives, which in clinical practice is often difficult to ensure. The rate method does not require urine to be collected until no more drug is excreted. (2) Ae_t values are usually obtained by summing the amount excreted in each collection period. Hence, assay errors are accumulated, while failure to obtain a complete urine collection produces a systematic error in all subsequent estimates of Ae_t. The excretion rate analysis does not contain these sources of error. (3) Smoothing out data can obscure important information. Urinary pH and urine volume fluctuate throughout the day. If the renal clearance of a drug is sensitive to these factors, it is readily apparent in an excretion rate plot but tends to be lost in the ARE plot. (4) When the drug is administered extravascularly, e.g., orally, delays in excretion caused by absorption produces distortions of the ARE plot, frequently making the analysis difficult. In contrast, the excretion rate plot can be readily analyzed.

Study Problem (See part (e) of Unifying Problem, Chapter 7.)

Appendix D. Estimation of the Absorption Half-Life from Plasma Concentration Data

Consider the plasma data in Table D-1, obtained following a 100-mg oral dose of a drug. Figure D-1 is a semilogarithmic plot of the same data. The half-life estimated from the linear portion of the decline phase is 5 hours. Giving the drug intravenously confirmed that this is the elimination half-life of the drug. Hence, disposition rate limits drug elimination.

A graphic procedure to test whether or not absorption is a first-order process, and if so to determine the absorption half-life, is known as the *method of residuals*. The procedure is simple to follow: (1) Back extrapolate the log linear portion of the decline phase. Let $\overleftarrow{C}$ denote the plasma concentration along this extrapolated line. (2) Subtract the observed plasma concentration (C) from the corresponding extrapolated value at each time point. These calculations are shown in Table D-1. (3) Plot the residuals ($\overleftarrow{C} - C$) against time on the same semilogarithmic graph paper.

If, as in this example, the residual plot is a straight line, then absorption is a first-order process. The absorption half-life,

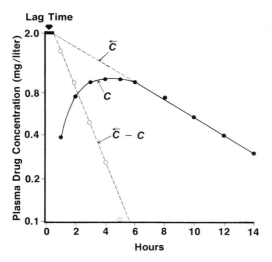

Figure D-1. *By the method of residuals, an estimate can be made of both the absorption half-life and the lag time following oral administration of a drug.*

taken as the time for the residual value to diminish by one-half, is 1.3 hours. The corresponding absorption rate constant, *ka*, is 0.7/1.3 or 0.53 hours^{-1}.

Theoretically, the absorption half-life can also be estimated from urinary excretion data. Assuming that the renal clearance of the drug is constant, the excretion rate parallels the plasma concentration. The

method of residuals should, therefore, be equally applicable to excretion rate data. In practice, however, estimates of absorption half-life from urinary data are usually poor. The half-life of many absorption processes is 30 min or less. Incomplete bladder emptying and the inability to collect samples frequently enough to characterize such absorption processes are two major sources of error. Consequently, analysis of plasma data is the preferred method for estimating absorption kinetics.

Let us examine the underlying basis of the method of residuals. At any time the plasma concentration following extravascular administration is given by:

$$C = \left(\frac{F \cdot \text{Dose} \cdot ka}{V(ka - k)}\right)(e^{-k \cdot t} - e^{-ka \cdot t}) \quad 1$$

where all terms are previously defined in the body of the book. The proof of Equation 1 is involved and beyond the scope of this book. When (as is most frequently the case) absorption is the more rapid process, the value of $ka \cdot t$ is always greater than $k \cdot t$ and hence $e^{-ka \cdot t}$ approaches zero more rapidly than does $e^{-k \cdot t}$. At some point past the peak plasma concentration, $e^{-ka \cdot t}$ is essentially zero, absorption is over, and the extrapolated line is given by:

Table D-1. Plasma Concentration-Time Data Following Oral Administration of a 100-mg Dose of a Drug

	Observation		Treatment of Data	
Time (hours)	Plasma Concentration C, (mg/liter)		Extrapolated Plasma Concentration $\bar{C}$, (mg/liter)	Difference in Concentration $\bar{C} - C$, (mg/liter)
1	0.38		1.90	1.52
2	0.73		1.65	0.92
3	0.91		1.40	0.49
4	0.97		1.23	0.26
5	0.97		1.07	0.10
6	0.92		0.95	0.03
8	0.71		0.71	—
10	0.53		0.53	—
12	0.40		0.40	—
14	0.30		0.30	—

$$\overleftarrow{C} = \left(\frac{F \cdot \text{Dose} \cdot ka}{V(ka - k)}\right) e^{-k \cdot t} \qquad 2$$

Subtracting C from $\overleftarrow{C}$, therefore, yields

$$\overleftarrow{C} - C = \left(\frac{F \cdot \text{Dose} \cdot ka}{V(ka - k)}\right) e^{-ka \cdot t} \qquad 3$$

and taking logarithms:

$$\log(\overleftarrow{C} - C) = \log\left(\frac{F \cdot \text{Dose} \cdot ka}{V(ka - k)}\right) - \frac{k_a \cdot t}{2.3} \qquad 4$$

Hence, if absorption is a first-order process, a semilogarithmic plot of the residual value against time yields a straight line of slope $-ka/2.3$. Occasionally, this residual line is not log linear, implying that absorption is not a simple first-order process. In those instances, other methods are available to calculate how absorption varies with time.

Lag Time: Examination of Equations 2 and 3 suggests a simple graphic method for estimating the lag time, that is, the time between administration and the start of absorption. By definition, absorption begins when the extrapolated and residual curves intersect. This must be so since only at that time, $t = 0$, when $e^{-ka \cdot t} = e^{-kt} = 1$, are the values of the two equations the same, and equal to $(F \cdot \text{Dose} \cdot ka)/[V(ka - k)]$. It is seen from Figure D-1 that in the present example the lag time is approximately 30 min.

Study Problems

1. The following plasma concentrations (Table D-2) were observed in a patient who took 10 ml of an elixir containing 10 mg/ml of a drug.

Table D-2.

Time (hours)	0.25	0.5	1	2	3	4	6	8	10	12
Plasma concentration (mg/liter)	1.6	2.7	3.7	3.5	2.7	2.0	1.02	0.49	0.26	0.12

(a) Prepare a semilogarithmic plot of the data and determine the rate constants for absorption and elimination.
(b) Estimate when absorption began.
(c) Assuming that absorption is complete (100 percent), calculate: (i) the total clearance of the drug; (ii) the volume of distribution of the drug.

2. The absorption kinetics of a drug, known to be acid labile, was studied in two groups: group A, patients with normal gastric function; group B, patients with achlorhydria (a condition in which little or no acid is secreted into the stomach). Each group received the same dose of drug. Analysis of the plasma concentration-time curve yielded the following estimates: Group A, $F = 0.30$, $ka = 1.15$ hour^{-1}; Group B, $F = 0.90$; $ka = 0.39$ hour^{-1}. The investigators proposed that the longer half-life for absorption of the drug in patients with achlorhydria was caused by a slower stomach emptying in this group. Suggest an alternative proposal that is consistent with all the observations.

Answers to Study Problems

1. (a) $ka = 1.4$ hour^{-1}, $k = 0.35$ hour^{-1}.
   (b) Absorption began immediately because there was no lag time.
   (c) (i) Clearance = 5.9 liters/hour:
         Assuming $F = 1$, Clearance = Dose/Area = 100 mg/(17.05 mg × hours/liter)
      (ii) V = Clearance/k = 17 liters
         Note: Assuming that absorption is the rate-limiting step, $V = 5.9/1.4 = 4.2$ liters. This is an unlikely value.

2. Observations can be explained entirely by a competing reaction. With a competing reaction, the observed absorption rate constant $ka = ka' + kc$, and $F = ka'/ka$, where ka' is the true rate constant defining the absorption process and kc is the rate constant of the competing reaction. For both groups $ka' = ka \cdot F = 0.35$ hour^{-1}. Both the lower availability and the apparent faster absorption of the drug in group A are due to more extensive degradation in the acidic gastric contents. Lesson: Be careful in interpreting the value of the absorption rate constant when a competing reaction is likely.

Appendix E. Amount of Drug in the Body on Accumulation to the Plateau

Consider the situation in which a dose of drug is given as an intravenous bolus every dosing interval, τ. Recall that after each dose the fraction remaining at time, t, is e^{-kt}. The fraction of drug remaining at the end of a dosing interval τ therefore, is $e^{-k\tau}$. When time is equal to 2τ the fraction remaining is $e^{-2k\tau}$. Alternatively, these fractions may also be expressed as $(\frac{1}{2})^\epsilon$ and $(\frac{1}{2})^{2\epsilon}$, respectively, where ϵ equals $\tau/t_{1/2}$. The amount of drug in the body following multiple doses is simply the sum of the amounts remaining from each of the previous doses. The amount of drug in the body just after the next dose is shown in Table E-1 for four successive equal doses given every τ.

It is apparent from the table that the maximum amount of drug in the body just after the fourth dose, $Ab_{4,max}$, is the fourth dose plus the sum of the amount remaining from each of three previous doses (sum of terms in row 4). That is, letting $r = (\frac{1}{2})^\epsilon$,

$$Ab_{4,max} = \text{Dose} \,(1 + r + r^2 + r^3) \quad\quad 1$$

Just after the Nth dose the amount in the body is

$$Ab_{N,max} = \text{Dose} \,(1 + r + r^2 + r^3 \cdots + r^{N-2} + r^{N-1}) \quad 2$$

Multiplying by r,

$$Ab_{N,max} \cdot r = \text{Dose} \,(r + r^2 + r^3 + r^4 \cdots + r^{N-1} + r^N) \quad 3$$

Subtracting Equation 3 from Equation 2,

$$Ab_{N,max} \cdot (1 - r) = \text{Dose} \,(1 - r^N) \quad 4$$

Therefore,

$$Ab_{N,max} = \text{Dose} \,\frac{(1 - r^N)}{(1 - r)} \quad 5$$

At any time during a dosing interval, the fraction remaining is $(\frac{1}{2})^n$, where n is the time within a dosing interval expressed in half-life units, that is, $n = t/t_{1/2}$. Hence the amount of drug in the body during a dosing interval, after the Nth dose, $Ab_{N,t}$, is

$$Ab_{N,t} = Ab_{N,max} \cdot (\tfrac{1}{2})^n \quad 6$$

Table E-1. Drug in Body Just After Each of Four Successive Doses

Time	Amount Remaining in Body from Each Dose			
	1st Dose	2nd Dose	3rd Dose	4th Dose
0	Dose			
τ	Dose $\cdot (\frac{1}{2})^{\epsilon}$	Dose		
2τ	Dose $\cdot (\frac{1}{2})^{2\epsilon}$	Dose $\cdot (\frac{1}{2})^{\epsilon}$	Dose	
3τ	Dose $\cdot (\frac{1}{2})^{3\epsilon}$	Dose $\cdot (\frac{1}{2})^{2\epsilon}$	Dose $\cdot (\frac{1}{2})^{\epsilon}$	Dose

At the end of the dosing interval, when $t = \tau$, and $n = \epsilon$, it follows that the minimum amount in the body after the Nth dose, $Ab_{N,min}$, is

$$Ab_{N,min} = Ab_{N,max} \cdot r = \text{Dose} \frac{(1 - r^N) \cdot r}{(1 - r)} \quad 7$$

As the number of doses, N, increases, the value of r^N approaches zero, since r is always a value less than 1. The maximum and minimum amounts of drug in the body during each interval each approach a limit. At the limit the amount lost in each interval equals the amount gained, the dose. For this reason the drug in the body then is said to be at *steady state* or at *plateau*. At steady state, the maximum, $Ab_{ss,max}$, the minimum, $Ab_{ss,min}$, and the amount in the body at anytime during the dosing interval, $Ab_{ss,t}$, are readily obtained by letting $r^N = 0$ in Equations 5, 6, and 7

$$Ab_{ss,max} = \frac{\text{Dose}}{1 - r} \quad 8$$

$$Ab_{ss,min} = \frac{\text{Dose} \cdot r}{1 - r} = Ab_{ss,max} - \text{Dose} \quad 9$$

$$Ab_{ss,t} = \frac{\text{Dose}}{1 - r} \cdot (\tfrac{1}{2})^n \quad 10$$

or expressed in terms of the dose,

$$\frac{Ab_{ss,max}}{\text{Dose}} = \frac{1}{1 - r} = \frac{1}{1 - (\frac{1}{2})^{\epsilon}} \quad 11$$

$$\frac{Ab_{ss,min}}{\text{Dose}} = \frac{r}{1 - r}$$

$$= \frac{(\frac{1}{2})^{\epsilon}}{1 - (\frac{1}{2})^{\epsilon}} = \frac{1}{1 - (\frac{1}{2})^{\epsilon}} - 1 \quad 12$$

$$\frac{Ab_{ss,t}}{\text{Dose}} = \frac{(\frac{1}{2})^n}{1 - r} = \frac{(\frac{1}{2})^n}{1 - (\frac{1}{2})^{\epsilon}} \quad 13$$

Prove to yourself the identity of the two $(\frac{1}{2})^{\epsilon}$ functions in Equation 12.

A similar set of equations involving exponential terms can be developed by substituting $e^{-k\tau}$ for $(\frac{1}{2})^{\epsilon}$, and e^{-kt} for $(\frac{1}{2})^n$ in all the equations above.

Time to Reach Plateau: The time to approach the plateau, whether defined with respect to the maximum or minimum amount of drug in the body, depends solely upon the half-life of the drug. The proof of this statement is readily apparent by dividing the equations that define the respective amounts after the Nth dose, by the equations that define the respective amounts at plateau,

$$\frac{Ab_{N,max}}{Ab_{ss,max}} = \frac{Ab_{N,min}}{Ab_{ss,min}} = 1 - (\tfrac{1}{2})^{N\epsilon} \quad 14$$

Thus, in one half-life, $N\epsilon = 1$, half the plateau value is reached; in two half-lives, $N\epsilon = 2$, three-quarters of the plateau value is reached and so on. A similar conclusion is drawn when relating the average amount during each dosing interval with the average amount at plateau.

Appendix F.   I. Table of Exponential Functions

x	e^{-x}	$1 - e^{-x}$	$\dfrac{1}{1 - e^{-x}}$	x	e^{-x}	$1 - e^{-x}$	$\dfrac{1}{1 - e^{-x}}$
0.000	1.000	0.000	∞	0.22	0.803	0.198	5.064
0.001	0.999	0.001	1000	0.23	0.795	0.206	4.867
0.005	0.995	0.005	200.5	0.24	0.787	0.213	4.687
0.01	0.990	0.010	100.5	0.25	0.779	0.221	4.521
0.015	0.985	0.015	67.17	0.26	0.771	0.229	4.368
0.02	0.980	0.020	50.50	0.27	0.763	0.237	4.226
0.025	0.975	0.025	40.50	0.28	0.756	0.244	4.095
0.03	0.970	0.030	33.84	0.29	0.748	0.252	3.972
0.035	0.966	0.034	29.07	0.30	0.741	0.259	3.858
0.04	0.961	0.039	25.50	0.31	0.733	0.267	3.752
0.045	0.956	0.044	22.73	0.32	0.726	0.274	3.652
0.05	0.951	0.049	20.50	0.33	0.719	0.281	3.558
0.06	0.942	0.058	17.17	0.34	0.712	0.288	3.469
0.07	0.932	0.068	14.79	0.35	0.705	0.295	3.386
0.08	0.923	0.077	13.01	0.36	0.698	0.302	3.308
0.09	0.914	0.086	11.62	0.37	0.691	0.309	3.233
0.10	0.905	0.095	10.51	0.38	0.684	0.316	3.163
0.11	0.896	0.104	9.600	0.39	0.677	0.323	3.097
0.12	0.887	0.113	8.843	0.40	0.670	0.330	3.033
0.13	0.878	0.122	8.203	0.41	0.664	0.336	2.973
0.14	0.869	0.131	7.655	0.42	0.657	0.343	2.916
0.15	0.861	0.139	7.179	0.43	0.651	0.350	2.861
0.16	0.852	0.148	6.763	0.44	0.644	0.356	2.809
0.17	0.844	0.156	6.397	0.45	0.638	0.362	2.760
0.18	0.835	0.165	6.071	0.46	0.631	0.369	2.712
0.19	0.827	0.173	5.779	0.47	0.625	0.375	2.667
0.20	0.819	0.181	5.517	0.48	0.619	0.381	2.623
0.21	0.811	0.189	5.279	0.49	0.613	0.387	2.581

x	e^{-x}	$1 - e^{-x}$	$\dfrac{1}{1 - e^{-x}}$	x	e^{-x}	$1 - e^{-x}$	$\dfrac{1}{1 - e^{-x}}$
0.50	0.607	0.394	2.541	2.10	0.123	0.878	1.140
0.55	0.577	0.423	2.364	2.20	0.111	0.889	1.125
0.60	0.549	0.451	2.216	2.30	0.100	0.900	1.111
0.65	0.522	0.478	2.092	2.40	0.091	0.909	1.100
0.70	0.497	0.503	1.986	2.50	0.082	0.918	1.089
0.75	0.472	0.528	1.895	2.60	0.074	0.926	1.080
0.80	0.449	0.551	1.816	2.70	0.067	0.933	1.072
0.85	0.427	0.573	1.746	2.80	0.061	0.939	1.065
0.90	0.407	0.593	1.685	2.90	0.055	0.945	1.058
0.95	0.387	0.613	1.631	3.00	0.050	0.950	1.052
1.00	0.368	0.632	1.582	3.10	0.045	0.955	1.047
1.05	0.350	0.650	1.538	3.20	0.041	0.959	1.042
1.10	0.333	0.667	1.499	3.30	0.037	0.963	1.038
1.15	0.317	0.683	1.463	3.40	0.033	0.967	1.035
1.20	0.301	0.699	1.431	3.50	0.030	0.970	1.031
1.25	0.287	0.714	1.402	3.60	0.027	0.973	1.028
1.30	0.273	0.728	1.375	3.70	0.025	0.975	1.025
1.35	0.259	0.741	1.350	3.80	0.022	0.978	1.023
1.40	0.247	0.753	1.327	3.90	0.020	0.980	1.021
1.45	0.235	0.765	1.306	4.00	0.018	0.982	1.019
1.50	0.223	0.777	1.287	4.2	0.015	0.985	1.015
1.60	0.202	0.798	1.253	4.4	0.012	0.988	1.012
1.70	0.183	0.817	1.224	4.6	0.010	0.990	1.010
1.80	0.165	0.835	1.198	4.8	0.008	0.992	1.008
1.90	0.150	0.850	1.176	5.0	0.007	0.993	1.007
2.00	0.135	0.865	1.157				

Appendix F.   II. Table of $(\tfrac{1}{2})^n$ Functions

n	$(\tfrac{1}{2})^n$	$1 - (\tfrac{1}{2})^n$	$\dfrac{1}{1 - (\tfrac{1}{2})^n}$	$\dfrac{(\tfrac{1}{2})^n}{1 - (\tfrac{1}{2})^n}$	n	$(\tfrac{1}{2})^n$	$1 - (\tfrac{1}{2})^n$	$\dfrac{1}{1 - (\tfrac{1}{2})^n}$	$\dfrac{(\tfrac{1}{2})^n}{1 - (\tfrac{1}{2})^n}$
0.005	0.997	0.004	289.039	288.039	0.090	.940	.061	16.535	15.535
0.010	.993	.007	144.770	143.770	0.095	.936	.064	15.692	14.692
0.015	.990	.010	96.681	95.681	0.100	.933	.067	14.933	13.933
0.020	.936	.014	72.636	71.636	0.110	.927	.073	13.622	12.622
0.025	.983	.017	58.209	57.209	0.120	.920	.080	12.529	11.529
0.030	.979	.021	48.592	47.592	0.130	.914	.086	11.605	10.605
0.035	.976	.024	41.722	40.722	0.140	.908	.092	10.813	9.813
0.040	.973	.027	36.570	35.570	0.150	.901	.099	10.127	9.127
0.045	.969	.031	32.563	31.563	0.160	.895	.105	9.526	8.526
0.050	.966	.034	29.357	28.357	0.170	.889	.111	8.996	7.996
0.055	.963	.037	26.734	25.734	0.180	.883	.117	8.525	7.525
0.060	.959	.041	24.548	23.548	0.190	.877	.123	8.104	7.104
0.065	.956	.044	22.699	21.699	0.200	.871	.129	7.725	6.725
0.070	.953	.047	21.114	20.114	0.210	.865	.136	7.382	6.382
0.075	.949	.051	19.740	18.740	0.220	.859	.141	7.070	6.070
0.080	.946	.054	18.538	17.538	0.230	.853	.147	6.786	5.786
0.085	.942	.057	17.478	16.478	0.240	.847	.153	6.525	5.525

Appendix F. II. Table of $(\frac{1}{2})^n$ Functions (continued)

n	$(\frac{1}{2})^n$	$1-(\frac{1}{2})^n$	$\dfrac{1}{1-(\frac{1}{2})^n}$	$\dfrac{(\frac{1}{2})^n}{1-(\frac{1}{2})^n}$	n	$(\frac{1}{2})^n$	$1-(\frac{1}{2})^n$	$\dfrac{1}{1-(\frac{1}{2})^n}$	$\dfrac{(\frac{1}{2})^n}{1-(\frac{1}{2})^n}$
0.250	.841	.159	6.285	5.285	0.810	.570	.430	2.328	1.328
0.260	.835	.165	6.064	5.064	0.820	.566	.434	2.307	1.307
0.270	.829	.171	5.859	4.859	0.830	.563	.438	2.286	1.286
0.280	.824	.176	5.669	4.669	0.840	.559	.441	2.266	1.266
0.290	.818	.182	5.492	4.492	0.850	.555	.445	2.246	1.246
0.300	.812	.188	5.326	4.326					
0.310	.807	.193	5.172	4.172	0.860	.551	.449	2.227	1.227
0.320	.801	.199	5.027	4.027	0.870	.547	.453	2.208	1.208
0.330	.796	.205	4.891	3.891	0.880	.543	.457	2.190	1.190
0.340	.790	.210	4.763	3.763	0.890	.540	.460	2.172	1.172
0.350	.785	.215	4.642	3.642	0.900	.536	.464	2.155	1.155
0.360	.779	.221	4.528	3.528	0.910	.532	.468	2.138	1.138
0.370	.774	.226	4.421	3.421	0.920	.529	.472	2.121	1.121
0.380	.768	.232	4.319	3.319	0.930	.525	.475	2.105	1.105
0.390	.763	.237	4.222	3.222	0.940	.521	.479	2.089	1.089
0.400	.758	.242	4.130	3.130	0.950	.518	.482	2.073	1.073
0.410	.753	.247	4.042	3.042	0.960	.514	.486	2.058	1.058
0.420	.747	.253	3.959	2.959	0.970	.511	.490	2.043	1.043
0.430	.742	.258	3.880	2.880	0.980	.507	.493	2.028	1.028
0.440	.737	.263	3.804	2.804	0.990	.504	.497	2.014	1.014
0.450	.732	.268	3.732	2.732	1.000	.500	.500	2.000	1.000
0.460	.727	.273	3.663	2.663	1.050	.483	.517	1.934	0.934
0.470	.722	.278	3.597	2.597	1.100	.467	.534	1.875	0.875
0.480	.717	.283	3.533	2.533	1.150	.451	.549	1.820	0.820
0.490	.712	.288	3.473	2.473	1.200	.435	.565	1.771	0.771
0.500	.707	.293	3.414	2.414	1.250	.420	.580	1.726	0.726
0.510	.702	.298	3.358	2.358	1.300	.406	.594	1.684	0.684
0.520	.697	.303	3.304	2.304	1.350	.392	.608	1.646	0.646
0.530	.693	.307	3.253	2.253	1.400	.379	.621	1.610	0.610
0.540	.688	.312	3.203	2.203	1.450	.366	.634	1.577	0.577
0.550	.683	.317	3.155	2.155	1.500	.354	.646	1.547	0.547
0.560	.678	.322	3.109	2.109	1.550	.342	.659	1.519	0.519
0.570	.674	.326	3.064	2.064	1.600	.330	.670	1.492	0.492
0.580	.669	.331	3.021	2.021	1.650	.319	.681	1.468	0.468
0.590	.664	.336	2.979	1.979	1.700	.308	.692	1.445	0.445
0.600	.660	.340	2.939	1.939	1.750	.297	.703	1.423	0.423
0.610	.655	.345	2.900	1.900	1.800	.287	.713	1.403	0.403
0.620	.651	.349	2.863	1.863	1.850	.277	.723	1.384	0.384
0.630	.646	.354	2.826	1.826	1.900	.268	.732	1.366	0.366
0.640	.642	.358	2.791	1.791	1.950	.259	.741	1.349	0.349
0.650	.637	.363	2.757	1.757	2.000	.250	.750	1.333	0.333
0.660	.633	.367	2.724	1.724	2.100	.233	.767	1.304	0.304
0.670	.629	.371	2.692	1.692	2.200	.218	.782	1.278	0.278
0.680	.624	.376	2.661	1.661	2.300	.203	.797	1.255	0.255
0.690	.620	.380	2.631	1.631	2.400	.190	.811	1.234	0.234
0.700	.616	.384	2.601	1.601	2.500	.177	.823	1.215	0.215
0.710	.611	.389	2.573	1.573	2.600	.165	.835	1.198	0.198
0.720	.607	.393	2.545	1.545	2.700	.154	.846	1.182	0.182
0.730	.603	.397	2.518	1.518	2.800	.144	.856	1.168	0.168
0.740	.599	.401	2.492	1.492	2.900	.134	.866	1.155	0.155
0.750	.595	.405	2.467	1.467	3.000	.125	.875	1.143	0.143
0.760	.591	.410	2.442	1.442	3.100	.117	.883	1.132	0.132
0.770	.586	.414	2.418	1.418	3.200	.109	.891	1.122	0.122
0.780	.582	.418	2.394	1.394	3.300	.102	.899	1.113	0.113
0.790	.578	.422	2.372	1.372	3.400	.095	.905	1.105	0.105
0.800	.574	.426	2.349	1.349	3.500	.088	.912	1.097	0.097
					3.600	.082	.918	1.090	0.090

n	$(\frac{1}{2})^n$	$1 - (\frac{1}{2})^n$	$\dfrac{1}{1 - (\frac{1}{2})^n}$	$\dfrac{(\frac{1}{2})^n}{1 - (\frac{1}{2})^n}$	n	$(\frac{1}{2})^n$	$1 - (\frac{1}{2})^n$	$\dfrac{1}{1 - (\frac{1}{2})^n}$	$\dfrac{(\frac{1}{2})^n}{1 - (\frac{1}{2})^n}$
3.700	.077	.923	1.083	0.083	5.000	.031	.969	1.032	0.032
3.800	.072	.928	1.077	0.077	5.200	.027	.973	1.028	0.028
3.900	.067	.933	1.072	0.072	5.400	.024	.976	1.024	0.024
4.000	.063	.938	1.067	0.067	5.600	.021	.979	1.021	0.021
4.200	.054	.946	1.058	0.058	5.800	.018	.982	1.018	0.018
4.400	.047	.953	1.050	0.050	6.000	.016	.984	1.016	0.016
4.600	.041	.959	1.043	0.043					
4.800	.036	.964	1.037	0.037					

Appendix G. Answers to Problems

Answers to Study Problem (Chap. 2)

Pharmacokinetics—quantitation of the time course of a drug and its metabolites in the body.

Intravascular administration—parenteral injection of a drug directly into the blood, either arterial or venous.

Extravascular administration—administration by any route other than directly into the blood.

Absorption—process by which a drug proceeds from the site of administration to the site of measurement within the body.

Disposition—all the processes that occur subsequent to the absorption of a drug.

Distribution—reversible transfer of a drug to and from the site of measurement.

Metabolism—irreversible conversion to another chemical species.

Excretion—irreversible loss of the chemically unchanged drug.

First-pass effect—a drug must first cross the gastrointestinal membranes and pass through the liver to be absorbed. Removal of drug on this first passage into the general circulation is the *first-pass effect*.

Answers to Study Problems (Chap. 3)

1. (a) B; (b) C, D; (c) A, B, C, D; (d) A, B, C, D; (e) C, D.

2. (a) much faster (solubility of solid has greater effect than pH of medium); (b) at essentially the same rate (dissolution relatively insensitive to pH of solution); (c) in divided doses during the day (solubility problem); (d) A (solubility problem).

Answers to Study Problems (Chap. 4)

1. Lung > Kidneys > Liver > Heart > Skin: Note $k_P = t \cdot (Q/V_T)$

2. (a) 0.025 mg/liter; (b) 600 mg; (c) 99.9925 percent.

3. a, b, c.

4. (a) Salicylic acid might be bound in the plasma (which it is) and bound outside the plasma giving this volume of distribution.
   (b) True. The volume of the liver is 2.3 percent of body weight; therefore, at distribution equilibrium the minimum volume of distribution (consisting only of plasma and liver) $= V_P + 50\ V_T = [3 + (50 \times 1.6)]$ liters $= 83$ liters.
   (c) True. It would take much longer, if the drug primarily distributed into poorly perfused tissues.

5. (a) Fraction bound in tissues $(1 - fu_T) = 0.97$:

$$V(40 \text{ liters}) = V_P(3 \text{ liters}) + \left[\frac{fu(0.03) \cdot V_T\,(39 \text{ liters})}{fu_T}\right]$$

   (b) Digitoxin is more tightly tissue bound than digoxin; digoxin, $1 - fu_T = 0.95$.

Answers to Study Problems (Chap. 5)

1.
   Drug A. Filtered, reabsorbed, and perhaps secreted.
   Drug B. Filtered only or filtered with secretion and reabsorption exactly matched.
   Drug C. Filtered, secreted, and perhaps reabsorbed.

2. (a) *i* (b) *ii* (c) *i* (d) *iii*

3. Glucose must be actively reabsorbed. At concentrations above 200 mg/100 ml plasma the capacity of the reabsorption system is exceeded.

Plasma Glucose (mg/100 ml)	200	301	398	503	605 ·	708	799
Renal Clearance (ml/min)	2.5	22	38	51	66	73	79

4. (a) Probenecid competes with penicillin for a secretory process.
   (b) Yes—if the inhibition is competitive. The maximum rate of secretion of penicillin is the same in the presence or absence of probenecid.
   (c) Penicillin is a relatively polar molecule. The pKa is also at the lower limit of compounds showing pH sensitivity.

5. (a) Alcohol is reabsorbed in the nephron virtually to the same extent as water.
   (b) The excretion rate is calculated from urine flow times urine concentration. Thus, at a given plasma concentration the excretion rate is flow dependent. Because of the variability in urine flow the excretion rate will only roughly correlate with the plasma concentration.

Answers to Study Problems (Chap. 6)

1. (a) Major.

$$\text{Clearance by hepatic glucuronidation} = 110 \times \frac{50 \text{ ml}}{\text{hour}} = 5.5 \text{ liters/hour}$$

$$\text{Total blood clearance} = 0.7 \times \frac{100 \text{ liters}}{9 \text{ hours}} = 7.7 \text{ liters/hour}$$

Therefore, fraction of drug eliminated via glucuronidation $= 5.5/7.7 = 0.71$
    (b) 0.086

$$\text{Hepatic extraction ratio} = \frac{\text{Blood clearance}}{\text{Blood flow}} = \frac{7.7 \text{ liters/hour}}{90 \text{ liters/min}}$$

(c) Since the extraction ratio is low, clearance is more sensitive to changes in plasma protein binding than to changes in blood flow.
    (d) No, if biliary obstruction does not affect glucuronidation, a microsomal activity. Because its elimination is impaired, the plasma concentration of the glucuronide will be higher than normal.

2. (a) 43,000 liters.
    (b) (i) $E_H = 0.02$: $V = (1/0.7) \cdot Cl \cdot t_{1/2}$
$$= (1/0.7) \times (90 \text{ liters/hour}) \times (14 \times 24 \text{ hours})$$

$$\text{Hepatic extraction ratio} = \frac{\text{Blood clearance}}{\text{Blood flow}} = \frac{(90/50)\text{liters/hour}}{90 \text{ liters/hour}}$$

(ii) $F_H = 0.98$: $F_H = 1 - \text{Hepatic extraction ratio}$
    (iii) $V_b = 860$ liters

3. Minimum $t_{1/2} = 2.3$ min: $t_{1/2} = 0.7 \, V/Cl$; Blood volume (5 liters) is smallest volume; hepatic blood flow (1.5 liters/min) is highest clearance.

4. (a) Rate of elimination $= Cl_u \cdot Cu = Cl_b \cdot C_b$ therefore $Cl_b/Cl_u = Cu/C_b = fu_b$
    (b) $Ab = V \cdot C = Vu \cdot Cu = V_b \cdot C_b$ therefore $V/V_b = C_b/C = (Cu/fu_b)/(Cu/fu) = fu/fu_b$

Answers to Unifying Problems (Chap. 6)

1. (a) B (b) B (c) A (d) B (e) B (f) C

2. (a) increase (b) less (c) alkalinization

3. (a) false (b) metabolism (c) false (d) 99 percent

Answers to Study Problems (Chap. 7)

1. (a) Half-life $= 1.8$ hours.

(b) Area = 6 mg × hours/liter;   using   the   relationship,   Area = C_o/k.   Area = 6.3 mg × hours/liter, using the trapezoidal rule and remembering that at zero time the concentration is C_o. The slightly higher value using the trapezoidal rule arises because, at any time, the concentration along the straight line connecting two data points is always greater than the corresponding concentration on the declining exponential curve.

(c) Clearance = 6.2 liters/hour.

(d) Volume of distribution = 16 liters.

2. First determine the half-life ($0.7/0.347 = 2$ hours). Place a datum point of 0.9 mg/liter at zero time and another point, 0.45 mg/liter, at the half-life (2 hours). Connect and extend the line joining these two data points.

3. (b) Half-life = 3.3 hours
       Total clearance = 4.8 liters/hour:

    From: $Cl = \dfrac{Dose}{Area}$. For the intravenous bolus case only, Area = C_0/k.

    (c) Volume of distribution = 23 liters

Answers to Unifying Problem (Chap. 7)

1. (a) Volume of distribution = 15 liters or 0.18 liter/kg; half-life = 6.3 hours; clearance = 1.65 liters/hour or 20 ml/hour/kg.

    (b) Half-life = 6.5 hours. Note scatter in semilogarithmic plot of rate of excretion against midpoint time of urine collection.

    (c) $fe = 0.9$; $fe = Ae_\infty/Dose = 1800$ mg/2000 mg. Renal clearance = 1.5 liters/hour or 25 ml/min; $Cl_R = fe \cdot Cl = 0.9 \times 1.65$ liters/hour.

    (d) Yes. Contribution of glomerular filtration ($fu \cdot GFR$) = about 4 ml/min. Because the ratio, $Cl_R/fu \cdot GFR$, is greater than one, the drug must be secreted.

    (e) Half-life = 6.5 hours. Note that the semilogarithmic plot of the amount remaining to be excreted against time of urine collection is much smoother than the excretion rate plot.

Answers to Study Problems (Chap. 8)

1. 2.8 and 28 min. At the plateau, infusion rate (R_{inf}) = $k \cdot Ab_{ss}$, or $t_{1/2}$ is given by 0.7 Ab_{ss}/R_{inf}. For succinylcholine $Ab_{ss} = 20$ mg, so that when $R_{inf} = 0.5$ mg/min, $t_{1/2} = 28$ min, and when $R_{inf} = 5$ mg/min, $t_{1/2} = 2.8$ min. The wide range in the half-life of succinylcholine arises from differences in the amount of pseudocholinesterase, the enzyme responsible for its hydrolysis and inactivation. The longer half-life is only rarely encountered.

2. (a) $k = 0.06$ min^{-1}, $V = 10$ liters. From the plot of C versus time, a rapid but rough estimate of $t_{1/2}$ (and hence k) is given by the time taken to reach one-half (26 mg/liter) the plateau. Because this concentration lies between experimental values, the $t_{1/2}$ (12 min) must be determined by interpolation. The $t_{1/2}$ (and k) is determined more accurately from the slope of a semilogarithmic plot of $(C_{ss} - C)$ against time. The volume of distribution can be estimated in two ways: by dividing the amount of drug in the body at steady state $(Ab_{ss} = R_{inf}/k;$ 50 mg) by the plateau concentration; or by dividing the clearance $(Cl = R_{inf}/C_{ss};$ 600 ml/min) by the elimination rate constant. The answer is the same.

(b) 1.6 mg/liter. Knowing the half-life, the concentration 20 min after stopping the infusion either may be estimated as $5.18 \times (\frac{1}{2})^{1.73}$, or by plotting drug decay on a semilogarithmic plot. Alternatively, it is the difference between the plateau concentration and the value at 20 min during the infusion.

(c) Plasma concentrations at 20, 40, and 60 min are 7, 9.6, and 10.3 mg/liter, respectively. Doubling the infusion rate results in a doubling of the concentration at all times.

(d) Loading dose $= 70$ mg $(V \cdot C_o)$; infusion rate $= 4.2$ mg/min. The same answer for the infusion rate $\left[\left(\frac{7}{5.18}\right) \times 3 \text{ mg/min}\right]$ is calculated from the proportionality between infusion rate and plateau concentration.

(e) 7 mg/min; 60 min. Infusion rate (by proportionality) is $\left(\frac{12}{5.18}\right) \times 3$ mg/min. Time to reach new plateau depends solely on the half-life of the drug.

3. $V = 25$ liters, $k = 0.1$ hour^{-1}, $t_{1/2} = 7$ hours, $Cl = 2.5$ liters/hour.

$$V = \frac{\text{Dose}}{C_o} = \frac{250 \text{ mg}}{10 \text{ mg/liter}}, \quad Cl = R_{inf}/C_{ss} = (10 \text{ mg/hour})/(4 \text{ mg/liter})$$

$$k = \frac{Cl}{V} = (2.5 \text{ liters/hour})/(25 \text{ liters})$$

4. $V = 22$ liters, $t_{1/2} = 2.5$ hours, $Cl = 6.25$ liters/hour. From postinfusion data, $t_{1/2} = 2.5$ hours $(k = 0.28$ hours$^{-1})$. At $t_{1/2}$ during infusion:

$$C = \frac{R_{inf}}{2kV} = \frac{C_{ss}}{2} = 4 \text{ mg/liter}$$

$$Cl = \frac{R_{inf}}{C_{ss}} = \frac{50 \text{ mg/hour}}{2 \times 4 \text{ mg/liter}}$$

$$V = \frac{Cl}{k} = \frac{6.25 \text{ liters/hour}}{0.28 \text{ hour}^{-1}}$$

The answers might also have been obtained by estimating clearance from the relationship, $Cl = $ Dose/area, where Dose is 50 mg/hour $\times$ 7.5 hours and the total area under the curve is 60.4 mg $\times$ hours/liter.

5. (a) *During Infusion.* When renal clearance is constant, the half-life is the time at which the rate of excretion is one-half the excretion rate at the plateau. Excretion rate data are generally more scattered than plasma data. Estimates of the half-life from urine data, using the preceding simple rule are, therefore, usually poor. It is better to subtract excretion rate values from the value at the plateau, and plot the difference

on semilogarithmic paper against the midpoint time of the urine collection. This follows since multiplying Equation 10 by renal clearance and taking logarithms yields:

log (Excretion rate at plateau − excretion rate at midpoint time)

$$= \log \text{(Excretion rate at plateau)} - \frac{k}{2.3} \times \text{(midpoint time)}$$

Treatment of the urine data in this manner gives an estimate for the half-life of 1.7 hours. Note that, owing to the scatter in the data, difference values at times beyond 90 percent of the plateau should not be considered.

Postinfusion. A semilogarithmic plot of the excretion rate against the midpoint time of urine collection (Equation 12 multiplied by renal clearance) yields a straight line. The half-life estimated from the line is 1.6 hours. Note that these data superimpose upon the difference data obtained during the infusion, indicating that the half-life is the same throughout the period of study.

(b) The cumulative amount excreted unchanged is 143 mg. The dose administered ($R_{inf} \times$ duration of infusion) is 480 mg, so that *fe* = 143 mg/480 mg or 0.3.

Answers to Study Problems (Chap. 9)

1.

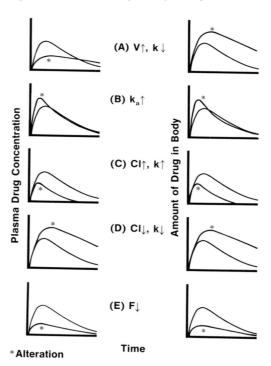

(A) V↑, k↓

(B) k_a↑

(C) Cl↑, k↑

(D) Cl↓, k↓

(E) F↓

Plasma Drug Concentration

Amount of Drug in Body

Time

Figure G-1   *Alteration

2. (a) Absorption rate-limits griseofulvin elimination for 30 to 40 hours. This time corresponds to the normal transit time of food in the gut. Thereafter unabsorbed drug is expelled from the gut and the plasma concentration of griseofulvin then falls parallel to that following the intravenous dose.

(b) Griseofulvin is poorly available in this subject. A cursory examination of the data plotted on regular graph paper indicates that, based on area corrected for dose, griseofulvin is poorly available (F approximately 0.4). Griseofulvin, sparingly soluble in water (10 mg/liter), is difficult to dissolve.

3. Let Bz denote benzylpenicillin and Pm denote penamecillin.
    (a) Relative availability $= 0.66$.

$$\text{Dose of Pm expressed in Bz equivalents} = 25 \text{ mg/kg} \times \left(\frac{334}{406}\right) = 20.6 \text{ mg/kg}$$

$$\begin{array}{l}\text{Relative amount} \\ \text{of Bz entering} \\ \text{the body following} \\ \text{Pm and Bz}\end{array} = \text{Area}_{Pm}/\text{Area}_{Bz} = \frac{(5.6 \text{ mg} \times \text{hours/liter})/(20.6 \text{ mg/kg})}{(10.3 \text{ mg}) \times \text{hours/liter})/(25 \text{ mg/kg})}$$

(b) $F_{Pm} = 0.13$, $F_{Bz} = 0.2$. Availability $= \text{Area} \cdot Cl/\text{Dose}$

$$F_{Pm} = \frac{(8 \text{ ml/min/kg}) \times (5.6 \text{ mg} \times \text{hours/liter})}{20.6 \text{ mg/kg}} = 0.13$$

Similarly, $F_{Bz} = 0.20$. Hence even Bz is poorly absorbed primarily due to hydrolysis in the gastrointestinal lumen.

(c) As only Bz is measured in plasma, the slower decline of Bz following Pm administration, compared to Bz administration, indicates that the elimination of Bz following Pm administration is absorption rate-limited.

$t_{1/2}$ associated with absorption following Pm $= 2.4$ hours.

Either dissolution of Pm (sparingly soluble) or intestinal hydrolysis of Pm to Bz is the rate-limiting step.

4. (a) Relative availability $= 0.55$.

$$\text{Relative availability} = \frac{Ae_{\infty,A}}{Ae_{\infty,B}} = 22 \text{ mg/40 mg}.$$

Method assumes that fe is constant.
(b) fe, as $F = Ae_\infty/fe \cdot \text{Dose}$.
(c) Possibly dissolution is hampered in the intestinal fluid lumen. Food, by delaying stomach emptying, promotes retention and greater dissolution in the stomach. The microcrystalline drug, having a greater surface, dissolves more rapidly than the larger crystals and, therefore, is less affected by differences in stomach emptying time.

Answers to Unifying Problems (Chap. 9)

1. **Table G-1**

Figure	Elimination Half-life	Volume of Distribution	Total Clearance	Renal Clearance	Availability
a. Dapsone	✔			✔	
b. Penicillins	✔	✔	✔		✔

2. (a) Independent of route of drug administration,

$$\text{Rate of excretion} \left(\frac{dAe}{dt}\right) = \text{Renal clearance} \times C$$

Integrating between time zero and time infinity

$$\int_0^\infty dAe = \text{Renal clearance} \int_0^\infty C \cdot dt$$

or

$$Ae_\infty = \text{Renal clearance} \times \text{Area}$$

(b) Following intravenous administration:

$$\text{Renal clearance} = (Ae_\infty/\text{Area}) = 152 \text{ mg}/(7.6 \text{ mg} \times \text{hours}/\text{liter})$$
$$= 0.33 \text{ liter}/\text{min}$$

The same value for the renal clearance is obtained from the intramuscular and oral data.

Answers to Study Problems (Chap. 10)

1. Only the clearance associated with the formation of N-acetylprocainamide and the total clearance of N-acetylprocainamide: this follows from Equation 11, $Cm_{ss}/C_{ss} = Cl_m/Cl(m)$. Note that in all patients in whom the ratio is greater than 1, the clearance of N-acetylprocainamide must be less than the total clearance of procainamide.

2. The rate of excretion of salicyluric acid can be taken to be its rate of formation from salicylic acid; the rate of elimination of salicyluric acid is rate limited by, and hence essentially equal to, its rate of formation. However, the rate of elimination of salicyluric acid is its rate of excretion.

3. Fraction of acetohexamide converted to hydroxyhexamide $= 1$. Disposition kinetics of hydroxyhexamide: $t_{1/2} = 3.8$ hours, $k = 0.18$ hours^{-1}, $Cl = 3.8$ liters/hour, $V = 20$ liters.

4. **Table G-2**

Plasma Metabolite Concentration	Rate-Limiting Step	
	A. Drug Elimination	B. Metabolite Elimination
Time to peak	↑	↑
Peak height	↑	↑
Area	↑	↑
Terminal $t_{1/2}$	↔	↑

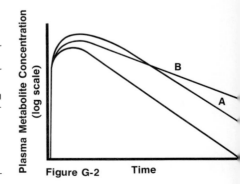

Figure G-2

Answers to Study Problems (*Chap. 11*)

1. Because propranolol is a drug of a relatively high extraction ratio, the changes in protein binding affect the volume of distribution but not the total blood clearance. The half-life, therefore, is shorter when the plasma protein binding is greater (*fu* smaller).

2. See Figure G-3.

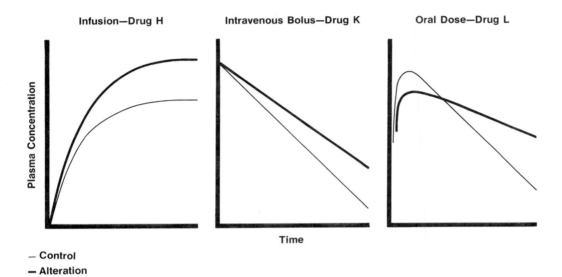

Infusion—Drug H   **Intravenous Bolus—Drug K**   **Oral Dose—Drug L**

Plasma Concentration

Time

— **Control**
— **Alteration**

Figure G-3

3. **Table G-3**

Hepatic Extraction Ratio	Hepatic Blood Flow	Fraction in Blood Unbound	Fraction in Tissue Unbound	Total Clearance[a]	Volume of Distribution[a]	Half-life	Oral Availability
High	↑	↔	↔	↑	↔	↓	↑
High	↔	↓	↔	↔	↓	↓	↑
High	↔	↔	↑	↔	↓	↓	↔
Low	↑	↔	↔	↔	↔	↔	↔
Low	↔	↔	↑	↔	↓	↓	↔
Low	↔	↑	↑	↑	↔	↓	↔

[a]Based on drug concentration in blood.

4. **Table G-4**

Total Clearance[a] (ml/min)	Fraction Excreted Unchanged	Total Clearance[a]	Renal Clearance[a]	Half-life	Fraction in Blood Unbound	Fraction in Tissue Unbound	Urine Flow
Drug A 24	0.5	↓	↓	↔	↔	↑	↓
Drug B 100	0.01	↑	↑	↓	↑[b]	↑[b]	↔
Drug C 1400	0.005	↔	↑	↑	↑	↔	↔

[a] Based on drug concentration in blood.
[b] By same factor.

Answers to Unifying Question (Chap. 11)

1. (a) $Cl = 171$ liters/hour; $Cl_b = 86$ liters/hour; $V_b = 120$ liters; $t_{1/2} = 1$ hour.
   (b) Yes; tissue binding is decreased;

   $$\frac{fu_T(\text{uremic})}{fu_T(\text{normal})} = 5.2.$$

   (c) A sixfold increase. Blood clearance should not change, therefore the total plateau concentration is unaltered, but the unbound concentration increases from 0.5 percent to 3 percent of the total.

Answers to Study Problems (Chap. 12)

1. (a) $Ab_{min} = 0.38$ mg/kg, from a plot of t_D versus log dose.
   (b) Data consistent; Ab_{min} still in body when second dose of 1 mg/kg is given; i.e., total effective dose is 1.38 mg/kg. This total dose, 1.38 mg/kg, on t_D versus log dose graph, gives t_D of about 8 min.

   Same answer by calculation, $t_D = \frac{2.3}{k} \log \left(\frac{\text{Dose}}{Ab_{min}} + 1 \right)$

2. (a) 11.4 hours [$Ab_{min} = 320$ mg; substitute into Eq. (3)].
   (b) 18.3 hours (11.4 hours + half-life)
   (c) (1) 22.8 hours (2) 8.9 hours
   (d) Doubling the dose increases the duration by one half-life. The effect of doubling the half-life depends upon the mechanism of the change. A decreased clearance leads to a doubling of the duration of effect, whereas in this example duration is decreased when the cause of the increased half-life is a doubling of the volume of distribution.

3. (a) Plot readily drawn using same C_0 and appropriate half-lives.
   (b) Statement valid; assuming $C_0 = 100$ in each species, relative plasma concentration at which each animal awoke, mouse = 64, rabbit = 57, rat = 64.
   (c) Dose ratio (mouse/rat): 1.5 ($t_D = 12$ min); 17 ($t_D = 90$ min).
   Note: 1700 mg/kg hexobarbital calculated to produce $t_D = 90$ min in mouse exceeds the dose that kills 50 percent of the population.

4. Initial dose = 20 mg; maintenance dose = 5 mg every 12 hours: By interpolation between data in inset of Figure 12-15, 20 mg is needed to immediately reduce MAP by 85 mm Hg and 15 mg is needed to reduce MAP by 75 mm Hg. As response wears off at 10 mm Hg/12 hours, 20–15 or 5 mg is needed every 12 hours to maintain MAP values between 95 and 105 mm Hg.

Answers to Study Problems (Chap. 13)

1. (a) 49
    (b) 11 days
    (c) Maximum—485 milliequivalents (49.5 grams sodium bromide);
        Minimum—475 milliequivalents (48.5 grams sodium bromide).
        Estimated from $Ab_{av} \pm \text{Dose}/2$.
    (d) 10.4 milliequivalents/liter (1.06 grams sodium bromide/liter).
        Calculated using Equation 2 and dividing by volume of distribution (extracellular volume).

2. There is no single answer. The regimen is appropriate as long as Ab remains within the limits proposed. Possibilities are:
    (a) 500 mg every 8 hours.
    (b) 500 mg initially, 350 mg every 6 hours.
    (c) 500 mg initially, 250 mg every 4 hours (inconvenient).
    Note: Since absorption is required, fluctuation will not be as large as calculated for intravenous doses.

3. (a) **Table G-5**

Dose	1	2	3	4	5	6	7	8
Chlorpropamide								
Ab_{max}(mg)	250	408	507	569	609	633	649	659
Ab_{min}(mg)	158	257	319	359	383	399	409	415
Tolbutamide								
Ab_{max}(mg)	500	625	656	664	666	666	667	667
Ab_{min}(mg)	125	156	164	166	166	167	167	167

    (b) Chlorpropamide, Ab_{av} = 540 mg; tolbutamide, Ab_{av} = 360 mg.

4. (a) 70 mg, from Equation 24.
    (b) Immediately. Loading dose (50 mg) + sustaining dose (70 mg).
    (c) Total dose for day one = 260 mg; total dose for day two = 210 mg.

    (d) **Table G-6.** Amount in Body

Time (hours):	0	4	8	12	16	20	24	28	32	36
Regimen										
Every 4 hours	0	25	63	81	91	95	98	99	99.5	100
Every 8 hours	0	25	38	44	47	49	49	50	50	50
Every 12 hours	0	25	38	19	34	42	21	36	43	22

Answers to Unifying Problem (Chap. 13)

1. (a) 337 mg to be given every 6 hours:

   Clearance = 72 ml/min × 60 min/hour = 4.32 liters/hour:

   D/τ = 4.32 (liters/hour) × 13 mg/liter = 56.2 mg/hour

   Note: if clearance had been calculated from V and $T_{1/2}$, its value would have been 4.53 liter/hour. The six-hourly dose would then have been 353 mg. This apparent discrepancy occurs because the mean clearance is not the same as the value obtained from the average half-life and the average volume of distribution.

   (b) $C_{ss,min}$ = 8.5 mg/liter:

   $C_{ss,min}$ = Dose · $(\frac{1}{2})^\epsilon$ / $[V \cdot (1 - (\frac{1}{2})^\epsilon)]$;

   ϵ = 360 min/312 min = 1.15.

   (c) Regimen seems reasonable; $C_{ss,max}$ = 18 mg/liter (I.V. assumed). Oral administration would give less fluctuation because it does take some time to absorb the drug.

   (d) Rate of infusion = 126 mg/hour.

   R_{inf} = 56.2 mg/hour × (13 mg/liter)/(5.8 mg/liter)

   (e) Half-life = 2.3 hours:

   $$t_{1/2} = \left(\frac{312}{60}\ \text{hours}\right) \times \left(\frac{5.8\ \text{mg/liter}}{13\ \text{mg/liter}}\right)$$

   (f) 500 mg orally every 4 hours. Every 6 hours is too infrequent in this person. A much shorter interval is inconvenient. If absorption smooths the fluctuations, every 4 hours may be appropriate. A prolonged-release preparation is another approach. One might question whether or not this drug is appropriate for this patient.

Answers to Study Problems (Chap. 14)

1. Availability, due to variable hepatic drug extraction on the first pass. Estimates of the ratio Cl/F (from Dose/τ · C_{av}) range from 0.25 to 2.5 liter/min. Therefore either high clearance, low F, or both are responsible. Since nortriptyline is stable in the gastrointestinal tract and lipophilic, high clearance in the liver is a probable explanation. Most variability is in F, due to first-pass effect. See Table 3-3.

2. Either the patient population sampled was biased, or this patient represents an extreme of the whole patient population. Recall that the patient was not part of the patient population from which the population pharmacokinetic values were obtained.

3. Wide differences in hepatic metabolic activity. Propranolol is highly cleared by the liver. Accordingly, differences in hepatic enzyme activity do not produce much variability in clearance, which is perfusion rate limited; but these small differences in clearance may cause wide differences in availability ($F_H = 1 - E_H$).

4.   (a) Most variable is fu_T, least variable is Cl_u.

Table G-7

Subject	1	2	3	4	5	Range Mean
Cl_u (liters/hour)	40	42	38	42	40	0.10
fu	0.1	0.15	0.09	0.16	0.11	0.57
fu_T	0.05	0.12	0.18	0.07	0.09	1.27

(b) The lack of variability in the unbound clearance means that the unbound concentration and presumably the drug effect at plateau are highly predictable from the rate of administration. There will, however, be differences in the total concentration. Also, the time to achieve the plateau will be variable because of large differences in the half-life. This is primarily a result of variability in tissue binding.

Answers to Study Problems (Chap. 15)

1.   24 mg (1.6 mg/kg) gentamicin, administered intramuscularly every 8 hours. Calculation based on surface area considerations alone. *Note:* The manufacturer's recommended dose of gentamicin for a child is 2–2.5 mg/kg every 8 hours. The age of the adult patient population was not given. If, as likely, those adults with severe infections requiring gentamicin are more elderly, then assuming a mean age of 55 years is reasonable. In that case, the additional correction for the 28 percent diminished renal function between a young adult and the adult patient, would suggest that the child's maintenance dose should be $1.6/(1 - 0.28)$ or 2.2 mg/kg.

2.   (a) **Table G-8**

Age:	6 days	6 months	4 years	Adult (55 years)
1. Based on weight	4	4	4	4
2. Based on surface area (Adult = 1.8 m²)	9.8(13.0)[a]	7.8(10.4)	6.2(8.3)	4
3. Based on observed clearance	4	15	9	4

[a] The values in parentheses incorporate the correction made for the diminished kidney function between a young and a 55-year-old adult.

(b) The considered therapeutic objective is to maintain the same C_{av}.
   (1) The higher calculated values based on surface area, rather than body weight, take into account the higher weight-normalized clearance with decreasing weight and age.
   (2) The lower needs in the newborn, calculated from observed clearance rather than surface area, are explained by immaturity of kidney function.
   (3) The higher needs in the infant and the child, calculated from observed clearance rather than surface area, may be due to a higher than anticipated metabolic clearance.
(c)   0.125 mg digoxin.

Answers to Study Problems (Chap. 16)

1. (a) b, e, c, a, d.
    (b) b and e, possibly c if Drug C has a low therapeutic index.
    (c) (*i*) All drugs have the same therapeutic index.
       (*ii*) Doubling of the half-life required before seriously considering adjustment.
       (*iii*) No active metabolites present.

2. (a) Corrected for surface area, $KF = 0.17$; $t_{1/2}$ is increased about 6 times.
       Possible dosage regimens:
       (*i*)   20 mg/kg every 72 hours
       (*ii*) 20 mg/kg initially, 7 mg/kg every 24 hours
       (*iii*) 20 mg/kg initially, 3.5 mg/kg every 12 hours

    (b) **Table G-9.** Maximum and Minimum Amounts of Vancomycin
       in Body (mg/kg)

	Normal Regimen in Normal Patient		Patient					
			Regimen 1		Regimen 2		Regimen 3	
Dose	Max	Min	Max	Min	Max	Min	Max	Min
1	20	5	20	5	20	12.6	20	15.6
2	25	6.3	25	6.3	19.6	12.3	19.4	15.4
3	26.4	6.6	26.4	6.6	19.3	12.2	18.9	15.0
4	26.7	6.6	26.7	6.6	19.2	12.1	18.5	14.7
5	26.7	6.7	26.7	6.7	19.1	12.0	18.2	14.4

3.   *Digitoxin*   *Digoxin*
    (a) 11.6 microgram/liter   0.037 microgram/liter
    (b) 16.5 microgram/liter   0.18 microgram/liter
    (c) The contribution of digoxin to the effect of digitoxin would be negligible in the
       anuric patient as well as in a patient with normal renal function.

Answers to Unifying Problems (Chap. 16)

1. (a) (*i*) 1.6 grams.

$$Cl_{Li}/Cl_{Cr} = 0.2$$
$$Cl_{Li} = 0.2 \times 124 \text{ (ml/min)} = 25 \text{ ml/min or } 35.7 \text{ liters/day}$$

$$\text{Rate in} = \frac{35.7 \text{ liters}}{\text{day}} \times \frac{1.2 \text{ mEq}}{\text{liter}} = 43 \text{ mEq/day}$$

Eq. wt. = 37. Therefore daily dose = 1.6 grams
    (*ii*) 0.8 grams/day.
$$Cl_{Li}/Cl_{Cr} = 0.1$$

$$\text{Daily dose} = \frac{0.1}{0.2} \times 1.6 \text{ grams} = 0.8 \text{ grams}$$

(b) Dosage regimen = 0.8 grams lithium twice daily; $t_{1/2} = 0.7 \times (0.7 \times 70$ liters)/(35.7 liters/day) = 0.96 days

Table G-10. Amount of Lithium in Body (grams)

Dose	1	2	3	4	5	6	7	8	9	∞
Maximum	0.8	1.37	1.77	2.05	2.25	2.39	2.49	2.56	2.61	2.73
Minimum	0.57	0.97	1.25	1.45	1.59	1.69	1.76	1.81	1.85	1.93

(c) (*i*) 0.14 grams/12 hours.

$$\text{Dosing rate} = \frac{21 \text{ ml/min}}{124 \text{ ml/min}} \times 1.6 \text{ gram/day} = 0.27 \text{ gram/day}$$

(*ii*) 6 days for plasma lithium to fall below therapeutic range; $C_{av} = 1.2$ mEq/liter, $t_{1/2} = (124 \text{ ml/min}/21/\text{ml/min}) \times 0.96$ day = 5.7 days. Time to fall from 1.2 to 0.6 mg/liter is one half-life.

2. (a) (*i*) *Maximum*   *Minimum*
       20 mg/liter   10 mg/liter

   (*ii*) Half-life = 5 days

Table G-11. Blood Drug Concentration (mg/liter)

Dose	1	2	3	4	5	6	∞
Maximum	20	27.4	34	39.5	44.4	48.6	77.3
Minimum	17.4	23.9	29.5	34.4	38.6	42.3	67.3

(b) (*i*) Drug A   1 mg initially, 0.1 mg daily
       Drug B   240 mg initially, 24 mg daily
       Drug C   No change
       Drug D   No change

   (*ii*) Assumed: metabolites inactive, and F, V, and metabolic clearance do not change.

(c) 22 micrograms/liter:
    Blood clearance $(0.7 \times V/t_{1/2}) = 1.3$ liters/min
    Hepatic clearance $(0.9 \times$ blood clearance) = 1.17 liters/min
    Hepatic blood flow (assumed) = 1.5 liters/min
    $F = 1 - E_H = 1 - 1.17/1.5 = 0.22$
    Maximum possible blood concentration = F · Dose/V

$$= \frac{0.22 \times 90 \text{ mg}}{900 \text{ liters}} = 0.022 \text{ mg/liter}$$

Answers to Study Problems (Chap. 17)

1. 100 mg initially and 50 mg twice daily or 100 mg once daily.

The metabolic clearance becomes 20 percent of normal value, which is 80 percent of the normal total clearance value. Renal clearance is 20 percent of the normal total clearance. By sum, the total clearance becomes 36 percent of its normal value. The maintenance dosing rate should, therefore, be adjusted by a factor of 0.36.

2. See Figure G-4.

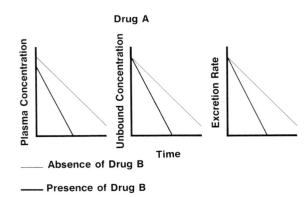

Figure G-4

_____ Absence of Drug B

▬▬▬ Presence of Drug B

Answers to Unifying Problem (Chap. 17)

3. (a) Drug A is secreted and reabsorbed. Renal clearance/($fu \cdot GFR$) is 2.1 in the absence and 0.3 in the presence of Drug B.
    (b) Displacement from plasma and tissue binding sites and either inhibition of tubular secretion or enhanced tubular reabsorption, e.g., by a change in urine pH. The threefold increase in the unbound fraction of Drug A in the presence of Drug B should increase the renal clearance threefold; instead the renal clearance decreased from 1.5 liters/hour to 0.6 liters/hour.

    The extrarenal clearance increased approximately threefold. For Drug A alone

$$Cl \text{ (extrarenal)} = \frac{25 \text{ mg/hour}}{10 \text{ mg/liter}} - 1.5 \text{ liter/hour}$$

$$= 1.0 \text{ liter/hour}$$

and in the presence of Drug B,

$$Cl \text{ (extrarenal)} = \frac{25 \text{ mg/hour}}{6.7 \text{ mg/liter}} - 0.60 \text{ liter/hour}$$

$$= 3.1 \text{ liter/hour}$$

Being a low extraction ratio drug and having a volume of distribution of 52 liters, by calculation, the displacement from plasma protein should not have materially altered the half-life. If anything the half-life should have increased because the renal clearance decreased. Thus, displacement from tissue is also evident.
    (c) The plateau unbound concentration ($fu \cdot C$) of Drug A increases from 1 mg/liter in the absence to 2 mg/liter in the presence of Drug B, suggesting that the response to it is increased, perhaps excessively. No information is given on A → B.

Answers to Unifying Problem (Chap. 17)

Table G-12

		Observation			
	Clearance	Volume of Distribution	Half-life	Availability	Fraction Excreted Unchanged
Drug A	↓	↔	↑	↔	↓
Drug B	↑	↔	↓	↔	↔
Drug C	↔	↔	↔	↔	↔
Drug D	↔	↑	↑	↑	↑
Drug E	↔	↓	↓	↔	↔
Drug F	↑	↑	↔	↔	↔
Drug G	↔	↔	↔	↔	↔

Answers to Study Problems (Chap. 18)

1. Answers in section on target concentration strategy (pages 269–271).

2. (a) Either a regimen of 3 100-mg aminophylline tablets every 12 hours or a regimen of 2 100-mg tablets every 8 hours. With a half-life of 16 hours and a clearance of 1.4 liters/hour, the maintenance rate of theophylline administration is 21 mg/hour (1.4 liters/hour × 15 mg/liter). Thus, either 252 mg every 12 hours or 168 mg every 8 hours would be appropriate. Since each 100-mg tablet contains 85 mg of theophylline, the preceding regimens are suggested.
    (b) Three 100-mg aminophylline tablets every 6 hours. Using a volume of distribution of 0.5 liters/kg, $F = 0.85$, and Equation 3, the calculated clearance for a trough sample obtained on a regimen of 3 tablets every 12 hours is 2.54 liters/hour; for a regimen of 2 tablets every 8 hours, it is 2.89. Thus, in either case the rate of administration required to maintain an average concentration of 15 mg/liter is about 40 mg/hour.

3. 4.6 liters/hour and 5.3 hours. The value of the elimination rate constant is calculated by iteratively solving Equation 8, that is,

$$C = \frac{0.85}{35} (400 \times e^{-24k} + 200 \times e^{-20k} + 300 \times e^{-10k} + 300 \times e^{-6k})$$

until $C = 6$ mg/liter.

k	C
0.1	8.2
0.13	6.12
0.15	5.10

The clearance is then $k \cdot V$ and the half-life, $0.7/k$.

4. Using Equation 6 and the usual parameter values, the predicted plasma theophylline concentrations are 3.5, 10.9, and 12.9 mg/liter in the three patients, respectively. Clearly, patient 2 has a lower than average value of clearance and patient 3 has a much higher than average value. By an iterative procedure and using Equation 6, the values of clearance in the three patients are 0.052, 0.012, and 0.113 liters/hour per kg, and the values of the half-life are 7, 29, and 3 hours, respectively. In patient 1 the sampling time is so short that one has virtually no confidence in the clearance or half-life estimate; a wide range of clearance values gives essentially the same concentration. In patient 2, the clearance is low, and indeed from the estimated clearance and half-life, the value of 18 is far from the estimated steady-state concentration, 57 mg/liter. Clearly, the rate of administration of aminophylline in this patient should be reduced, probably about fourfold. A subsequent sample, obtained about 48 to 72 hours later, would then be appropriate. In patient 3, the estimated value of the half-life is such that a good estimate of clearance is obtained. Here, the rate of administration must be doubled to achieve a concentration within the therapeutic range of 10 to 20 mg/liter.

index

Page numbers in *italics* refer to illustrations; page numbers followed by t refer to tables. When more than one section is referred to, the major reference is in **boldface type**.

319